POPE PIUS XII LIBRARY, ST. JOSEPH COL.

3 2528 09343 7061

D1714734

Health and Behavior
in Childhood
and Adolescence

Laura L. Hayman, PhD, RN, FAAN, is a Professor in the Division of Nursing, The Steinhardt School of Education, New York University and Adjunct Professor, Integrative and Behavioral Cardiovascular Health Program, Mount Sinai School of Medicine, New York. Dr. Hayman received her MSN in Nursing of Children and PhD in Interdisciplinary Studies in Human Development from the University of Pennsylvania. She was a member of the University of Pennsylvania faculty (in Nursing and later Medicine) for nearly 20 years, and served as Chair of the Nursing of Children Division. Following this, she was the Carl W. and Margaret Davis Walter Professor of Nursing at Case Western Reserve University. Her research focuses on primary prevention of cardiovascular disease (CVD) and includes a twelve-year study of genetic and environmental determinants of risk for CVD in twins as they advance through childhood and adolescence. Dr. Hayman is a Fellow of the American Academy of Nursing, the American Heart Association, and the Society of Behavioral Medicine. She has co-edited five previous books and has served on numerous expert panels and editorial boards, including (currently) *American Journal of Health Behavior, MCN: The Journal of Maternal-Child Nursing,* and *Annals of Behavioral Medicine.*

Margaret M. Mahon, PhD, RN, FAAN, is Clinical Nurse Specialist, End-of-Life Care, Hospital of the University of Pennsylvania, and Senior Fellow, University of Pennsylvania Center for Bioethics. Dr. Mahon's major research has focused on children's concepts of death, bereaved siblings, and bereaved parents' experiences and responses. Her clinical experience with children and families includes advanced practice nursing roles in pediatric trauma, intensive care, and chronic illness. Dr. Mahon has worked with bereaved children and families in hospital, hospice, home, school, and other community settings. She is a regular guest on the award winning "Kid's Corner" radio program designed to provide children and the adults in their lives with information and counsel on issues in child and family health care. Dr. Mahon is a Fellow in the American Academy of Nursing.

J. Rick Turner, PhD, is an experimental psychologist who has spent 15 years conducting research in the field of Cardiovascular Behavioral Medicine. His research has focused on the effects of stress on the cardiovascular system, and the possible role of stress-induced responses in the development of cardiovascular disease. He has published 50 scientific papers describing his collaborative research, two textbooks, and two previous edited volumes. His authored text entitled *Cardiovascular Reactivity and Stress: Patterns of Physiological Response* (1994) introduced the research methodology and findings of cardiovascular reactivity research to undergraduate and graduate students. Dr. Turner has received research awards from the Society for Psychophysiological Research and the American Psychosomatic Society. He is Founding Editor of the Sage Publications Series in Behavioral Medicine and Health Psychology, and a Fellow of the Society of Behavioral Medicine. He lives in Chapel Hill, North Carolina, where he works as a Medical Editor in the pharmaceutical industry.

Health and Behavior
in Childhood
and Adolescence

Laura L. Hayman, PhD, RN, FAAN
Margaret M. Mahon, PhD, CRNP, FAAN
J. Rick Turner, PhD
Editors

 Springer Publishing Company

Copyright © 2002 by Springer Publishing Company, Inc.

All rights reserved

No part of this publication may be reproduced, stored in a retrieval system, or transmitted in any form or by any means, electronic, mechanical, photocopying, recording, or otherwise, without the prior permission of Springer Publishing Company, Inc.

Springer Publishing Company, Inc.
536 Broadway
New York, NY 10012-3955

Acquisitions Editor: Ruth Chasek
Production Editor: Jeanne W. Libby
Cover design by Joanne E. Honigman

01 02 03 04 05/5 4 3 2 1

Library of Congress Cataloging-in-Publication Data

Hayman, Laura Lucia.
  Health and behavior in childhood and adolescence / Laura L. Hayman, Margaret M. Mahon, J. Rick Turner
    p. cm.
  Includes bibliographical references and index.
  ISBN 0-8261-3852-7 1. Health behavior in children. 2. Health behavior in adolescence. 3. Health promotion. I. Mahon, Margaret M. II. Turner, J. Rick III. Title.
  RA776.9 .H395 2002
  613'.0432—dc21
                                    2002020928
                                          CIP

Printed in the United States of America by Maple-Vail.

Children are messages we send to a time that we will not see.

Neil Postman

This book is dedicated to my son, David Joseph Louis Hayman.

LLH

Contents

Contributors

Kristi Alexander, PhD
Associate Professor
Alliant International University
San Diego, CA

Emma J. Brown, PhD, RN, CS
Associate Professor
University of Central Florida
School of Nursing
College of Health and Public
  Affairs
Orlando, FL

Oscar G. Bukstein, MD, MPH
Associate Professor of Psychiatry
Department of Psychiatry
School of Medicine
University of Pittsburgh and
Western Psychiatric Institute and
  Clinic
Pittsburgh, PA

Sean D. Cleary, Psy. D
Assistant Professor
Department of Epidemiology and
  Biostatistics
George Washington University
School of Public Health & Health
  Services
Washington, DC

Ori Shinar, Psy. D
Assistant Professor
Department of Social and
  Behavioral Sciences
Mercy College
Dobbs Ferry, NY

Marnie Fegan, PhD
Private Practice
Monmouth County, NJ

**Loretta Sweet Jemmott, PhD,
  RN, FAAN**
Professor and Director
Center for Urban Health Research
University of Pennsylvania
School of Nursing
Philadelphia, PA

John B. Jemmott, III, PhD
Kenneth B. Clark Professor of
  Communications
Annenberg School of
  Communications
University of Pennsylvania
Philadelphia, PA

Han C.G. Kemper, PhD
Institute of Research in Extramural
  Medicine (EMGO)
Faculty of Medicine
Vrije Universiteit
Van der Boechorststraat 7
Amsterdam, The Netherlands

Jennifer Moore, RN, BSN, MSN
Director of Government Affairs
Michigan Nurses Association
Doctoral Student
University of Michigan
Ann Arbor, MI

Nola J. Pender, PhD, RN, FAAN
Professor and Associate Dean for
  Research
University of Michigan
School of Nursing
Ann Arbor, MI

Michael C. Roberts, PhD, ABPP
Professor and Director
Clinical Child Psychology Program
University of Kansas
Lawrence, KS

Julie Sochalski, PhD, RN, FAAN
Associate Director and Assistant
  Professor
Center for Health Outcomes and
  Policy Research
University of Pennsylvania
Philadelphia, PA

Karen Farchaus Stein, PhD, RN
Associate Professor
University of Michigan
School of Nursing
Ann Arbor, MI

Andrew M. Tershakovec, MD, MPH
Associate Professor, Department of
  Pediatrics
University of Pennsylvania School
  of Medicine
Division of Gastroenterology and
  Nutrition
Children's Hospital of Philadelphia
Philadelphia, PA

Linda Van Horn, PhD, RD
Professor
Department of Preventive Medicine
Northwestern University
School of Medicine
Chicago, IL

Thomas A. Wills, PhD
Professor
Department of Epidemiology and
  Social Medicine
Albert Einstein College of
  Medicine
Bronx, NY

Introduction

Throughout the past two decades, considerable multidisciplinary research has focused on the complex relationships between health and behavior in childhood and adolescence. This text was designed to address this information with emphasis on the state-of-the art and science and contemporary issues relevant to behavioral health in childhood and adolescence. Conceptualized within a developmental–systems framework, content focuses on individual characteristics as well as broader contextual/system factors that influence health-related behaviors in childhood and adolescence. Considerable attention is also devoted to the implications of this information for promoting health-related behaviors and preventing behaviorally linked morbidities.

The contributors to this volume are scholars and expert clinicians from several disciplines including nursing, psychology, medicine, epidemiology, and public health. The target audience is researchers, clinicians, and students from these disciplines and other professionals who work with children in health, developmental, and educational settings. A major goal of this collaborative effort is to inform the interdisciplinary practice of health promotion and disease prevention and future research focused on the links between health and behavior in childhood and adolescence.

Section I of this text focuses on recent advances in our understanding of health and behavior in childhood and adolescence. In chapter 1, Wills and colleagues present a developmental model outlining potential links between temperament dimensions and health status. Results from several lines of inquiry including recent research of Wills and colleagues suggest that dimensions of temperament assessed in childhood or early adolescence have implications for an individual's health risk status during other phases of the life span. The importance of context is illustrated by Pender and Stein (chapter 2) in their comprehensive and insightful examination of social support, self-concept, and adolescent health behaviors. These authors view social support as a dynamic reciprocal process between individuals or aggregates in a particular social context. Emphasis is placed on characteristics of social support resources including family, peers, educators, health professionals, religious organizations, neighborhoods, and communities. Pender and Stein suggest that the adolescent's evolving self-definition is both a product of the network of social support and a determinant of health and health behavior lifestyle choices. In advancing the need for intervention research incorporating social support and self system constructs, they offer suggestions for intervention based on theoretical analysis and available descriptive data.

Section II of this text addresses recent advances in our understanding of health promoting behaviors and highlights the importance of nutrition and physical activity. Tershakovec and Van Horn (chapter 3) present a comprehensive overview of the preventive health aspects of nutrition interventions in children and youth. Emphasis is placed on the evidence linking dietary intake and health risk as well as implications for implementing developmentally appropriate health-promoting dietary interventions. Kemper (chapter 4) reviews the development of physical activity patterns in youth, outlines developmental trends and gender differences in this health behavior, and indicates the need to consider developmental processes in assessment and intervention strategies.

Section III of this text addresses the major behaviorally linked morbidities of childhood and adolescence. In chapter 5, Alexander and Roberts provide an overview of the epidemiology of childhood injuries, outline suggestions for prevention and intervention strategies, and detail population-based approaches targeting environmental and public policy issues in injury prevention and control. Bukstein (chapter 6) describes family, peer, and community-neighborhood risk factors as important contextual influences relevant to the initiation and continued use of addictive or illegal substances. He acknowledges the likely contribution of genetic and constitutional factors as an important component of individual risk for substance use and suggests the need for additional research focused on individual differences in response to substances using a gene-environment interaction paradigm.

Obesity is a highly prevalent chronic condition that results from an imbalance in energy intake and expenditure. The current epidemic of obesity in the United States indicates an urgent need for effective high-risk and population-based approaches to prevention and management with emphasis on the potentially modifiable influences including health behaviors and the contexts/environments in which they develop and are maintained. Toward that goal,

Hayman (chapter 7) identifies characteristics of developmental contexts such as the family, school, and community environment as important determinants of health behaviors associated with obesity including patterns of dietary intake and physical activity. Consistent with suggestions for future research offered by other contributors to this volume, Hayman emphasizes interdisciplinary initiatives focused on both individual and population-based approaches to primary prevention.

The past decade has witnessed substantial progress in the treatment of AIDS; however, prevalence and trend data indicate the need for continued emphasis on behaviorally focused prevention strategies for AIDS and other sexually transmitted diseases (STDs). Toward this goal, Jemmott and colleagues (chapter 8) present an epidemiologic overview of STDs, describe a cognitive behavioral approach for reducing adolescents' risk for STDs, detail evidence-based intervention strategies for reducing STD risk, and outline implications for screening, management, and treatment of STDs among adolescents.

Concluding this volume (chapter 9), Villarruel and Sochalski persuade us that strategies to reduce rates of behaviorally based morbidity and mortality among children and adolescents cannot ignore the social and environmental contexts that influence health behaviors and health outcomes. Health and social policies designed to support healthy environments, communities, and families are advocated with the ultimate goal of promoting optimal health for all our children.

PART 1

Understanding Behavior and Health in Childhood and Adolescence

CHAPTER 1

Temperament Dimensions and Health Behavior: A Developmental Model

Thomas A. Wills, Sean D. Cleary, Ori Shinar, and Marnie Fegan

This chapter outlines a developmental model of how temperament dimensions are related to health status. Several types of research indicate that measures of temperament dimensions, assessed in childhood or early adolescence, have implications for an individual's health risk status at other parts of the life span: late adolescence, young adulthood, and later adulthood. The purpose of this chapter is to discuss evidence indicating that temperament is related to health over time, and to suggest mechanisms for how this may occur.

The theoretical concepts in this chapter are related to research linking adult personality variables and health status (Friedman & Booth-Kewley, 1987; Friedman, 1990; Siegman, 1994). Research with adults has usually been based on broad band personality dimensions, notably the Big Five system (Goldberg, 1993). A person at the high end on each dimension would be characterized as follows.

- *Neuroticism*: nervous, excitable, anxious, unstable, jealous;
- *Extraversion*: sociable, energetic, talkative, cheerful, assertive;
- *Agreeableness*: cooperative, considerate, adaptable, courteous, easygoing;

- *Conscientiousness*: organized, dependable, self-disciplined, decisive, persistent; and
- *Openness to Experience*: intellectual, creative, intelligent, insightful, nonconforming.

Recent research has suggested some convergence between Big Five scales and dimensions of temperament, which are presumed to have a psychobiological basis (Angleitner & Ostendorf, 1994; John et al., 1994; Molfese & Molfese, 2000). There are alternative systems for adult personality, which include different dimensions such as *novelty seeking* or *sensation seeking* (e.g., Cloninger, Svrakic, & Przybeck, 1993; Zuckerman, 1994). We will discuss how temperament dimensions may be related to constructs from the Big Five system and constructs from alternative systems (Almagor, Tellegen, & Waller, 1995; Zuckerman et al., 1993).

Theoretical papers have noted that some risk factors for adult substance abuse are conceptually similar to dimensions of temperament studied in developmental research (e.g., Tarter, 1988). This theoretical work has had considerable impact on our research with adolescents (e.g., Wills, Sandy, & Yaeger, 2000). Evidence shows substantial heritability for both temperament dimensions and adult personality traits (e.g., Bouchard, 1994; Heath, Cloninger, & Martin, 1994; Plomin, Owen, & McGuffin, 1994), so the idea that there is some continuity between childhood characteristics and adult personality traits should be taken seriously (Caspi, Moffitt, Newman, & Silva, 1996). This line of thinking suggests that the basis for linkages of personality and health status may begin in childhood.

In considering mechanisms of temperament-health relationships, we have taken a multivariate approach. Previous research has tended to take a dichotomous approach to the question, such as comparing a behavioral explanation (e.g., personality related to health status through effect on smoking) or a social mechanism (e.g., personality related to health status through influence on social support) versus a direct effect mechanism. Rather than assuming that a dispositional characteristic acts through a single mechanism, we inquire about multiple pathways and test empirically which of these are implicated in mediating relationships between temperament and health behavior. We have tested structural models in which temperament constructs may be related to a health-relevant behavior (e.g., smoking) through several processes: linkage to emotional support from parents, to patterns of self-regulation, to patterns of life stress, or to patterns of peer group social affiliation. The question then becomes: How are temperament characteristics translated into behaviors and situational exposures that may ultimately place a person at risk for disease?

In this chapter, first the nature of temperament dimensions is described and the tenets of epigenetic theories, which link temperament and behavioral development, are explained. In the next sections, a range of research is reviewed that suggests how temperament dimensions may be related to health, and studies of the authors that have tested various mechanisms with children and adolescents are presented. Finally, implications for further research on relationships of temperament dimensions to behavior and health in adulthood are considered.

TEMPERAMENT DIMENSIONS AND EPIGENETIC THEORY

The study of temperament originated with child psychologists who were interested in describing consistencies in infant and child behavior (Rothbart & Derryberry, 1981; Thomas & Chess, 1977). It was found that temperament measures predicted outcomes, including behavior problems (Caspi, Henry, McGee, Moffitt, & Silva, 1995) and substance use (Lerner & Vicary, 1984; Wills, Cleary, Filer, Shinar, Mariani, & Spera, 2001), and that they were implicated in resiliency effects (Werner, 1986; Wills, Sandy, Yaeger, & Shinar, 2001). The recent progress of this area is now represented in a number of volumes and review articles (e.g., Molfese & Molfese, 2000; Rothbart & Bates, 1998; Tarter, Vanyukov, Giancola, Dawes, Blackson, Mezzich, & Clark, 1999; Wills, Sandy, & Yaeger, 2000).

Temperament can be defined as *characteristics that manifest early and show reasonable stability over time.* Temperament dimensions measured at early ages are relatively simple in form. For example, activity level is how often the individual moves around physically. In this sense, temperament represents the style rather than the content of behavior. A high activity level would be reflected in different ways in various situations (e.g., reading in a classroom versus playing games on a playground), but individual rankings in activity are expected to show consistency over situations. It is thought that temperamental characteristics had some type of survival value during evolution (Super & Harkness, 1986) and became represented in the structure of neurological systems (Cloninger et al., 1993; Nelson, 1994). Evidence of heritability for temperament dimensions is indicated for humans through observational behavior/genetic studies (Buss & Plomin, 1984; Heath et al.,

1994) and for other species through experimental studies (Bardo, Donohew, & Harrington, 1997). Some dimensions represent emotional reactions (e.g., negative emotionality); some represent information processing characteristics (e.g., attentional orientation); and some represent orientations toward conspecifics (e.g., sociability).

The manifestations of a temperament dimension may change over the period from infancy to later childhood. For example, negative emotionality could be manifested as crying in early childhood, temper tantrums and oppositional/defiant behavior in middle childhood, and aggressive behavior in adolescence. However, when age-appropriate measures are used, temperament dimensions show reasonable stability over time (Hagekull, 1989; Pedlow, Sanson, Prior, & Oberklaid, 1993). It is expected also that environmental factors have a substantial influence on the expression of temperament characteristics (see Loehlin, 1992; Katainen, Räikkönen, Keskivaara, & Keltikangas-Järvinen, 1999). Thus, within limits, it is possible that individuals with similar initial temperament characteristics could show divergence at later ages depending on factors such as parent-child relationship and socioeconomic context (Kochanska, 1995; Tarter, Moss, & Vanyukov, 1995).

Structure of Temperament Dimensions

At present there is general agreement on several dimensions of temperament that are replicable across studies (Rothbart & Ahadi, 1994; Rothbart & Bates, 1998). Three dimensions are usually construed as risk factors, though this designation is not absolute.[1]

Activity level. Activity level is the tendency to be physically active. An individual high on the dimension is often moving around and feels restless after sitting still for a time.

Negative emotionality. Negative emotionality is the tendency to be easily and intensely distressed. An individual high on this dimension is readily irritated and shows a strong emotional reaction. This is distinguished from a dimension reflecting inhibitory tendency with consequent anxiety and depressive symptomatology (Wills, Windle, & Cleary, 1998).

Rigidity. This dimension reflects the tendency to have an inhibitory response to new situations. An individual high on rigidity would show hesitation or withdrawal when confronted with a novel situation, would dislike environmental changes, and would have difficulty in adapting to change. Variants represent social anxiety, labeled as *shyness*, or a high sensitivity to stimuli interpreted as threatening, labeled as anxiety or *fearfulness*.

Several dimensions are construed as protective factors. The designation again is not absolute, as some dimensions may have complex effects.

Attentional orientation (also termed *persistence* or *task orientation*). This dimension reflects the ability to focus attention and concentrate on a task. An individual high in this dimension would be able to focus on a task (versus being easily distracted) and would persist at the task until finished. This temperament characteristic is conceptually different from I.Q., which is a higher-order construct based on a number of cognitive systems that develop at different ages (Fulker, Cherny, & Cardon, 1993; Stuss, 1992).

Positive emotionality. This dimension reflects the tendency to easily and frequently experience positive mood. A person high on this dimension would laugh and smile frequently and would show indications of enjoyment in many situations. It should be noted that positive emotion is not simply the absence of negative emotion (Rothbart & Bates, 1998). Rather, the dimensions of positive and negative emotionality are not strongly correlated empirically (Diener, 1984; Wills, Sandy, Shinar, & Yaeger, 1999).

Approach. This dimension reflects the tendency to approach things. An individual high on this dimension would show approach toward new situations or people, would be interested in new things, and would adapt quickly in new situations. The distinction between social and nonsocial aspects of approach tendency is complex and not well understood at present (Windle, 1995; Wills, Windle, & Cleary, 1998). The tendency to enjoy being around people is often defined as a separate dimension of *sociability* (Buss & Plomin, 1984).

Theory of Behavioral Epigenesis

Temperament dimensions are simple characteristics that are observable at younger ages (e.g., Kochanska et al., 1997, 2000), whereas complex personality traits such as conscientiousness are complex and manifest later. Theoretical approaches under the rubric of *behavioral epigenesis* provide a developmental approach to this issue, asking whether there are underlying principles that describe the way in which simple temperament dimensions are related to complex behaviors (Rothbart & Ahadi, 1994; Wills, Sandy, & Yaeger, 2000).

Epigenetic approaches have been developed by investigators from different disciplines including behavior genetics, developmental psychology, and neuropsychology (Moffitt, 1993; Scarr, 1991; Tarter, Moss, & Vanyukov, 1995). While having somewhat different emphases, they present a common set of postulates. Epigenetic models propose that behaviors are organized systems and that organization of behavior at one point in time provides a basis for organization of behavior at a subsequent point in time (Cairns & Ornstein, 1979). Temperament characteristics are predicted to influence the development of behavior patterns in early childhood, and the organization of these behavior patterns then provides a basis from which more complex patterns of behavior emerge in later childhood and adolescence (Rothbart & Ahadi, 1994; Wills et al., 2001). Some models posit that a phenotype of behavioral characteristics emerges through a continuing series of genotype X environment interactions, such that parent-child relationships and socioeconomic factors have a continuing impact on the development of behavior (Tarter, Moss, & Vanyukov, 1995; Wills et al., 2001; Zucker, 1994). It is postulated that in the progression from simple to more complex behaviors, temperament characteristics exert a systematic influence on development so that within limits, termed the *range of reaction* (Tarter et al., 1995), individuals with certain temperament characteristics will tend toward certain behavioral outcomes.

For example, consider the dimension of attentional orientation. The epigenetic model suggests that a child with good attentional control would have better initial experiences in dealing with problem situations and would be better able to calm him/herself in upsetting situations, through shifting attention from unpleasant stimuli. This is predicted to produce better ability for regulating emotion and selecting appropriate responses in problem situations (Eisenberg, Fabes, Guthrie, & Reiser, 2000; Kochanska et al., 2000; Rothbart et al., 1994). As individuals experience repeated instances of coping with problem situations and elicit similar feedback from the environment, behavior is predicted to become more crystallized and dispositional over time (Tarter et al., 1995). In this manner, the temperament characteristic shapes the way in which children and adolescents learn to cope with problem situations, so that when a person high on the dimension of attentional orientation is observed at school age, he/she is predicted to have better skills for coping with problem situations.

The relation of temperament dimensions to self-control is proposed as a major aspect of the process of behavioral development. In part this is because some dimensions present an inherent barrier to development of self-control.

For example, an individual with high negative emotionality is more reactive to situations and experiences emotional distress more frequently. The greater affective burden and the lesser likelihood of reinforcement from reduction of negative affect would make it more difficult for the child to learn self-control of emotional responses (Tarter et al., 1995). Therefore, by later childhood the person would have less ability to control emotions. In addition, temperament dimensions may affect the quality of interpersonal relationships that contribute to self-control development. For example, a child with high activity level is more difficult for some parents to deal with and may provide fewer rewards in daily contact with parents, whereas a child with high positive emotionality may form better attachment with parents (see Maunder & Hunter, 2001; Rothbart & Ahadi, 1994). Hence it is predicted that temperament dimensions will be correlated with the quality of the parent-child relationship, and this will influence the development of self-control ability occurring through socialization processes (Wills, Windle, & Cleary, 1998; Wills et al., 2001). This is particularly relevant for prediction of preventive health behaviors, as these typically depend on good self-regulation and effective planning and organization, whereas many health risk behaviors may result from poor self-control and ineffective emotion regulation (Wills, 2001).

Temperament and Adult Personality

The relation between temperament dimensions and adult personality characteristics has been a focus of research (see Angleitner & Ostendorf, 1994; Digman & Inouye, 1986; John et al., 1994; Molfese & Molfese, 2000). The question of how the constructs are related does not have a simple answer (e.g., temperament dimension X = Big Five dimension X). This is demonstrated by examining the content of the measures. For example, the Dimensions of Temperament Survey (DOTS-R) measure for attentional orientation consists of simple questions indicating that a person can focus attention on a task. In contrast, a Big Five scale such as Conscientiousness may contain upward of 60 items that are parceled into 10–12 subscales representing complex attributes including logic, efficiency, organization, dependability, persistence, reliability, punctuality, and thrift (see Goldberg & Rosolack, 1994). Though these constructs have some intuitive similarity, the question is: how does a person get from A to B? Application of the epigenetic approach suggests a position based on three issues.[2]

First is the concept of *isomorphism*: a similarity in form. At a basic level, a core aspect should be observable both in a simple childhood attribute and in a complex adult personality trait. For example, the ability to complete a task is common to both attentional orientation and conscientiousness, so it could be argued that they are similar in form. For another example, the temperament dimension of negative emotionality, indicating that one is easily irritated, is correlated in adolescence with items on anger-proneness (e.g., dealing with problems through blaming and criticizing other people) which in turn shares essential content with terms such as *quarrelsome*, and *explosive*, which are markers for the Big Five trait of (low) Agreeableness. Hence, one can observe similarity in core content for these dimensions, though the Big Five measure of Agreeableness is considerably more complex.

A second issue for the linkage of temperament and personality is termed *accretion of socialized content*. Certain facets of behavior may become incorporated in adult personality because of the correlation of temperament with social interaction processes (Rothbart & Ahadi, 1994; Wills, Sandy, & Yaeger, 2000). For example, a child with good attentional orientation can finish tasks that he/she begins and accordingly would receive positive social reinforcement for projects conducted with other persons. Hence, when the individual promises to do something the promise will likely be fulfilled, so this person will acquire a social reputation for being dependable and reliable. For another example, a child with high negative emotionality will not easily form communal relationships with other persons, and the child will have to deal with the social environment through threats, tantrums, and deceitful behavior. As the child acquires additional cognitive skills and uses them to pursue these aims, then he or she would come to be regarded as bossy, manipulative, or devious. In each case it should be noted that the adult characteristics are not inherent in the core content of the temperament dimension, but may occur as correlated attributes because of a systematic impact of the temperament characteristic on the social environment.

The third issue for the linkage of temperament and personality is the concept of good self-control and poor self-control as *higher-order organized systems*. For example, good self-control in everyday situations is a complex behavior that is based on learning of social rules and moral standards and involves use of cognitive behavioral strategies to delay gratification and cue appropriate problem-solving responses (Mischel et al., 1989; Rothbart, Derryberry, & Posner, 1994). In theory, achieving mastery of some aspects will facilitate learning and performance of other aspects, so there should be correlations among different aspects of good self-control. This predicts that various indices of good self-control will be internally consistent, that is, they represent an organized system. Conversely, children with initial difficulty in achieving an expected level of control may come to rely more on approaches that impose impulsive, emotional response and coercion on others, and will learn to have an impact on other persons through opposition and defiance rather than through cooperative responses. Therefore, it is predicted that various indices of poor self-control (including impulsiveness and angry responses to problem situations) also will be intercorrelated. These arguments lead to a perspective suggesting that good self-control and poor self-control will be relatively independent systems, and will be related to different aspects of temperament. Supportive data for these predictions have been reported in several places (Martin, Earleywine, Blackson, Vanyukov, Moss, & Tarter, 1994; Wills, Sandy, & Shinar, 1999; Wills et al., 2001).

EVIDENCE ON EARLY DISPOSITIONAL FACTORS AND HEALTH RISK

Evidence from different types of studies has suggested a linkage of early dispositional factors with adult health status. These variables are referred to here as *dispositional factors* rather than temperament because the initial assessments in several studies were conducted long before current temperament theories were developed, so it is not always clear how the measures map onto particular dimensions of temperament. However, the mapping is sometimes fairly clear and inferences can be made about what dimensions were measured.

Follow-Up Study of the Terman Cohort

Evidence from a long-term follow-up study has linked two dispositional factors with longevity (Friedman et al., 1993, 1995a, 1995b; Schwartz et al., 1995). This project was based on data from a study of bright middle-class students in California, begun in 1922 by Lewis Terman and colleagues. The initial assessment involved ratings on 25 personality traits by parents and teachers, obtained when the participants had a mean age of 11 years. The original sample of 856 males and 672 females has been followed over time and reassessed at 5- to 10-year intervals. In recent reports, over 90% of the sample had been successfully followed; 63% of the participants were still alive, and mortality status was verified for the other 37% of the sample.

The research by Friedman and colleagues (1993) used constructed scales derived from the original 25 personality ratings, with most groupings based on their presumed resemblance to traits in the Big Five model. For example, a scale termed *Conscientiousness-Social Dependability* was derived from four ratings indicating at the high pole that the participant was *prudent, free from vanity, conscientious,* and *truthful*. This constructed scale was inferred to represent the Big Five dimension of *Conscientiousness*. A measure labeled *Cheerfulness* was based on the ratings *cheerful-optimistic* and *has sense of humor*. Other scales were labeled Sociability (e.g., popularity, leadership, preference for being in groups), High Energy (e.g., physical energy, preference for playing outdoors), High Motivation (e.g., self-confidence, desire to excel), and Permanency of Moods (one item).

Predictive analyses used longevity as the criterion. The strongest finding was a protective effect for Conscientiousness, found for both males and females. Participants who had high conscientiousness scores as children lived longer (Friedman et al., 1993) and were less likely to die from cancer, cardiovascular disease, or accidental injury (Friedman et al., 1995b). This represents a 30% greater mortality risk among low-conscientious participants, comparable to the risk associated with physiological measures such as high serum cholesterol (Friedman et al., 1995b). Control analyses included indices for obesity, alcohol consumption, and cigarette smoking, obtained through retrospective reports by participants or their survivors. The data indicated that conscientious children were less likely to be smokers or heavy drinkers as adults. Mediation analyses showed that including smoking and alcohol consumption variables reduced the effect for the dispositional measure, but the effect of conscientiousness on longevity remained significant. The authors suggested that the effect of conscientiousness was not mediated through smoking or drinking, but they did recognize that retrospective reports and missing data reduced the sensitivity of these analyses.

Predictive analyses showed the scale for Cheerfulness was *inversely* related to longevity, and people with high cheerfulness scores in childhood were more likely to smoke, drink, and take risks as adults (Friedman et al., 1995b). So again there is support for relation of a dispositional characteristic to substance use. Control analyses showed the effect of cheerfulness remained significant when alcohol use was included in the model, but became nonsignificant when smoking was included, suggestive of mediation.[3] The finding that the scale for cheerfulness was a risk factor was surprising to the authors, who suggested several interpretations for this effect (Friedman et al., 1995b). It is possible this scale was a proxy for the temperament dimension of sociability, which has some of the same correlates among adolescents (Tarter, 1988; Wills, Sandy, & Yaeger, 2000).

Long-Term Effects of Hostility

Measures of hostility may be related to the temperament dimension of negative emotionality. Longitudinal studies have shown that measures of hostility predict incidence of cardiovascular disease in adulthood (e.g., Barefoot, Dahlstrom, & Williams, 1983), and researchers have obtained measures of some intermediate risk factors. For example, Siegler and colleagues (1992) analyzed data for a sample of 7038 participants who were originally assessed as undergraduates at Duke University. A 25-year follow-up included blood lipid measures and self-reports of health behavior. Results showed that hostility score at age 19 was significantly related to cigarette smoking, larger body mass index, and unfavorable ratio of total cholesterol/high density lipoproteins (HDL) as measured at follow-up. Cross-sectional analyses for data from age 42 also indicated significant relationships of hostility to hypertension and heavy drinking. This study provides evidence on how hostility is related to known risk factors for cardiovascular disease.

Similar findings were noted in the CARDIA (Coronary Artery Risk Development in Young Adults) study (Scherwitz et al., 1992), in which a representative sample of 5115 young adults (ages 18–30 years) was assessed and measures of physiological risk factors were obtained through direct examination. Results indicated that hostility was related to cigarette and marijuana use, to alcohol intake, and to a high waist/hip ratio (an index of central body-fat distribution). Although relationships to blood lipids were nonsignificant in this study, hostility was related to a clustering of factors that place an individual at risk for cardiovascular disease, including physiological variables, low social support, and more negative life events (Scherwitz et al., 1991). There is evidence that hostility and anger-proneness are relatively stable during childhood and adolescence (Matthews, Woodall, Kenyon, & Jacob, 1996), so these findings imply that risk status accruing from hostility may begin before adulthood.

Longitudinal Studies on Prediction of Substance Use

Longitudinal studies are of interest because they obtain measures of dispositional characteristics at early ages, follow the subjects over time, and examine whether early characteristics predict substance abuse. Four consistent findings from earlier studies have been noted for prediction of alcoholism assessed at ages 30–47 years (see Tarter, 1988; Zucker & Gomberg, 1986). First, people who became alcoholic were likely to have been highly active as children, sometimes being described as hyperactive; this suggests a link to the temperament dimension of activity level. Second, a history of poorly controlled behavior was predictive of adult alcoholism; this dimension was variously characterized as irritability, aggressiveness, or school behavior problems. Though temporal relationships are unclear (because many of these variables were retrospective), this suggests a linkage between negative emotionality and poor self-control. The third finding is that, although early I.Q. was similar for alcoholics and nonalcoholics, evidence of learning difficulties was predictive of alcohol abuse. This suggests a linkage to attentional and self-control problems that affect school performance. The fourth convergence was that individuals who became alcoholic were not closely tied to others interpersonally; they were more likely to have parents who displayed lack of affection, and were more likely to have distant relationships with siblings.

In the Oakland Growth Study (Jones, 1968), a representative sample was assessed with multiple methods at ages 12–14 years, and participants were followed into adulthood and classified for drinking behavior in their middle 40s. Though the longitudinal sample of 66 people was relatively small, findings indicated that several variables from adolescent assessments discriminated the future problem drinkers. Elevations were noted on ratings such as *rapid tempo*, markers for activity level; rating of *direct hostility*, which may be a marker for negative emotionality; and ratings such as *undercontrolled* and *self-indulgent*, which may be markers for poor self-control. Future problem drinkers had low scores on ratings on being *dependable* and *objective*, which appear to be markers for conscientiousness, and on items such as *doesn't seek reassurance from others* and *not considerate of others*, which seem to reflect distancing from interpersonal relationships.

A prospective study by Block and colleagues was based on a sample of 105 participants recruited from a university nursery school and measured from 3–4 years of age through multiple assessments conducted by trained examiners. Follow-up data obtained at age 14 years (Block, Block, & Keyes, 1988) indicated that drug users were characterized in early assessments as high on activity and restlessness, *negativism* and hostility, reactivity to frustration, independence and rebelliousness. The future drug users were also characterized early on as low on *planfulness* and ability to concentrate, dependability, ability to delay gratification, cooperativeness and consideration for others, and closeness to others. The similarity of predictive variables to temperament dimensions and self-control is evident in these data, and the convergence with findings from Jones's (1968) study is striking.

A notable investigation conducted in Finland was based on a sample of 292 children who were first assessed at 8–9 years of age (Pulkkinen &

Pitkänen, 1994). The sample was followed into young adulthood, and alcohol usage status at 26–27 years was determined from self-report and official arrest records. Results indicated that problem drinking was predicted by early ratings of poor concentration ability, high aggressiveness, low prosociality, and poor school performance. A gender difference was noted for ratings of social anxiety; *low* anxiety predicted alcohol abuse among males, whereas *high* anxiety predicted alcohol abuse among females. In this study the measure of *prosociality* was based on items about being reliable, keeping promises, and acting reasonably in problem situations, so this seems more like a scale of good self-control than an index of gregariousness or sociability.

Temperament and Hostility in Relation to the Metabolic Syndrome

A study of a cohort of 3596 Finnish children and adolescents (ages 3–18 years at baseline) by Keltikangas-Järvinen and colleagues has provided evidence on how temperament dimensions and related constructs are linked to physiological variables. Somatic risk indicators in this research include systolic blood pressure (SBP) and diastolic blood pressure (DBP); serum lipid levels based on measures such as low density lipoproteins (LDL) and high-density lipoproteins (HDL); and body mass index, the ratio of weight/height. These researchers have examined relationships of predictors to components of the metabolic syndrome, which comprises insulin resistance, high blood pressure, and an atherogenic plasma lipid profile together with central body-fat distribution (Björntorp, 1991, 1992).

The metabolic syndrome is of relevance to health status for two reasons (Epel et al., 2000; Schneiderman & Skyler, 1995). One is that the components of the syndrome are consistently observed to be intercorrelated among adults (Haffner, Ferrannini, Hazuda, & Stern, 1992; Niaura et al., 2000) as well as in children (Chu, Rimm, Wang, Liou, & Shieh, 1998), and a high score on the syndrome places individuals at risk for heart disease (Lindblad, Langer, Wingard, Thomas, & Barrett-Connor, 2001; Nelson, Palmer, & Pederson, 2001; Vitaliano et al., 2002). A second reason is that syndrome scores are moderately stable from childhood/adolescence into young adulthood (Bao, Srinivasan, Wattingney, & Berenson, 1994; Katzmarzyk, Perusse, Malina, Bergeron, Despres, & Bouchard, 2001; Raitakari, Porkka, Räsänen, Rönnemaa, & Viikari, 1994). Thus early levels of the physiological variables may be prognostic for adult health status.

Data have been reported on relations of several indices of hostility to behavioral and somatic risk factors within the metabolic syndrome. Räikkönen and Keltikangas-Järvinen (1991) analyzed data from two assessments with a selected group of 2938 participants who were 12–21 at the first examination and were followed up 3 years later. Hostility was indexed with a three-item measure (e.g., "I get angry easily"). Results showed people with higher hostility were more likely to smoke heavily at the time of the second interview, and also reported physical inactivity more frequently (cf. Scherwitz et al., 1991). A relationship of hostility to alcohol use was found for males. Longitudinal findings on aggression, indexed by the Hunter-Wolf (HW) inventory, showed aggressiveness related among males to increases in triglyceride values, serum insulin concentration, and body mass index (Ravaja, Keltikangas-Järvinen, & Keskivaara, 1996). For females a subscale termed Energy (e.g., "I eat too fast") was the only variable related to change in metabolic syndrome score.

Data on Type A personality attributes were obtained using a measure that factored into several scales (see Keltikangas-Järvinen & Räikkönen, 1989). One scale, which is conceptually similar to high activity level and poor self-control, included items such as "I can't sit still for long," "When I have to wait for others I become impatient," and "I get easily irritated;" this was termed *Impatience-Aggression*. The second scale included favorable items such as "Other children look to me for leadership," "I am hard-driving and competitive," and "When working or playing I try to do better than others." This was termed *Leadership-Sense of Responsibility*. These characteristics are related in opposite directions to coronary disease risk factors (Keltikangas-Järvinen & Räikkönen, 1990; Räikkönen, Keltikangas-Järvinen, & Solakivi, 1990). Subjects with high scores on Impatience-Aggression had more unfavorable lipid profiles and higher blood pressure, though findings were not totally consistent across age-sex groups. People scoring high on Sense of Responsibility tended to have more favorable status, for example, lower cholesterol levels.

These researchers have also investigated relationships of several temperament measures to indicators of the metabolic syndrome. Keltikangas-Järvinen, Räikkonnen, and Lehtimäki (1993) examined relationships of temperament to six phenotypes of apolipoprotein E (apoE) that have a known ranking in relation to risk for cardiovascular disease. Temperament was assessed through two sources, mother's ratings for younger subjects and self-reports for older subjects; and through two methods, Likert scales and semantic-differential scales. Activity level was related to apoE phenotypes in the predicted order, with highest activity among participants with the highest risk phenotype. The result for activity is conceptually similar to a previous finding that hyperactivity, impatience, and aggressiveness were related to higher levels of apolipoprotein B (apoB), also a risk factor for heart disease (Keltikangas-Järvinen, Räikkonnen, & Solakivi, 1990).

The relation of temperament dimensions from mothers' reports to components of the metabolic syndrome was studied by Rajava and Keltikangas-Järvinen (1995) in a sample of 1589 participants who were 6–15 years of age at baseline and 9–18 years at follow-up. A number of significant relationships of temperament dimensions to syndrome components were observed, consistent across cross-sectional and longitudinal analyses. High motor activity level and negative emotionality were clearly risk factors, related to most of the syndrome components (e.g., higher blood pressure, insulin and body mass, lower HDL). In contrast, two semantic-differential measures termed mental vitality (alert, full of energy) and emotionality (friendly, happy) were clear protective factors, related to lower levels of risk on all the syndrome components in a multivariate analysis.[4] Results for sociability measures were perplexing. A measure termed "responsivity to others" (e.g., sociable, talkative) was positively related in univariate analyses to higher insulin, higher triglycerides, and lower HDL. Though social interaction is associated with positive mood (Diener, 1984), these correlations seem to indicate the temperament measure as positively related to risk status.

STUDIES OF TEMPERAMENT AND ADOLESCENT SUBSTANCE USE

Studies conducted by the present authors with adolescents have focused on substance use as a behavioral mechanism through which dispositional factors may be related, over the long-term, to health risk. It was hypothesized that temperament dimensions may be relevant for early onset of substance use (ca. 11 years). The research was designed to test an epigenetic model of the relationship between temperament and substance use, proposing that effects of temperament are primarily indirect ones, mediated through self-control.

Theoretical Model

The essence of the predictions is outlined in Figure 1.1. The first part of the model, indicated graphically at the left side of the figure, proposes that effects of temperament will be mediated through self-control ability (Rothbart & Ahadi, 1994; Tarter et al., 1995). From epigenetic theory it is predicted that

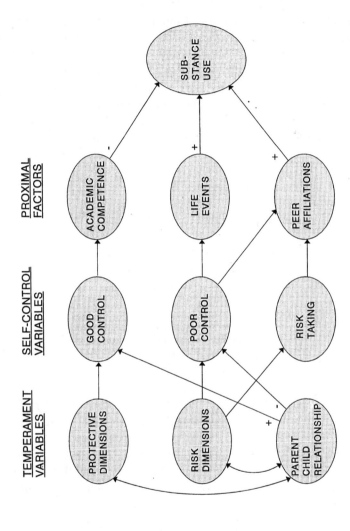

FIGURE 1.1 Theoretical model of mediational process for relationship between temperament dimensions and adolescent substance use. Distal factors (temperament and parental variables) are at left side of figure, mediating variables (self-control and risk-taking) are in center, and proximal factors are at right. Double-headed arrows represent correlations, single-headed arrows represent causal effects. + symbol indicates hypothesized positive effect, – symbol represents hypothesized inverse effect.

some temperament dimensions, such as attentional control, will be related to good self-control ability, whereas other dimensions such as activity level will be related to poor self-control. The parent-child relationship is included as a variable in the epigenetic model: A correlation is predicted between temperament and parent-child relationship variables, and this effect should be observable in adolescence.

The second part of the model, indicated in the center of the figure, specifies how self-control is related to proximal risk factors for substance use. It is known that variables such as low academic competence, negative life events, and affiliation with peer substance users are risk factors for adolescent substance use (e.g., Hawkins, Catalano, & Miller, 1992; Wills, 1990). The epigenetic approach suggests that these factors will be related to self-control variables; specifically, good control will contribute to better academic competence (a protective factor), whereas poor control could be predisposing to experiencing negative life events and affiliating with deviance prone peers (risk factors).

The third part of the model, indicated at the right-hand side of the figure, posits that negative life events and deviant peer affiliations are proximal risk factors for substance use. It is possible that experiencing many negative life events is an independent risk factor because of concomitant emotional distress and feelings of helplessness and meaninglessness in life (Newcomb & Harlow, 1986; Wills, 1994). Affiliation with peer substance users is predicted to be a proximal factor because friends who smoke or drink provide modeling of the behavior, communicate favorable attitudes and norms about substance use, and may actually be a source of cigarettes or alcohol that they get from family members or older peers (Mosbach & Leventhal, 1988). In addition, being part of a substance-using group means becoming immersed in an environment where a group attitude develops with increasing tolerance for deviance (Patterson, DeBaryshe, & Ramsey, 1989; Wills, McNamara, Vaccaro, & Hirky, 1996). Thus, it was predicted that life events and peer affiliations would be pathways through which other variables operate.

Methods

The authors have conducted several studies in school-based research with samples from the New York metropolitan area, obtaining data through questionnaires administered by trained research staff to students in classrooms. The samples of participants range from 11–16 years. The samples are multiethnic, including approximately 30% African Americans, 25% Hispanics, and 35%

Caucasians. In terms of socioeconomic status the samples are generally representative of the New York State population. Across five studies, sample sizes ranged from about 900 subjects to around 1800 subjects.

The temperament measures have included the Revised Dimensions of Temperament Survey (DOTS-R, Windle & Lerner, 1986), the Emotionality, Activity, and Sociability Inventory (EAS, Buss & Plomin, 1984), and the Adolescent Temperament Survey (Capaldi & Rothbart, 1992). This was done because no single inventory included all the scales that have been discussed as theoretically relevant to prediction of substance use.

Temperament and Early Onset

One aim of this research program was to determine whether temperament dimensions are predictive for early onset of tobacco/alcohol use, which is known to be of prognostic significance for liability to substance abuse in adulthood (Kandel & Davies, 1992; Robins & Przybeck, 1985). In one study a sample of 1810 students who were in sixth grade (mean age 11.5 years) was surveyed using scales for five dimensions of temperament and related self-control variables. For the criterion construct, measures of cigarette, alcohol, and marijuana use were combined in a composite score representing involvement in substance use.

The results showed significant relationships of temperament to substance use even at this young age (Wills et al., 2001). Activity level and negative emotionality were positively related to substance use, attentional orientation, and positive emotionality were inversely related to substance use, and these were all independent effects. Thus, temperament was related to early onset. Correlations with self-control measures were consistent with the model: Activity level and negative emotionality were related to poorer self-control abilities, whereas attentional orientation and positive emotionality were related to better self-control abilities. Hence, the predictions for the first stage of the theoretical model were supported.

Structural modeling analysis was tested whether the effects of temperament on proximal risk factors were mediated in the predicted manner. The paths were quite close to those hypothesized in Figure 1.1. Temperament dimensions had paths to the self-control constructs. These in turn had effects to negative life events and deviant peer affiliations; for example, poor self-control was related to more negative life events. Finally, peer affiliations had a strong path to participants' substance use. There were no direct effects from temperament to substance use. Thus, the analysis showed the effects of temperament were mediated through self-control, as predicted by epigenetic theory.

Temperament and Risk Taking

Another set of studies has examined how temperament is related to risk-taking tendency. This is relevant for health behavior because constructs labeled as risk-taking (Wills, Vaccaro, & McNamara, 1994) or sensation-seeking (Zuckerman, 1994) have been related to adolescent substance use and other health risk behaviors, but it is not clear whether they reflect a temperamentlike dimension or some epigenetic derivative.

A study conducted with 1225 older adolescents (mean age 15.5 years) provided a direct test of whether risk-taking represented an independent pathway for substance use etiology (Wills, Sandy, & Shinar, 1999). Confirmatory analyses demonstrated that a construct of risk-taking tendency was distinct from poor self-control, and structural modeling analysis indicated risk-taking tendency was related to deviant peer affiliations and coping motives for substance use. Risk-taking is related to activity level and novelty seeking, so studies suggest that it is a derivative from simpler temperament dimensions (Wills, Windle, & Cleary, 1998). It should be noted that family measures (e.g., parent-child conflict) also made contributions to risk-taking, so it is evident that risk-taking is a construct with multiple determinants, some more temperamental and some more familial in nature.

Rigidity and Risk Behavior

The dimension of rigidity has been construed as indexing the behavioral inhibition system as outlined in Gray's theory (Gray, 1991; Rothbart et al., 1994). Results for rigidity emphasize the need for careful construal of dimensions related to anxiety, social withdrawal, and other indicators of negative affect. Zero-order correlations typically show rigidity *positively* related to substance use, with significant but modest correlations. However, in multivariate analyses that include other dimensions, rigidity may be *inversely* related to substance use.

Structural modeling analyses clarified the basis for this complexity, showing rigidity related both to indices of good control and to indices of poor control (e.g., Wills et al., 2001). In one study (Wills, Windle, & Cleary, 1998) rigidity was related to Cloninger's scale of harm avoidance, which, in turn, was inversely related to adolescent substance use, probably because of the aspects of inhibition and social anxiety that are parts of this dimension. These results suggest that there is a common element of negative affect associated with several temperament dimensions, and only when this element is partialled do the unique effects of inhibition become evident.

Approach Dimensions and Risk Behavior

Results for dimensions representing social approach were complex. In various studies we have used the Sociability scale from the EAS, which has items such as "I like to be around people," and the Approach dimension from the DOTS-R, which has items such as "I approach new situations and people." Sociability and approach are related to measures of positive mood; individuals with high scores also endorse items such as "I am a cheerful person." So sociability would appear to be a protective attribute. It also shows some positive correlation with activity level, so one can see here the beginnings of the typical adult Extraversion dimension that includes facets for gregariousness, energy, and positive mood.

The zero-order correlation of sociability (or approach) with substance use is usually nonsignificant; in fact the correlations are close to zero. When these are included in multiple regression models with other dimensions, however, they are significantly and *positively* related to substance use. So in this sense approach tendency appears more like a risk dimension. This type of relationship (technically termed a suppression effect) is typical for social competence measures, and has been found in several studies (e.g., Chassin et al., 1993; Wills, Mariani, & Filer, 1996).

Third, sociability and approach dimensions have complex effects in structural models. Approach has paths to good self-control and task reward dependence, which are protective effects, but it also has independent effects to novelty seeking, poor self-control, and risk taking—definitely risk-promoting effects. The complexity of effects may help to explain why approach considered alone has no significant correlation with substance use: the complex effects tend to cancel each other out. When the total effects for sociability and approach through multiple pathways are computed, these temperament dimensions have positive effects on substance use because of their indirect effects through novelty seeking and poor control.

Findings from Other Samples

Though there has been little investigation of cultural differences in how temperament is related to outcomes (Rothbart & Bates, 1998), there have been questions about the predominance of Caucasian samples in previous temperament research. One recent study has investigated effects of temperament and self-control in a sample of 889 rural African American children (mean age 10.5 years) who lived in two different geographic areas of the U.S., Iowa and Georgia. This study showed significant effects for risk-promoting temperament dimensions (e.g., activity level) and protective dimensions (e.g., task orientation) that were similar to those found in other studies. In addition, indirect effects of temperament, through self-control, were found in relation to predisposing factors for early onset; these included protective factors such as resistance efficacy, and risk factors such as willingness to try cigarettes or alcohol.

For physiological variables, clustering of metabolic-syndrome indicators and prospective relations of hostility and Type A personality measures to metabolic syndrome indicators have been found in U.S. samples with African American adolescents (Davis, Kapuku, Goldberg, Kumar, & Treiber, 2001; Räikkönen, K., personal communication, 16 August 2001). Thus, effects for dispositional characteristics have been found in several different samples, and have been demonstrated to be relevant for early onset of substance use as well as for development of other risk factors.

GENERAL DISCUSSION

In this chapter the proposition has been advanced that temperament dimensions, measured at relatively early ages, may be related to health status at later ages. This perspective was used to discuss evidence for behavioral and physiological mechanisms, and findings from our studies that tested a mediational model of temperament/substance use relationships were presented. The results were generally supportive of our theoretical perspective: They show that temperament dimensions are related to substance use in predicted ways, and demonstrate that effects of temperament are mediated through more complex attributes: self-control and risk-taking tendency. The form of our findings is consistent with evidence from studies on personality predictors of adult health status.

Findings from the authors' research show that dimensions of temperament may operate as risk factors or as protective factors. The strongest evidence for a protective effect is for the dimension of attentional orientation, which has several types of desirable effects. This seems to be a precursor for the personality dimension of Conscientiousness, which has been related to health behavior and health status in several studies (Friedman et al., 1995a; Jones, 1968). Evidence of risk-factor status is clear for two dimensions. Negative emotionality appears to be a precursor for hostility at later ages, a trait that has been consistently linked to risk for heart disease in adulthood (Scherwitz et al., 1992; Siegler et al., 1992). In addition there is definite evidence for activity level as a risk factor (e.g., Rajava & Keltikangas-Järvinen, 1995; Wills, Windle, & Cleary, 1998). This dimension has no clear analogue in the Big Five system, but is linked to the constructs of novelty seeking and sensation seeking, which have been demonstrated in other personality systems (Cloninger et al., 1993; Zuckerman, 1994).[5]

For a dimension defined as either general approach tendency or social approach tendency (i.e., sociability), the evidence is perplexing. Our studies show that while approach dimensions are correlated with positive mood, they also represent a risk factor for substance use. This is because approach tendency is related to novelty seeking and risk-taking tendency (cf. Cloninger, 1994). These findings need to be considered together with evidence showing a measure labeled Cheerfulness to be positively related to mortality (Friedman et al., 1995b). The exception is a study reporting a measure labeled as Positive Emotionality to be inversely related to the metabolic syndrome (Rajava & Keltikangas-Järvinen, 1995). This suggests that positive emotionality is a protective factor, but approach tendency has risk-promoting effects when its correlation with positive mood is partialled.

The theoretical model suggested that temperament dimensions have indirect effects in relation to substance use. The authors' research has consistently supported this model, showing effects of temperament to be indirect ones, through pathways to self-control. The position of self-control as a central factor in health behavior is increasingly suggested by theoretical work deriving both from clinical research (Miller & Brown, 1991) and from basic research in psychopharmacology (Koob & LeMoal, 1997). This perspective has been useful for elucidating how the effects of dispositional factors occur through impact of self-control on competencies (e.g., academic performance), stressors (e.g., negative life events), and social relationships (e.g., affiliation with deviant peers).

Substance Use and Other Possible Mechanisms

In this chapter, we have outlined an argument that temperament dimensions are related to health status through their relation to substance use. Evidence from studies of adolescents shows that temperament dimensions are related to cigarette smoking and alcohol use, and collateral evidence from other parts of the life span is consistent with this perspective (Scherwitz et al., 1992; Siegler et al., 1992). So we think there is a strong case for temperament/ substance use relationships as a significant mechanism linking dispositional factors and health status. Some analyses have failed to find evidence for complete mediation of personality effects through smoking and alcohol use (Friedman et al., 1995a&b), but these analyses were conducted for adult samples and were based on retrospective third-party reports, which may be relatively insensitive. Furthermore, studies of hostility consistently show relationships to substance use. Additional research may help to clarify this issue through investigating factors such as the quantity and extent of substance use, or the duration of exposure, and by giving consideration to gender differences.

While the substance use mechanism is a promising one, we do not suggest that this is the only possible mechanism through which temperament could be related to health status.A linkage of temperament characteristics to health status through relationships to preventive health behaviors that involve planning and self-control is plausible (Kirscht, 1983). For example, the dimension of attentional orientation and its derivative, Conscientiousness, involve ability for planning, gathering information, organizing and evaluating alternative courses of action. These executive functions would likely be of significant value for preventive behaviors that involve planning, such as engaging in regular exercise and making choices about diet. Some aspects of our research also indicate that *soothability*, the ability to calm oneself down when emotionally distressed, is a facet of good self-control (cf. Rosenbaum, 1990; Tarter et al., 1995), so a protective effect through emotional stabilization is also possible. In contrast, several temperamental derivatives under the rubric of poor self-control (impulsiveness, lack of foresight, risk-taking tendency, unwise choice of companions) are likely to increase the likelihood of accidents or disease exposures. Hence both protective and risk-promoting temperament characteristics may have ramifications beyond their linkage to substance use, because they may contribute to effective coping and problem solving (or the lack of these) across a variety of domains.

A third model would propose that a temperament dimension such as negative emotionality is associated with greater sympathetic nervous system (SNS) reactivity (i.e., elevation of heart rate and blood pressure), which is a risk factor for cardiovascular disease (see, e.g., Siegman, 1994), and this would constitute a direct physiological mechanism. This is a complex issue because even at younger ages, negative emotionality has a number of facets besides overt anger: greater irritability to all kinds of stimuli, lower feelings of control, beliefs about the hostile intentions of others, and attributions about events. Research is suggested to investigate how temperament dimensions are related in psychophysiological paradigms to reactivity variables that may play a role in cardiovascular disease. At the same time, addressing the question of how adverse effects of negative emotionality and hostility occur requires attention to cognitive/behavioral self-regulation mechanisms as well as to physiology (Friedman, 1992; Rosenbaum, 1990).

Finally, serious consideration should be given to the concept that a metabolic dysregulation may underlie some of the observed effects. One reason this model is plausible is that a heritable deficit in glucose metabolism may contribute to the metabolic syndrome (DeFronzo & Ferrannini, 1991), and this has been suggested as the starting point for effects on the syndrome involving body fat distribution, blood lipids, and hypertension (Björntorp, 1992). Although the causal priority among pathways to observed physiological effects has not been settled (Schneiderman & Skyler, 1995), the research of Keltikangas-Järvinen and colleagues (1993, 1995) has shown temperament dimensions to be related to the components of the metabolic syndrome, and this is suggestive of a linking mechanism. Moreover, recent neurobiological research on drug abuse liability has suggested that a dysregulation of the hypothalamic-adrenal-pituitary axis is associated with drug self-administration through a higher sensitivity to the behavioral and dopamine-activating effects of glucocorticoids (Piazza & Le Moal, 1996). The implication for human research is that drug abuse liability may be related to deficits in emotional or behavioral regulation, and the relationship of some temperament dimensions to substance use may occur through this kind of mechanism (Koob & Le Moal, 1997). This suggests attention to research focused on the linkage of temperament characteristics to neurobiological systems involved in self-regulation.

Immutable Attributes or Modifiable Mechanisms?

What message does this research send for prevention research? Some might think that if temperament dimensions and personality traits have significant heritability, then prevention efforts would be futile. Nothing could be further from the truth. For one thing, characteristics such as activity level or attentional ability are subject to many types of influences. For example, it has been observed that children's temperament characteristics are related to parental substance abuse (e.g., Rajava & Keltikangas-Järvinen, 2001; Windle, 1990), and recent research has shown that early exposure to lead is a significant influence on subsequent levels of these characteristics (Minder, Das-Small, Brand, & Orlebeke, 1994; Winneke, Lilienthal, & Kramer, 1996). Hence reducing environmental exposures is a tenable goal for prevention. Another consideration is the finding of genotype X environment interactions, which show that the expression of heritable characteristics is markedly influenced by the social environment in which a child develops (see Loehlin, 1992; Wills, Sandy, Shinar, & Yaeger, 2001). Hence, the appropriate concept for prevention research is not the idea that temperament characteristics are immutable, but rather that risk status can be reduced through modification of early physical and social environments.

The other message involves the concept that dispositional factors operate by steering individuals toward certain *social niches*, such as affiliating with peers who have a proclivity for risky behavior (Scarr & McCartney, 1983; Wills & Cleary, 1999). Because this is a mechanism of temperament effects as we see them, the message is that the focus of prevention efforts should be on training to improve self-control ability and academic performance and interventions that teach skills for avoiding high-risk situations. Hence, understanding the mechanism of temperament effects expands, not contracts, the range of options for prevention of adverse outcomes.

CONCLUSIONS

The temperament model provides a useful perspective for research on the determinants of behavior and health. There is evidence that temperament dimensions have long-term predictive value for health status, and studies with adolescents provide evidence of mechanisms for these effects. Epigenetic theory provides a framework for understanding how abstract dispositional constructs become translated into concrete behaviors that are relevant for health. The results from these studies help to clarify the multiple pathways to health risk behavior. The concepts and findings from this research may be useful for design of new studies that test theoretical mechanisms of relationships between dispositional factors and health status throughout the life span.

FOOTNOTES

[1]For example, Super and Harkness (1986) discuss observational studies indicating how temperament dimensions usually regarded as difficult were related to survival in extreme conditions such as famine.

[2]This discussion should not obscure the fact that there is still vigorous debate among researchers about the structure of adult personality. Cloninger and colleagues have advanced a system that distinguishes between more biological temperament dimensions and more socialized adult personality traits (Cloninger et al., 1993). Several investigators have marshalled evidence for additional dimensions not found in the Big Five (see Almagor, Tellegen, & Waller, 1995; Zuckerman et al., 1993).

[3]Three other scales did not show general predictive effects. Sociability was nonsignificant. The measure for Permanency of Moods, which the authors interpreted as a marker for the Big Five dimension of Neuroticism, was positively related to longevity for males only. Measures of psychological adjustment assessed when the subjects were around 40 years of age indicated that maladjustment was inversely related to longevity, but these data are not prospective.

[4]The results for Positive Emotionality seem contradictory to findings on apoE from Keltikangas-Järvinen, Räikkonnen, and Lehtimäki (1993). However, this lipoprotein is not part of the metabolic syndrome.

[5]It remains unclear how temperament dimensions map onto other health-relevant constructs such as optimism (Scheier & Carver, 1987) or perceived control (Wills, 1994). Are they primary attributes or complex derivatives from simpler dimensions? We think the evidence favors the latter interpretation. For example, a recent study found task reward dependence correlated with optimism and internal control, whereas novelty seeking and harm avoidance were correlated with pessimism and lack of control (Wills, Sandy, & Shinar, 1999). Further research is necessary to determine the linkage between these constructs.

REFERENCES

Almagor, M., Tellegen, A., & Waller, N. G. (1995). The Big Seven Model: A cross-cultural replication. *Journal of Personality and Social Psychology, 69,* 300–307.

Angleitner, A., & Ostendorf, F. (1994). Temperament and the Big Five factors of personality. In C. Halverson, G. Kohnstamm, & R. Martin (Eds.), *The developing structure of temperament and personality from infancy to adulthood* (pp. 69–90). Hillsdale, NJ: Erlbaum.

Bao, W., Srinivasan, S., Wattingney, W., & Berenson, G. S. (1994). Persistence of multiple cardiovascular risk clustering related to syndrome X from childhood to young adulthood: The Bogalusa Heart Study. *Archives of Internal Medicine, 154,* 1842–1847.

Bardo, M. T., Donohew, R. L., & Harrington, N. G. (1997). Psychobiology of novelty seeking and drug-seeking behavior. *Behavioural Brain Research, 77,* 23–43.

Barefoot, J. C., Dahlstrom, G., & Williams, R. B. (1983). Hostility, CHD incidence, and mortality: A 25-year follow-up study of physicians. *Psychosomatic Medicine, 45,* 59–64.

Björntorp, P. (1991). Metabolic implications of body fat distribution. *Diabetes Care, 14,* 1132–1143.

Björntorp, P. (1992). Abdominal obesity and the metabolic syndrome. *Annals of Medicine, 24,* 465–468.

Block, J., Block, J., & Keyes, S. (1988). Foretelling drug use in adolescence: Early personality and environmental precursors. *Child Development, 59,* 336–355.

Bouchard, T. (1994). Genes, environment, and personality. *Science, 264,* 1700–1701.

Buss, A., & Plomin, R. (1984). *Temperament: Early developing personality traits.* Hillsdale, NJ: Erlbaum.

Cairns, R. B., & Ornstein, P. A. (1979). Developmental psychology. In E. Hearst (Ed.), *The first century of developmental psychology.* Hillsdale, NJ: Erlbaum.

Capaldi, D. M., & Rothbart, M. K. (1992). Development and validation of an early adolescent temperament measure. *Journal of Early Adolescence, 12,* 153–172.

Caspi, A., Henry, B., McGee, R. O., Moffitt, T. E., & Silva, P. A. (1995). Temperamental origins of adolescent behavior problems. *Child Development, 66,* 55–68.

Caspi, A., Moffitt, T., Newman, D., & Silva, P. (1996). Behavioral observations at age 3 years predict adult psychiatric disorders. *Archives of General Psychiatry, 53,* 1033–1039.

Chassin, L. A., Pillow, D. R., Curran, P. J., Molina, B., & Barrera, M. (1993). Relation of parental alcoholism to early adolescent substance use: A test of three mediating mechanisms. *Journal of Abnormal Psychology, 102,* 3–19.

Chu, N-F., Rimm, E. B., Wang, D-J., Liou, H-S., & Shieh, S-M. (1998). Clustering of cardiovascular disease risk factors among obese school children: The Taipei Children's Heart Study. *American Journal of Clinical Nutrition, 67,* 1141–1146.

Cloninger, C. R. (1994). Temperament and personality. *Current Opinion in Neurobiology, 4,* 266–273.

Cloninger, C. R., Svrakic, D. M., & Przybeck, T. R. (1993). A psychobiological model of temperament and character. *Archives of General Psychiatry, 50,* 975–990.

Davis, C. L., Kapuku, G., Goldberg, R., Kumar, M., & Treiber, F. A. (2001, March). Insulin resistance syndrome and left ventricular mass in healthy adolescents. Paper presented at the meeting of the American Psychosomatic Society, Monterey, CA.

DeFronzo, R. A., & Ferrannini, E. (1991). Insulin resistance: A multifaceted syndrome responsible for NIDDM, obesity, hypertension, dyslipidemia, and atherosclerotic cardiovascular disease. *Diabetes Care, 14,* 173–194.

Diener, E. (1984). Subjective well-being. *Psychological Bulletin, 95,* 542–575.

Digman, J. M., & Inouye, J. (1986). Further specific of five robust factors of personality. *Journal of Personality and Social Psychology, 50,* 116–123.

Eisenberg, N., Fabes, R. A., Guthrie, I. K., & Reiser, M. (2000). Dispositional emotionality and regulation: Their role in predicting quality of social functioning. *Journal of Personality and Social Psychology, 78,* 136–157.

Epel, E. S., McEwen, B., Seeman, T., Matthews, K., Castellazzo, G., Brownell, K. D., Bell, J., & Ickovics, J. R. (2000). Stress and body shape: Stress-induced cortisol secretion is greater among women with central fat. *Psychosomatic Medicine, 62,* 623–632.

Friedman, H. (Ed.) (1990). *Personality and disease.* New York: Wiley.

Friedman, H. (Ed.) (1992). *Hostility, coping, and health.* Washington, DC: American Psychological Association.

Friedman, H. S., & Booth-Kewley, S. (1987). The 'disease-prone personality': A meta-analytic view of the construct. *American Psychologist, 42,* 539–555.

Friedman, H. S., Tucker, J. S., Schwartz, J. E., Martin, L. R., Tomlinson-Keasey, C., Wingard, D. L., & Criqui, M. H. (1995a). Childhood conscientiousness and longevity: Health behaviors and cause of death. *Journal of Personality and Social Psychology, 68,* 696–703.

Friedman, H. S., Tucker, J. S., Schwartz, J. E., Tomlinson-Keasey, C., Martin, L. R., Wingard, D. L., & Criqui, M. H. (1995b). Psychosocial and behavioral predictors of longevity. *American Psychologist, 50,* 69–78.

Friedman, H. S., Tucker, J. S., Tomlinson-Keasey, C., Schwartz, J. E., Wingard, D. L., & Criqui, M. H. (1993). Does childhood personality predict longevity? *Journal of Personality and Social Psychology, 65,* 176–185.

Fulker, D. W., Cherny, S. S., & Cardon, L. R. (1993). Continuity and change in cognitive development. In R. Plomin & G. E. McClearn (Eds.), *Nature, nurture, and psychology* (pp. 77–97). Washington, DC: American Psychological Association.

Goldberg, L. R. (1993). The structure of phenotypic personality traits. *American Psychologist, 48,* 26–34.

Goldberg, L. R., & Rosolack, T. K. (1994). The Big Five structure as an integrative framework: An empirical comparison with Eysenck's P-E-N model. In C. F. Halverson, G. A. Kohnstamm, & R. P. Martin (Eds.), *The developing structure of temperament and personality from infancy to adulthood* (pp. 7–35). Hillsdale, NJ: Erlbaum.

Gray, J. A. (1991). The neuropsychology of temperament. In J. Strelau & A. Angleitner (Eds.), *Explorations in temperament: Perspectives on theory and measurement* (pp. 105–128). New York: Plenum Press.

Haffner, S. M., Ferrannini, F., Hazuda, H. P., & Stern, M. P. (1992). Clustering of cardiovascular risk factors in prehypertensive individuals. *Hypertension, 20,* 38–45.

Hagekull, B. (1989). Longitudinal stability of temperament within a behavioral style framework. In G. A. Kohnstamm, J. E. Bates, & M. K. Rothbart (Eds.), *Temperament in childhood* (pp. 283–297). New York: Wiley.

Hawkins, J. D., Catalano, R. F., & Miller, J. Y. (1992). Risk and protective factors for alcohol and other drug problems in adolescence and early adulthood. *Psychological Bulletin, 112,* 64–105.

Heath, A. C., Cloninger, C. R., & Martin, N. G. (1994). Testing a model for the genetic structure of personality: A comparison of the personality systems of Cloninger and Eysenck. *Journal of Personality and Social Psychology, 66,* 762–775.

John, O. P., Caspi, A., Robins, R. W., Moffitt, T. E., & Stouthamer-Loeber, M. (1994). The "Little Five": Exploring the nomological network of the five-factor model of personality in adolescent boys. *Child Development, 65,* 160–178.

Jones, M. C. (1968). Personality correlates and antecedents of drinking patterns in adult males. *Journal of Consulting and Clinical Psychology, 32,* 2–12.

Kandel, D., & Davies, M. (1992). Progression to regular marijuana involvement: Phenomenology and risk factors. In M. Glantz & R. Pickens (Eds.), *Vulnerability to drug abuse* (pp. 211–253). Washington, DC: American Psychological Association.

Katainen, S., Räikkönen, K., Keskivaara, P., & Keltikangas-Järvinen, L. (1999). Maternal child-rearing attitudes and children's temperament as antecedents of adolescent depressive tendencies. *Journal of Youth and Adolescence, 28,* 139–163.

Katzmarzyk, P. T., Perusse, L., Malina, R. M., Bergeron, J., Despres, J-P., & Bouchard, C. (2001). Stability of indicators of the metabolic syndrome from childhood and adolescence to young adulthood. *Journal of Clinical Epidemiology, 54,* 190–195.

Keltikangas-Järvinen, L., & Räikkönen, K. (1989). Pathogenic and protective factors of Type A behavior in adolescents. *Journal of Psychosomatic Research, 33,* 591–602.

Keltikangas-Järvinen, L., Räikkönen, K., & Solakivi, T. (1990). Type A factors as predictors of somatic risk factors of coronary heart disease in young Finns—A six-year follow-up study. *Journal of Psychosomatic Research, 34,* 89–97.

Keltikangas-Järvinen, L., Räikkönen, K., & Lehtimäki, T. (1993). Dependence between apolipoprotein E phenotypes and temperament in children, adolescents, and young adults. *Psychosomatic Medicine, 55,* 155–163.

Kirscht, J. (1983). Preventive health behavior. *Health Psychology, 2,* 277–301.

Kochanska, G. (1995). Children's temperament, mother's discipline, and security of attachment: Multiple pathways to emerging internalization. *Child Development, 66,* 597–615.

Kochanska, G., Murray, K., & Coy, K. C. (1997). Inhibitory control as a contributor to conscience in childhood: From toddler to school age. *Child Development, 68,* 263–277.

Kochanska, G., Murray, K. T., & Harlan, E. T. (2000). Effortful control in early childhood: Continuity and change, antecedents, and implications for social development. *Developmental Psychology, 36,* 220–232.

Koob, G. F., & Le Moal, M. (1997). Drug abuse: Hedonic homeostatic dysregulation. *Science, 278,* 52–58.

Lerner, J. V., & Vicary, J. R. (1984). Difficult temperament and drug use. *Journal of Drug Education, 14,* 1–8.

Lindblad, U., Langer, R. D., Wingard, D. L., Thomas, R. G. & Barrett-Connor, E. L. (2001). Metabolic syndrome and ischemic heart disease in elderly men and women. *American Journal of Epidemiology, 153,* 481–489.

Loehlin, J. C. (1992). *Genes and environment in personality development.* Newbury Park, CA: Sage.

Martin, C. S., Earleywine, M., Blackson, T. C., Vanyukov, M. M., Moss, H. M., & Tarter, R. E. (1994). Aggressivity, inattention, hyperactivity, and impulsivity in boys and high and low risk for substance abuse. *Journal of Abnormal Child Psychology, 22,* 177–203.

Matthews, K. A., Woodall, K. L., Kenyon, K., & Jacob, T. (1996). Negative family environment as a predictor of boys' future status on measures of hostile attitudes, interview behavior, and anger expression. *Health Psychology, 15,* 30–37.

Maunder, R. G., & Hunter, J. J. (2001). Attachment and psychosomatic medicine: Developmental contributions to stress and disease. *Psychosomatic Medicine, 63,* 556–567.

Miller, W. R., & Brown, J. M. (1991). Self-regulation as a conceptual basis for the prevention of addictive behaviours. In N. Heather, W. R. Miller, & J. Greeley (Eds.), *Self-control and the addictive behaviours* (pp. 3–79). Sydney, Australia: Maxwell Macmillan.

Minder, B., Das-Small, E. A., Brand, E. F., & Orlebeke, J. F. (1994). Exposure to lead and specific attentional problems in school children. *Journal of Learning Disabilities, 27,* 393–399.

Mischel, W., Shoda, Y., & Rodriguez, M. L. (1989). Delay of gratification in children. *Science, 244,* 933–938.

Moffitt, T. E. (1993). The neuropsychology of conduct disorder. *Development and Psychopathology, 5,* 135–151.

Molfese, V. J., & Molfese, D. L. (Eds.) (2000). *Temperament and personality across the life span.* Hillsdale, NJ: Erlbaum.

Mosbach, P., & Leventhal, H. (1988). Peer group identification and smoking. *Journal of Abnormal Psychology, 97,* 238–245.

Nelson, C. A. (1994). The neurobiology of temperament. In J. E. Bates & T. D. Wachs (Eds.), *Temperament: Individual differences at the interface of biology and behavior* (pp. 47–82). Washington, DC: American Psychological Association.

Nelson, T. L., Palmer, R. F., & Pedersen, N. L. (2001, April). Syndrome X mediates the relationship between cynical hostility and cardiovascular disease: A prospective study. Paper presented at the meeting of the Society of Behavioral Medicine, Washington, DC.

Newcomb, M. D., & Harlow, L. L. (1986). Life events and substance use among adolescents. *Journal of Personality and Social Psychology, 51,* 564–577.

Niaura, R., Banks, S. M., Ward, K. D., Stoney, C. M., Spiro, A., Aldwin, C. M., Landsberg, L., & Weiss, S. (2000). Hostility and the metabolic syndrome in older males: The Normative Aging Study. *Psychosomatic Medicine, 62,* 7–16.

Patterson, G. R., DeBaryshe, B. D., & Ramsey, E. (1989). A developmental perspective on antisocial behavior. *American Psychologist, 44,* 329–335.

Pedlow, R., Sanson, A., Prior, M., & Oberklaid, F. (1993). Stability of maternally reported temperament from infancy to 8 years. *Developmental Psychology, 29,* 998–1007.

Piazza, P. V., & Le Moal, M. (1996). Pathophysiological basis of vulnerability to drug abuse: Interaction between stress, glucocorticoids, and dopaminergic neurons. *Annual Review of Pharmacology and Toxicology, 36,* 359–378.

Plomin, R., Owen, M. J., & McGuffin, P. (1994). The genetic basis of complex human behaviors. *Science, 264,* 1733–1739.

Pulkkinen, L., & Pitkänen, T. (1994). A prospective study of the precursors to problem drinking in young adulthood. *Journal of Studies on Alcohol, 55,* 578–587.

Räikkönen, K., & Keltikangas-Järvinen, L. (1991). Hostility and its association with behavioral and somatic coronary risk indicators in Finnish adolescents and young adults. *Social Science and Medicine, 10,* 1171–1178.

Räikkönen, K., & Keltikangas-Järvinen, L. (1992). Childhood hyperactivity and the mother-child relationship as predictors of risk Type A behaviour in adolescence: A six year follow-up. *Personality and Individual Differences, 13,* 321–337.

Räikkönen, K., Keltikangas-Järvinen, L., & Solakivi, T. (1990). Behavioral coronary risk indicators and apolipoproteins A-I and B in young Finnish children: Cross-sectional and predictive associations. *Preventive Medicine, 19*, 656–666.

Raitakari, O. T., Porkka, K. V. K., Räsänen, L., Rönnemaa, T., & Viikari, J. S. A. (1994). Clustering and six year cluster-tracking of serum total cholesterol, HDL-cholesterol and diastolic blood pressure in children and young adults: The Cardiovascular Risk in Young Finns Study. *Journal of Clinical Epidemiology, 47*, 1085–1093.

Ravaja, N., & Keltikangas-Järvinen, L. (1995). Temperament and metabolic syndrome precursors in children: A three-year follow-up. *Preventive Medicine, 24*, 518–527.

Ravaja, N., & Keltikangas-Järvinen, L. (2001). Cloninger's temperament and character dimensions in young adulthood and their relation to parental alcohol use and smoking. *Journal of Studies on Alcohol, 62*, 98–104.

Rajava, N., Keltikangas-Järvinen, L., & Keskivaara, P. (1996). Type A factors as predictors of changes in metabolic syndrome precursors in adolescents and young adults: A 3-year follow-up study. *Health Psychology, 15*, 18–29.

Robins, L. N., & Przybeck, T. R. (1985). Age of onset of drug use as a factor in drug and other disorders. In C. L. Jones & R. J. Battjes (Eds.), *Etiology of drug abuse* (pp. 178–192). Rockville, MD: National Institute on Drug Abuse.

Rosenbaum, M. (1990). The role of learned resourcefulness in self-control of health behavior. In M. Rosenbaum (Ed.), *Learned resourcefulness: On coping skills, self-control, and adaptive behavior* (pp. 3–30). New York: Springer.

Rothbart, M. K., & Ahadi, S. A. (1994). Temperament and the development of personality. *Journal of Abnormal Psychology, 103*, 55–66.

Rothbart, M. K., & Bates, J. E. (1998). Temperament. In W. Damon (Series Ed.) & N. Eisenberg (Vol. Ed.), *Handbook of child psychology (Vol. 3, pp. 105–176): Social, emotional, and personality development* (5th ed.). New York: Wiley.

Rothbart, M. K., & Derryberry, D. (1981). Development of individual differences in temperament. In M. E. Lamb & A. L. Brown (Eds.), *Advances in developmental psychology* (Vol. 1, pp. 37–86). Hillsdale, NJ: Erlbaum.

Rothbart, M. K., Derryberry, D., & Posner, M. J. (1994). A psychobiological approach to the development of temperament. In J. E. Bates & T. D. Wachs (Eds.), *Temperament: Individual differences at the interface of biology and behavior* (pp. 83–116). Washington, DC: American Psychological Association.

Scarr, S. (1991). Developmental theories for the 1990s: Development and individual differences. *Developmental Psychology, 63*, 1–19.

Scarr, S., & McCartney, K. (1983). How people make their own environments: A theory of genotype environment effects. *Child Development, 54*, 424–435.

Scheier, M. F., & Carver, C. S. (1987). Dispositional optimism and physical well-being: The influence of generalized outcome expectancies on health. *Journal of Personality, 55*(2), 169–210.

Scherwitz, L. W., Perkins, L. L., Chesney, M. A., et al. (1991). Cook Medley Hostility Scale: Relationship to psychosocial characteristics in young adults in the CARDIA study. *Psychosomatic Medicine, 53*, 36–49.

Scherwitz, L. W., Perkins, L. L., Chesney, M. A., Hughes, G. H., Sidney, S., & Manolio, T. A. (1992). Hostility and health behaviors in young adults: The CARDIA study. *American Journal of Epidemiology, 136*, 136–145.

Schneiderman, N., & Skyler, J. S. (1995). Insulin metabolism, sympathetic nervous system regulation, and coronary heart disease prevention. In K. Orth-Gomer & N. Schneiderman (Eds.), *Behavioral medicine approaches to cardiovascular disease prevention* (pp. 105–133). Mahwah, NJ: Erlbaum.

Schwartz, J. E., Friedman, H. S., Tucker, J. S., Tomlinson-Keasey, C., Wingard, D. L., & Criqui, M. H. (1995). Sociodemographic and psychosocial factors in childhood as predictors of adult mortality. *American Journal of Public Health, 85,* 1237–1245.

Siegler, I. C., Peterson, B. L., Barefoot, J. C., & Williams, R. B. (1992). Hostility during late adolescence predicts coronary risk factors at mid-life. *American Journal of Epidemiology, 136,* 146–154.

Siegman, A. W. (1994). From Type A to hostility and anger: Reflections on the history of research on coronary-prone behavior. In A. Siegman & T. Smith (Eds.), *Anger, hostility, and the heart* (pp. 1–21). Hillsdale, NJ: Erlbaum.

Stuss, D. T. (1992). Biological and psychological development of executive functions. *Brain and Cognition, 20,* 8–23.

Super, C. M., & Harkness, S. (1986). Temperament, development and culture. In R. Plomin & J. Dunn (Eds.), *The study of temperament* (pp. 131–162). Hillsdale, NJ: Erlbaum.

Tarter, R. E. (1988). Are there inherited behavioral traits that predispose to substance abuse? *Journal of Consulting and Clinical Psychology, 56,* 189–196.

Tarter, R. E., Moss, H. B., & Vanyukov, M. M. (1995). Behavior genetic perspective of alcoholism etiology. In H. Begleiter & B. Kissin (Eds.), *Alcohol and alcoholism* (Vol. 1, pp. 294–326). New York: Oxford University Press.

Tarter, R. E., Vanyukov, M., Giancola, P., Dawes, M., Blackson, T., Mezzich, A., & Clark, D. (1999). Etiology of early age onset substance use disorder: A maturational perspective. *Development and Psychopathology, 11,* 657–683.

Thomas, A., & Chess, S. (1977). *Temperament and development.* New York: Brunner-Mazel.

Vitaliano, P. P., Scanlan, J. M., Zhang, J., Savage, M. V., Hirsch, I. B., & Siegler, I. C. (2002). A path model of chronic stress, the metabolic syndrome, and coronary heart disease. *Psychosomatic Medicine, 64,* 418–435.

Werner, E. E. (1986). Resilient offspring of alcoholics: A longitudinal study from birth to age 18. *Journal of Studies on Alcohol, 47,* 34–40.

Wills, T. A. (1990). Stress and coping factors in the epidemiology of substance use. In L. T. Kozlowski, H. M. Annis, H. D. Cappell, F. B. Glaser, M. S. Goodstadt, Y. Israel, H. Kalant, E. M. Sellers, & E. R. Vinglis (Eds.), *Research advances in alcohol and drug problems* (Vol. 10, pp. 215–250). New York: Plenum.

Wills, T. A. (1994). Self-esteem and perceived control in adolescent substance use: Comparative tests in concurrent and prospective analyses. *Psychology of Addictive Behaviors, 8,* 223–234.

Wills, T. A. (2001). Adolescent health and health behaviors. In N. J. Smelser and P. B. Baltes (Series Editors), R. Schwarzer and J. House (Section Editors), *International encyclopedia of the social and behavioral sciences* (Vol. 4). Oxford: Elsevier Science.

Wills, T. A., & Cleary, S. D. (1999). Peer and adolescent substance use among 6th–9th graders: Latent growth analyses of influence versus selection mechanisms. *Health Psychology, 18,* 453–463.

Wills, T. A., Cleary, S. D., Filer, M., Shinar, O., Mariani, J., & Spera, K. (2001). Temperament related to early-onset substance use: Test of a developmental model. *Prevention Science, 2,* 145–163.

Wills, T. A., DuHamel, K., & Vaccaro, D. (1995). Activity and mood temperament as predictors of adolescent substance use: Test of a self-regulation mediational model. *Journal of Personality and Social Psychology, 68,* 901–916.

Wills, T. A., & Filer, M. (1996). Stress-coping model of adolescent substance use. In T. H. Ollendick & R. J. Prinz (Eds.), *Advances in clinical child psychology* (Vol. 18, pp. 91–132). New York: Plenum.

Wills, T. A., Gibbons, F. X., Gerrard, M., & Brody, G. (2000). Protection and vulnerability processes for early onset of substance use: A test among African-American children. *Health Psychology, 19,* 253–263.

Wills, T. A., Mariani, J., & Filer, M. (1996). The role of family and peer relationships in adolescent substance use. In G. R. Pierce, B. R. Sarason, & I. G. Sarason (Eds.), *Handbook of social support and the family* (pp. 521–549). New York: Plenum.

Wills, T. A., McNamara, G., Vaccaro, D., & Hirky, A. E. (1996). Escalated substance use: A longitudinal grouping analysis from early to middle adolescence. *Journal of Abnormal Psychology, 105,* 166–180.

Wills, T. A., Sandy, J. M., & Shinar, O. (1999). Cloninger's constructs related to substance use level and problems in late adolescence: A mediational model based on self-control and coping motives. *Experimental and Clinical Psychopharmacology, 7,* 122–134.

Wills, T. A., Sandy, J. M., Shinar, O., & Yaeger, A. (1999). Contributions of positive and negative affect to adolescent substance use: Test of a bidimensional model in a longitudinal study. *Psychology of Addictive Behaviors, 13,* 327–338.

Wills, T. A., Sandy, J. M., & Yaeger, A. (2000). Temperament and adolescent substance use: An epigenetic approach to risk and protection. *Journal of Personality, 68,* 1127–1152. (Special Issue on Personality and Problem Behavior)

Wills, T. A., Sandy, J. M., Yaeger, A., & Shinar, O. (2001). Family risk factors and adolescent substance use: Moderation effects for temperament dimensions. *Developmental Psychology, 37,* 283–297.

Wills, T. A., Vaccaro, D., & McNamara, G. (1994). Novelty seeking, risk taking, and related constructs as predictors of adolescent substance use: An application of Cloninger's theory. *Journal of Substance Abuse, 6,* 1–20.

Wills, T. A., Windle, M., & Cleary, S. D. (1998). Temperament and novelty-seeking in adolescent substance use: Convergence of dimensions of temperament with constructs from Cloninger's theory. *Journal of Personality and Social Psychology, 74,* 387–406.

Windle, M. (1990). Temperament and personality attributes of children of alcoholics. In M. Windle & J. S. Searles (Eds.), *Children of alcoholics: Critical perspectives* (pp. 129–167). New York: Guilford.

Windle, M. (1995). The approach-withdrawal concept: Associations with salient constructs in contemporary theories of temperament and personality development. In K. Hood, G. Greenberg, & E. Tobach (Eds.), *Behavioral development: Concepts of approach-withdrawal and integrative levels* (pp. 329–370). New York: Garland Press.

Windle, M., & Lerner, R. M. (1986). Assessing the dimensions of temperamental individuality across the life span: The Revised Dimensions of Temperament Survey. *Journal of Adolescent Research, 1,* 213–229.

Winneke, G., Lilienthal, H., & Kramer, U. (1996). The neurobehavioural toxicology and teratology of lead exposure. *Archives of Toxicology, 18*(Suppl.), 57–70.

Zucker, R. A. (1994). Pathways to alcohol problems: A developmental account of the evidence for contextual contributions to risk. In R. A. Zucker, J. Howard, & G. M. Boyd (Eds.), *The development of alcohol problems* (pp. 255–289). Rockville, MD: National Institute on Alcohol Abuse and Alcoholism.

Zucker, R., & Gomberg, E. (1986). Etiology of alcoholism reconsidered: The case for a biopsychosocial process. *American Psychologist, 41,* 783–793.

Zuckerman, M. (1994). *Behavioral expressions and biosocial bases of sensation seeking.* New York: Cambridge University Press.

Zuckerman, M., Kuhlman, D. M., Joireman, J., Teta, P., & Kraft, M. (1993). A comparison of three structural models of personality: The Big Three, the Big Five, and the Alternative Five. *Journal of Personality and Social Psychology, 65,* 757–768.

ACKNOWLEDGMENTS

This work was supported by a Research Scientist Development Award #K02-DA00252 and grant #RO1-DA08880 from the National Institute on Drug Abuse. We thank Catherine Davis and Peter Vitaliano for their comments.

CHAPTER 2

Social Support, the Self System, and Adolescent Health and Health Behaviors

Nola J. Pender and Karen Farchaus Stein

In western culture adolescence is viewed as a period of transition during which the child develops into an adult. Transition is marked by a myriad of dramatic changes. Biological changes include rapid increases in height and body weight, development of secondary sex characteristics, and sexual maturity. Psychological changes include increased strivings for independence, identity formation, and cognitive changes. Social changes encompass increased independence from family and increased reliance on friends, peers, and other nonfamilial adults for supportive relationships.

Adolescence is also a period of transition in health behaviors and lifestyle choices. Health-related behavioral patterns established during adolescence are of critical importance because they profoundly affect the quality of life during adolescence and serve as the foundation for adult health-related lifestyles. Adolescence provides the opportunity for youth to evolve along their life courses, encounter new realities, develop new skills and competencies, enjoy their own emergence, and lay the foundation for a positive, satisfying, productive and healthy life.

Because adolescence is a phase of development characterized by experimentation with various adult behaviors, both positive and negative, many youth will experiment with risky behaviors such as tobacco use, alcohol use, and sexual activity. Unfortunately, positive behaviors such as physical activity may decrease dramatically during adolescence, with the adoption of sedentary lifestyles that persist into adulthood and contribute to the risk of cardiovascular and other chronic diseases. The prevalence of disordered eating behaviors that impact emotional well-being, school performance, and stamina for daily living also increases and can lead to serious diagnosable eating disorders.

Despite the potential for risky behaviors, health care providers must capitalize on the potential for positive development during the adolescent years. Health care providers can promote positive development by enhancing the health promotion competencies of adolescents, fostering positive family relationships and healthy family lifestyles, encouraging positive peer and peer group affiliations, and creating health-strengthening school, neighborhood, and community environments during the adolescent years.

Within the adolescent literature, health behaviors are increasingly recognized as social products (Barrera & Prelow, 2000; Hawkins, Catalano, & Miller, 1992). Decisions to participate in sports, eat healthily, use tobacco or drugs, or be sexually active are not made in isolation. Rather, health behavior choices are a product of a dynamic and complex interaction between the social environment and the individual. In this chapter, the focus is on the self-concept as an important mediator between social influences, particularly social support, and the adolescent's resilience and health behavior choices. Based on the cognitive model of the self-concept, the authors propose that social support plays a central role in shaping the adolescent's emerging self-definition, and, in doing so, contributes emotional and behavioral resources that enable healthy lifestyle choices. In this chapter the relationships among social support, the self-concept, and adolescent health behaviors, will be explored by:

(1)   defining social support and examining characteristics that are unique to adolescents,

(2)   briefly reviewing the schemas model of the self-concept and describing the role of social support in shaping current and future-oriented self-conceptions, and

(3)   exploring the role of support and the self in the promotion of adolescent resilience and well-being, and in shaping of their health behaviors.

SOCIAL NETWORK AND SOCIAL SUPPORT RESOURCES

Social support is a dynamic, reciprocal process between individuals or aggregates in a particular social context directed toward providing assistance, encouragement, enhancement of esteem, and/or a sense of being valued by caring individuals. Social support is best conceptualized as a process of negotiated interactions in personally valued, socially embedded relationships rather than as a static set of behaviors or a commodity for exchange (Gottlieb & Sylvestre, 1994). The relational and situational contexts determine whether interactions are viewed as meaningful and supportive. Recognizing the social embeddedness of supportive relationships requires that the role of social support in promoting the health and health behaviors of adolescents be considered within a developmental perspective and in the relevant sociopolitical, historical, and cultural contexts.

The concepts of social networks and social support resources are not interchangeable. *Social networks* are structural components of support and are made up of persons that an adolescent knows and interacts with (Pierce, Lakey, Sarason, & Sarason, 1997). Both number of individuals and frequency of interactions vary highly across social networks. Cairns and Cairns (1995) found that adolescents' social networks frequently change configuration, and are dynamic rather than static structures. *Social support resources*, the primary focus of this chapter, refer to social interactions within a network that are sensed as being available and supportive or that actually provide support to the adolescent. These are individuals to whom adolescents believe they can turn for informational, instrumental, emotional, or other assistance when needed. The types of persons in the social network greatly influence the quality of social support available (Pender, Murdaugh, & Parsons, 2002; Underwood, 2000).

The social support resources for adolescents generally include the family, peers, educators and health professionals, religious and other organizations, and neighborhoods or communities. *Parental social support*, defined as behavior manifested by a parent that makes a child feel comfortable in the parents' presence, and confirms basic acceptance and approval as a person, significantly influences the health of adolescents (Raja, McGee, & Stanton, 1992). A family's ability to foster positive interactive styles among its members may relate to the extent to which the family has its own social network of long-term supportive relationships, and the extent to which the family is accorded respect within the community.

At the onset of adolescence, parents are central to their child's support network. School and role transitions can result in qualitative shifts in social support needs and resources throughout adolescence. Gradually, friends become more integral to the support network. This is viewed as an essential step in healthy adolescent development (Allender, 1998). Overall, peer relationships and the social support derived from them contribute positively to adolescent adjustment and development of future potential. The influence of the social group or crowd with which they affiliate or hang out is particularly unique to adolescence. Although crowds are relatively large and loosely organized and not all adolescents belong to them, these groups exert considerable influence over the behavior of youth and often serve as a source of identity and social support (Urberg, Degirmencioglu, Tolson, & Halliday-Scher, 1995).

Helping professionals such as educators, counselors, youth workers, and health care providers can enhance the positive effects of family and peer social support on emerging self-systems of adolescents by presenting multiple opportunities for students to elaborate their knowledge and competencies in particular domains valued by the individual adolescent and the wider community (Cauce, Hannan, & Sargeant, 1992). An increasing number of youth are becoming involved in personal development programs and sports ministries sponsored by religious or other organizations. These programs allow for exposure to differing adult role models and provide opportunities to observe positive lifestyles and to practice various behaviors admired in others.

Neighborhoods, particularly in African American communities, are often outstanding models of care structures for adolescents. The totality of the neighborhood and community become involved in the welfare of *their* adolescents. They communicate to youths that they are valued by patrolling the neighborhood to keep adolescents out of trouble. Watching for problem behaviors, community residents act to prevent escalation of problems or report misbehavior to parents so that appropriate counseling or disciplinary steps can be taken. Caring, supportive communities that facilitate authoritative parenting instill a sense of hope for the future among youth and provide a protective environment in which to develop toward responsible adulthood.

The multilevel structure of social support comprises a matrix of interpersonal relationships within which adolescent development occurs. Family, friends, health providers, and even the neighborhood and broader community provide the opportunities, challenges, and resources necessary for adolescents to move from their childhood self-definitions into personally meaningful, socially relevant and coherent adult identities. In this chapter, it is proposed that the adolescent's evolving self-definition is, both a *product* of the network of social support and a *determinant* of health and health behavior lifestyle choices. The schemas model of the self-concept provides an empirically-based theoretical framework for considering the complex pattern of relationships between social support, the self, and adolescent health and health behavior.

THE SCHEMAS MODEL OF THE SELF-CONCEPT

Self-concept refers to the person's total collection of mental representations or memory structures about the self that are stored in long-term memory

(Markus, 1977; Markus, Hamill, & Sentis, 1987). It is a complex and multifaceted memory structure that is comprised of individual units of information about the self, referred to as self-schemas and possible selves (Markus & Wurf, 1987). Self-schemas are rich, highly elaborated organizations of knowledge about the self in specific content domains. They are constructed through experience in the domain and reflect the categorizations and evaluations of behavior made by the self and others. For adolescents, parents, peers, and the wider social network are likely to play an important role in shaping the emerging self-schemas. Self-schemas emerge from relevant information input, targeted skills training, and feedback from others. Studies have documented self-schemas in a variety of domains in adolescent and young adult populations including body weight (Markus, Hamill, & Sentis, 1987; Stein & Hedger, 1997), exercise and fitness (Kendzierski, 1990), independence (Markus, 1977), and academic performance (Garcia & Pintrich, 1994; Stein, 1994).

Researchers have shown that self-schemas play an important role in motivating and regulating goal directed behavior. Self-schemas include not only descriptive information about who the self is but also procedural knowledge—action-based memories in the form of motoric skills, habits, rules, and strategies that enable competent and efficient behavior in the domain (Cantor, 1990; Markus & Wurf, 1987). People are more likely to: (1) direct their attention to information that is consistent with an established self-schema, (2) process consistent information more quickly, and (3) recall more schema-consistent versus schema-irrelevant information (Markus, 1977). Self-schemas play an important regulatory role in the emotional and behavioral responses in the domain (Froming, Nasby, & McManus, 1998; Kendzierski, 1990; Kendzierski & Whitaker, 1997; Stein, Roeser, & Markus, 1998).

Possible selves are the future-oriented component of the self-concept (Markus & Nurius, 1986). They are well-elaborated, detailed, and personalized beliefs that represent individuals' ideas of what they expect to become (anticipated), what they wish to become (hoped for), and what they fear becoming (feared). Like self-schemas, possible selves serve important self-regulatory functions including motivating and organizing behavior and regulating affect (Markus & Ruvolo, 1989).

SOCIAL SUPPORT AND THE DEVELOPMENT OF SELF-SCHEMAS

Competence in a domain requires not only knowledge, skills, and ability but also an elaborated mental representation of one's capacities in the domain

(Markus, Cross, & Wurf, 1990). According to Markus and colleagues, it is the mental representation of ability that allows an individual actually to use abilities and have a sense of control over them. A self-schema with elaborated procedural knowledge facilitates competent performance through mental rehearsals and simulations. Requisite behaviors that are mentally practiced, adjusted, and coordinated with the desired goals have been shown to enhance the level of performance in the domain (see Markus, Cross, & Wurf, 1990 for review).

Harter (1985; 1999) described 5 domains of competence: (1) scholastic, (2) athletic, (3) social acceptance, (4) physical appearance, and (5) behavioral conduct. Self-attributions of differing levels of competence in these domains have implications for both personal behavior and group or crowd affiliation. For example, adolescents' skills and perceptions of competencies may shape their opportunities to affiliate with different crowds. Athletic youth are more likely to have opportunities to play sports, make friendships and be part of the jock crowd. Those with scholastic competence may be in special classes with other similarly talented peers and be part of the smart crowd. Those who see themselves as having a high level of social acceptance will likely gravitate toward the socially elite, or popular group. Group affiliation may reinforce the development of relevant self-schema through repetitive behaviors in the domain and exposure to group norms and expectations characteristic of other youth highly competent in that domain.

When considering a course of action in a given social context, individuals with a self-schema in the domain can call upon the associated procedural knowledge to organize and guide the behavioral response (Cantor & Kihlstrom, 1987). For example, procedural knowledge of how to be a friend is an accumulating repertoire of behaviors from supportive interactions that enables adolescents to function progressively more effectively in this domain. Cauce, Hannan, and Sargeant (1992) examined the relationship between social support and psychological adjustment among 120 predominantly White, middle class, sixth and eighth graders. Family social support was correlated positively with perceptions of general competence and competence in peer relationships. Individuals with higher social support scores were higher in their knowledge of socially skilled behavior. The authors of this chapter propose that one of the functions of socially supportive families is to help adolescents develop a socially relevant schema of how to function as a friend or source of support and how to behave in supportive and friendly ways in social situations.

Stein, Markus, and Roeser (1997) asked 160 American girls and boys between the ages of 13 and 15 to generate descriptors about themselves (now, next year, and 10 years from now). Interestingly, among the most common self-descriptors generated by the adolescents were the attributes of being *caring, nice,* and *connected to family*—characteristics typical of socially supportive individuals. Furthermore, when the sample was grouped according to level of self-esteem, adolescents with high esteem were more likely than those with low esteem to define themselves in terms of the socially supportive attributes. Stein and her colleagues concluded that in the population of adolescents studied, there was a socially shared or collective vision of the *right* self and that this self embodied the importance of being supportive to others.

Identity development as a supportive or caring person during adolescence is essential to the future establishment of mature, enduring intimate relationships. Adult members of a community play a unique role in socialization of youth by modeling and reinforcing socially supportive behaviors, thus shaping emerging self-identities as *caring* and *helpful*. These identities, in turn, seem to foster continuing enactment of supportive behaviors toward others, leading to increased skill and competence in social behavior domains.

It is important to note that adolescents differ in the extent to which the procedural information in their social schemas is elaborated and organized. Some adolescents are very adept at social relationships, while others are not. This is reflected in the lament sometimes heard from adolescents that "no matter how hard I try, nobody likes me." Because adolescence is a critical period for developing relationship-building skills that will provide the basis for success in later life, appropriate elaboration of social schema during this phase of development is critical. The schema of *friend or supportive other* develops only as adolescents experience support from others and can analyze why they feel comfort in particular relationships.

Dimensions of culture, race, ethnicity, social class, economic status, gender, religion, language, sexual orientation, and age are critical variables in the formation of socially relevant self-schema. Meeus and Dekovic (1995), who studied 2777 Dutch adolescents, found different processes of identity development for boys and girls. Boys derived their self-definition from both relational commitments and school and/or work involvement, whereas girls derived their identity primarily from relational commitments. These findings are supported by researchers who have found that adolescent girls typically have more intimate and supportive friendships than adolescent boys. Girls are willing to be more open, disclose more of self, and talk about their fears and worries with best friends (Bukowski, Hoza, & Boivin, 1994; Camarena, Sarigiani, & Petersen, 1990). These gender-specific interactional patterns may result from differences in early identity formation processes.

SOCIAL SUPPORT AND THE DEVELOPMENT OF POSSIBLE SELVES

It has been proposed that clear views of one's self in alternative future states can organize and energize current actions and drive changes in self-concept and behavior (Markus, Cross, & Wurf, 1990; Oyserman & Markus, 1990). A future goal needs to be represented as the individual approaches and realizes the goal. Without this personalized representation, goals are not effective regulators of behavior. The coordination of a current self-schema with an elaborated future self in the domain serves as a cognitive "bridge" to mediate goal attainment (Markus & Ruvolo, 1989, p. 211). Parental social support during adolescence assists youth in clearly articulating detailed successful possible selves. Furthermore, educators and health care providers may play an important role in helping youth elaborate success states (goal attainment) rather than failure states (lack of goal attainment) to enhance performance in a domain.

The existence of possible selves may play an important role in motivating the development of supportive relationships in adolescents. For example, because the adolescent is able to represent future states that are hoped for, the *supported* self and the *supportive* self, and future states that are feared, the *alone* self or the *alienated* self, the adolescent enacts behaviors to move toward the hoped for end states and away from the feared states. The alone self or alienated self may be particularly feared during adolescence, due to strivings to be independent yet remain attached to significant others such as parents and peers. Further complicating matters, parents and adolescent may sometimes hold divergent perspectives on the adolescent's desired future self. When this occurs, adolescents' desired end states may focus on subjective well-being and happiness, whereas parents may emphasize behavioral stability and conformity to social rules. Open communication about these divergent views of possible selves can foster adolescents' sensitivity to others and enhance social competence.

GIVING AND RECEIVING SOCIAL SUPPORT, RESILIENCE, AND HEALTH

Both giving and receiving social support are crucial behavioral domains in which adolescents need to develop competencies to function in an interactive world. Self-schemas and possible selves may be a means by which behaviors learned through social interactions, such as supportive behaviors, become internalized into potentially enduring aspects of self. For adolescents, building self-schema that enhance human functioning occurs in multiple social contexts. Children live with families, attend school, have friends, and often crowd affiliations and live their lives in specific neighborhoods, communities, and cultures. These interactive influences on cognitions of the self are just beginning to be explored (Eccles, Early, Frasier, Belansky, & McCarthy, 1997). In the following section, the authors propose an explanation for how both giving and receiving support can enhance the development of relevant self-schema, perceived social competencies, and in turn, resiliency and health.

Giving Social Support

Adolescents differ in their capacity and motivation to engage in supportive relationships. Further, there are individual and developmental differences in the ability of adolescents to read cues from others and provide the appropriate amount and type(s) of support needed or desired across situations. The potential mediating role of the self-concept in fostering competence in providing social support needs further exploration.

Families, in order to provide an appropriate support system for all members, must establish expectations of mutual help and assistance. Thus, the family is the primary context for learning about giving social support. Repeated acts of support given within the family and confirming feedback can facilitate incorporation of care-giving into the behavioral repertoire of current self-schema and into the anticipated and hoped for future selves.

Werner (1992) completed a longitudinal study of high risk children in Kauai who grew into resilient adults, defined as those who successfully adapted to life despite exposure to risk factors and stressful life circumstances. Those who emerged as resilient not only had more positive self-concept than those who suffered maladjustment, but they were also more appreciative, gentler, nurturant, and socially perceptive. Resilient youth and adults were characterized by a greater level of social maturity and social responsibility than their peers who suffered similar life insults and had difficulty coping with life's challenges. Werner also found that a large majority of the respondents reported a period during childhood and adolescence during which they were required to provide *support or helpfulness to another* to minimize the recipient's (often a family member) stress or discomfort. These youth often had to care for younger siblings, manage the household when a parent was ill or hospitalized, and/or work to support the family. Productive roles of responsibility, when associated with close ties with a parent or other caring adult, may be critical protective factors during adversity and foundational to a positive self-concept and healthy adjustment in later life.

These findings are in agreement with those studies of resilience in African American children. Connell, Spencer, and Aber (1994) operationalized self-concept as perceived competence/efficacy and perceived relatedness to self and others. They assessed whether self-concept was a mediator of school outcomes among 215 economically and educationally at risk African American youth in grades 6–8. They found that perceived relatedness to others manifested by subjects' reports that they felt connected to their classmates and peers in mutually supportive relationships, was associated with positive school outcomes despite impoverished economic family and neighborhood conditions. Bullerdick (2000) found that perceptions of social connectedness to family, friends, school, other adults, and the Indian community had a positive relationship with emotional well-being among 426 Indian youth aged 10–16 years.

Early experiences of giving social support to significant others, as well as receiving it, seem to emerge as critical to healthy adjustment and resilience, particularly among vulnerable children. This finding, if replicated, has fascinating implications for structuring resiliency-enhancing interventions for adolescents. Giving help may have positive effects on the well-being of adolescents for at least three different reasons: (1) the realization that one has helped an individual in need is a self-validating experience that can bolster self-esteem, (2) giving aid to others fosters intimacy and trust, thereby strengthening existing social bonds and elaborating procedural information in relevant self-schema, and (3) giving support to significant others increases the probability that one's own need for assistance will be met in the future, thereby realizing the goals of the supported self.

Receiving Social Support

Receiving social support through caring families, developmentally appropriate schools, and a positive organizational and media environment has been shown to promote positive adolescent development (Takanishi, 2000). Specific mechanisms through which this occurs may be: (1) by providing a growth-promoting environment in which hoped for possible selves can emerge, (2) by offering positive and confirming feedback on effective role performance as son/daughter or sibling, thus building robust domain-specific schema, (3) by providing an emotional climate in which youth feel comfortable exploring their worlds to acquire new competencies in specific behavioral domains (Eccles, Early, Frasier, Belansky, & McCarthy, 1997), and (4) by encouraging healthy lifestyle behaviors that become incorporated as procedural knowledge into a variety of schema (exerciser self, abstainer self, supportive self).

The Family

Kaltiala-Heino and colleagues (2001) found that adolescents' perceptions of parents as a source of social support was a key factor in protection from the onset of depression among 14–16 year-old adolescents. Supportive families who provide positive feedback may encourage a positive view of self in difficult and stressful circumstances, and foster resilience in adversity. In a sample of 5531 adolescents in California, lack of parental support was highly related to depressive symptoms. It was concluded that helping parents establish and maintain supportive relationships with their children may decrease the likelihood of depressive symptoms among adolescents (Patten et al., 1997; Pierce, Lakey, Sarason, & Sarason, 1997).

The specific ways in which social support from the family affects mental health is unclear. The work of Yarcheski, Mahon, and Yarcheski (2001) may shed some light on this issue. They explored whether there was a mediating role of hopefulness in the relationship between social support and general well-being among early adolescents. Hopefulness was defined as the degree to which an adolescent possesses a comforting belief that a personal, positive future exists. The researchers found significant mediation of the social support and general well-being relationship by hopefulness. Positive views of hoped for (possible) selves may create a generalized sense of hopefulness and a positive affect that can help adolescents cope in times of adversity.

Ethnic and racial differences in family social support transactions is an area of increasing interest to researchers and health practitioners alike. Studies of African American adolescents have indicated the importance of support from the family, including the extended family, in protecting children or helping children to cope with their sometimes hostile social environments (Smokowski, Reynolds, & Bezruczko, 1999; Zimmerman, Salem, & Maton, 1995). Taylor and Roberts (1995), who studied adolescent adjustment and well-being in African American families, concluded that kinship support from adult relatives outside the immediate family structure was significantly related to better adjustment and fewer problem behaviors.

In studying factors that foster resilience among children in adverse circumstances, that is, loss of a parent, physical and psychological abuse, or extreme poverty, critical protection was offered by caring parents who have high expectations for their children, family cohesion, and supportive relationships with grandparents, when absence or marital discord made parents unavailable to their children (Garmezy, 1993; Nettles, Mucherah, & Jones, 2000). External support, in the form of a maternal substitute (neighbor, teacher, parent of a peer) when the child's mother was unresponsive, also enhanced resilience. Social support from families and problem-focused coping predicted resiliency among low-income Appalachian adolescents (Markstrom, Marshall, & Tryon, 2000). Among 1427 African American and European-American adolescents aged 13–17 years old, social support prevented self-reported health from declining despite experience of violent and nonviolent traumatic events (Cheever & Hardin, 1999). In a review of the knowledge base on resilience among African American adolescents, Winfield (1995) identified the following ways in which a supportive social context can enhance resilience: (1) reduce exposure to risk or the impact of risk on adolescents; (2) reduce the negative chain reaction, such as escalating from difficulty in school to truancy to substance use and delinquency; (3) build self-esteem and self-efficacy of adolescents; and (4) create new opportunities for self-definition.

According to Markus, Cross, and Wurf (1990), possible selves motivate evolving competence. Positive possible selves in the areas of future family and peer relationships serve as incentives for adolescents to observe the interactional patterns of others, to internalize those actions deemed successful, and to channel increased energy into interpersonal interaction. This, in turn, can promote further competence.

Winfield (1995) reported that regardless of socioeconomic status, adolescents who come from supportive home environments in which education and academic success are valued are more likely to excel in academic programs, associate with motivated peers, receive more favorable reactions from teachers, experience increased feelings of competence, and seek opportunities for growth experiences. When one has a sense of competence, one will become competent, or approach competence, at least relative to a self lacking this feeling (Markus, Cross, & Wurf, 1990). Competence may develop when an adolescent has a particular ability and then builds a growth-enhancing self-structure around it or because a person develops a self-structure and then uses it to motivate behaviors that develop the ability.

Peers: Friends and Crowds

In the search for social support outside the family, adolescents often turn to their peers. Research indicates that adolescents are most influenced by the few peers that they consider best friends. Adolescents begin to regard one or two friends as especially close and others as more peripheral. Through these close relationships, they derive a sense of self-esteem and a sense of acceptance, which contributes to psychological adjustment. Hirsch and Du-Bois (1992) did a prospective study of 143 children, 27% of whom were African American. They concluded that the level of peer support (frequent interaction with friends) decreased reported psychological symptomatology, (e.g., anxiety, depression) across the elementary to junior high school transition. Thus, social support can have positive effects on the adjustment of youth during major life transitions.

Adolescents who are disliked by their peers often have relationships that offer low support. This is likely to contribute to the development of negative self-evaluations and poorly developed friend self-schema (Berndt, 1996). Researchers have found that social support from friends or peers is sometimes viewed by youth as less stable than social support from parents (Frey & Rothlisberger, 1996). Adolescent friends may have tenuous self-concepts with very elementary conceptions of the supportive self. Thus, friends may exhibit erratic behaviors, some supportive, some nonsupportive in interactions with others.

If adolescents affiliate with peers who engage in healthy behaviors, they are likely to develop healthy lifestyles. If adolescents affiliate with peers who engage in health compromising or deviant behaviors, they are more likely to incorporate these behaviors into relevant self-schema, leading to poor health outcomes and poor social outcomes. The choice of behaviors depends on the actions endorsed by the peers with whom the adolescents choose to associate (Cauce, Hannan, & Sargeant, 1992).

Middle adolescence (15–17 years) is a peak period in peer influence, when youth are more responsive to both the positive and negative influences of their friends. This is a crucial period in the evolution of the self-system, during which conformity to the culturally embedded consensual self endorsed by one's relevant crowd is particularly rewarded. Group affiliation or crowds become important aspects of the adolescent's social context. Crowds are often distinguished from one another by dress, grooming style, sociability, academic achievement, hangouts at school, typical weekend activities, participation in sports, or involvement in illegal activities (Dolcini & Adler, 1994). The most common crowd labels used are elite or cool (hotshots or popular students), jocks (students with athletic prowess), and dirts, dropouts or losers (students that engage in delinquent or deviant behaviors). Other groups identified are regulars (students conforming to adult standards), smarts (those with high academic achievement) and skaters (students focused on skateboarding or surfing) (Sussman, Dent, Stacy, Buriaga, Raynor, et al., 1990). Brown and Mounts (1989) found in multiethnic high schools that although ethnicity added another dimension to crowds in these schools, it did not replace reputation as the basis for crowd formation. The crowd of affiliation can markedly impact self-definitions through stereotypical labels and shared norms.

Educators and Health Professionals

Health professionals are seldom the first source of support or assistance for an adolescent. Family and close friends or peers are sought out initially for advice. It is often only when this source of help is unavailable, interrupted, or exhausted that health professionals enter the support scene. Even though adolescents describe proactive, supportive relationships with health care providers that are helpful and important to them, such as anticipatory guidance or health counseling, youths rarely consider health professionals as continuing sources of social support. Thus, health care providers should garner support for adolescents by working with families and school personnel to provide nurturance for adolescents in their natural environment. This does not negate the responsibility of all health care providers to be nurturant, but it does emphasize the reality of the limited amount of time that most health care providers spend in actual contact with adolescents. Colarossi (2000) found among 364 adolescents of both genders that support from mothers, teachers, and friends all emerged as important in lowering depression and raising self-esteem and self-confidence. Synergy is achieved when health professionals teach multiple individuals the skills needed to be supportive to adolescents rather than the professional taking on this responsibility in isolation.

Religious and Other Organizations

Barbaran (1993) in studying coping and resilience of African American youth, identified churches as community organizations playing a major role in promoting competence in social and cognitive domains. This appears to occur through youth development programs, social action programs, and sports ministries in churches. Religious communities provide support to adolescents who participate in them primarily because the congregation share a common value system, a common set of beliefs about the purpose of life, traditions of worship, and a set of guidelines for living. In other words, religious groups often share a consensual self or right self that their members espouse. Adopting aspects of the consensual self shared by a particular religious community is one way in which such affiliations impact the self-system of the adolescent and their perceptions of self-esteem and self-worth. The consensual self may derive from a deity or from religious beliefs about the rules that govern human interaction. Although the extent of church involvement is not well documented among adolescents, increasingly, communities are looking to religious groups for assistance in helping children grow into healthy and responsible adults.

Neighborhoods and Communities

The neighborhood or community contexts in which adolescents reside has the potential to offer a sense of safety and support, a sense of cultural or ethnic identity, and alternative adult role models within the culture of origin. Although families are the primary groups in which most adolescents have opportunities for adolescent/adult intimacy and meaningful communication, relationships with nonrelated adults can also play a critical role in the formation of schema of the supportive self. Desirable characteristics of supportive adults identified by adolescents are: intelligence, openmindedness, trustworthiness, friendliness, personally interested in them, and willing to spend time with them. Supportive adults offer alternative perspectives to consider without coercion to accept them, encourage self-understanding of motives indirectly by sharing their own past experiences and lessons learned, willingly disclose information about their own lives, and treat youth nonjudgmentally and as an equal capable of mature dialogue (Gottleib & Sylvestre, 1994). Thus, individually and collectively, adults in the neighborhood or community create valuable support structures for adolescents.

In summary, the constellation of social support for adolescents is multidimensional and dynamic. At various stages of adolescence and in different situations, a flexible and changing mix of support is likely to best meet their needs.

SOCIAL SUPPORT AND HEALTH-PROMOTING BEHAVIORS

In the schemas model of the self-concept, cognitive structures in specific domains are the means by which positive behaviors become structuralized and enduring components of the behavioral repertoire. While self-cognitions are proposed as shaping behavior, behavior also shapes self-cognitions (Stein, Roeser & Markus, 1998). It is not proposed that the effect of social support on health behaviors of adolescents is mediated through global self-esteem. In fact, Yarcheski, Mahon, and Yarchevski (1997) tested this hypothesis on 200 adolescents ages 15–21 years; their data did not support it. Although perceived social support was related to self-esteem, self-esteem was not related to positive health practices (exercise, nutrition, relaxation, safety, prevention, and substance use). Social support was the strongest direct predictor of positive health practices. Thus, mobilizing social support, enriching existing social ties, modifying social networks that are dysfunctional, and introducing new network members may well increase positive healthy behaviors (Barrera & Prelow, 2000).

The authors propose that measures of social support and self-concept must be behavior specific to allow possible relationships to emerge; that is, the effect of exercise specific social support on moderate to vigorous physical activity may be mediated by the physically active self-schema. These relationships need to be empirically tested. Physical activity will be used as an exemplar of this proposed interface between cognitions of self and health related behavior.

Physical Activity

A number of researchers have explored participation of adolescents in sports, recreational pursuits, and other leisure time physical activities and concluded that both parents and peers influence level and regularity of activity (Pender, 1998). Researchers have found that more active parents have more active adolescents (Sallis, Prochaska, & Taylor, 2000); however, factors mediating this relationship are not well understood. The authors propose that family support for exercise, and its impact on self-schema in the domain of physical activity, may mediate this relationship.

Cauce, Hannan, and Sargeant (1992) found that family support was correlated significantly with the self cognition of perceived physical competence among 120 European-American, middle-class sixth and eighth graders. In a cross-sectional study of gender and developmental differences in exercise beliefs and behaviors among 286 racially diverse fifth, sixth, and eighth grade youth (Garcia, Broda, Frenn, Coviak, Pender, & Ronis, 1995), data indicated that eighth grade adolescents reported less social support from friends and family to be physically active than sixth grade adolescents. Based on the schemas model of the self-system, less support to be active can decrease the salience of the physical activity schema in the overall self-concept and lead to inactivity. Girls in both grades were less schematic for exercise than boys when measured by a single item of perception of self as physically active; girls in both grades were also less active than boys. Girls who received social support for exercise perceived greater benefits and fewer barriers to participation in physical activity. In a 2-year longitudinal study, Garcia, Pender, Antonakos, and Ronis (1998) studied 132 of the original 286 study participants as they transitioned from elementary school to junior high school. Both boys and girls reported significant decreases in social support for exercise. Thus, a source of motivation that has been shown to be predictive of exercise was seriously compromised as youth progressed through the adolescent years.

Zakarian, Hovell, Hofstetter, Sallis, and Keating (1994) explored a number of possible determinants of vigorous exercise among 1634 ninth and eleventh graders (60% Latino, 21% European-American, 12% Asian, 4% African American, 3% other). They found gender differences in the contribution of social support to the explanation of variance in vigorous exercise. When vigorous exercise both outside of school and in school was the dependent variable, friend support was correlated with level of vigorous physical activity among boys. Friend support was defined as frequency with which friends encouraged exercise or offered to exercise with the adolescent. When the same relationships were examined for girls, family support emerged as the significant variable and friend support was insignificant. Family support was defined as the frequency with which the family encouraged, rewarded, or reminded adolescents to exercise or offered to exercise with them and did not criticize exercise behavior.

Social support building specific to physical activity may hold promise for increasing activity among adolescents (Sallis, Prochaska, & Taylor, 2000). Family support of children's physical activity is related to increased activity in minority youth (Zakarian, Hovell, Hofstetter, Sallis, & Keating, 1994) and physical activity leading to increased fitness in obese youth (Epstein, Paluch, Coleman, Vrro, & Anderson, 1996). It is not clear, however, how social support of varying types and within varying contexts (family, school, neighborhood, community) across the stages of adolescence influence regular physical activity. Further, the role of behavior-specific domains of the self-system in mediating the effects of social support on exercise needs further investigation. The following studies are an important step in this direction.

The role of self-schema in influencing exercise behavior was explored by Kendzierski (1988) in a cross-sectional study of 220 subjects in late adolescence. Based on questionnaire responses, exerciser schematics, nonexerciser schematics, and aschematics were identified. It was predicted that exerciser schematics would exercise most, nonexerciser schematics least, and aschematics would fall in between. Further, exercise-related cognitions such as commitment, interest, intention, and number of strategies used to facilitate exercise were also examined. Exerciser schematics reported more days of physical activity than did aschematics and both reported more than nonexerciser schematics. Exerciser schematics were more committed, more interested, and had more intentions and plans to exercise than the other two groups. There was a nonsignificant trend for exerciser schematics to report more strategies for getting themselves to exercise regularly even on days when it was difficult to do so. In a subsequent prospective study of 66 youth in late adolescence, Kenzierski (1990) compared individuals who were exerciser schematic with those who were nonexerciser schematic or aschematic; she found that persons who endorsed more words related to exercising as self-descriptive, took less time to make these judgments, recalled more instances of exerciser behavior, were more likely to report pro-exercise attitudes, and were more likely to report adopting an exercise program. These studies represent a first step in understanding the mediating role of the self in the regulation of exercise behavior, a repetitive health behavior critical to well-being.

SOCIAL SUPPORT AND RISKY BEHAVIORS

The role of self-schema in motivating risky behaviors was studied by Stein, Roeser, and Markus (1998). In a longitudinal study, they measured self-schema and possible selves in three behavioral domains—the popular, conventional, and deviant selves—among 137 eighth and ninth grade students that were predominantly European-American. Relationships among current self-schema, future oriented possible selves, and risky behaviors were examined across the transition to high school. Risky behaviors assessed included alcohol use, tobacco use, precocious sexual activity, and poor school performance. Deviant self-schema, conventional self-schema, and possible self scores of eighth graders were not predictive of the level of ninth grade risky behaviors; however, the eighth grade popular self-schema score was a significant predictor of the ninth grade risky behaviors score ($p < .05$). Furthermore, results showed that the eighth grade risky behaviors score was predictive of both the ninth grade deviant self-schema and deviant possible self score. Interestingly, these effects were stronger for the females.

The results of this study highlight the complex interactive relationship between the self-concept and adolescent behavior. For the adolescents in this study, the self-concept not only played a role in shaping risky behaviors but, in addition, was reciprocally influenced by involvement in the behaviors. Conceptions of the self as socially popular predicted engagement in a constellation of risky behaviors, while engagement in risky behaviors themselves contributed to the crystallization of conceptions of the self as currently deviant and the expectations that one will be deviant in the future. When taken together, these findings suggest that self-concept may play a role not only in the early stages of engagement in the behaviors, but may also be one means through which the behaviors become internalized into a potentially enduring aspect of the self (Stein, Roeser, & Markus, 1998).

The perceived behavior of friends or crowds appears to have a profound affect on behaviors incorporated into one's self-schemas and personal behavioral repertoires. Urberg, Shiang-Jeou, and Liang (1990) found that overestimation of friends and crowds frequency of risky behaviors was common. This may well encourage youth to engage in risky behaviors at a high level primarily to match a standard that they believe their friends or crowd set. If the behaviors are addictive or life altering, inflated norms of peer performance can lead youth down self-destructive paths.

Oyserman and Markus (1990) emphasized the importance of balance between positive possible selves and feared possible selves to avoid risky or deviant behavior. In a study of adolescents with an officially documented history of delinquent behavior, they found that those with a delinquent history had fewer balanced pairs of positive expected and feared possible selves when compared to adolescents with no delinquent history. Furthermore, they found that although the delinquent youth had elaborated feared selves relevant to their delinquent behaviors, they lacked positive selves relevant to personal competence and achievement. These findings raise the interesting possibility that the availability of both negative and positive possible selves are necessary to avoid involvement in risky behaviors. Although a feared negative possible self in the domain may function to deter the risky behavior, a desired positive possible self is needed to give direction and form to behaviors necessary to avoid the feared states.

Health-Compromising Nutritional Practices and Eating Disorders

Among adolescent girls, the prevalence of disordered eating behaviors and actual eating disorders of anorexia nervosa and bulimia nervosa are rising sharply. Although recent estimates suggest that approximately 1–5% of girls between the ages of 15–19 meet diagnostic criteria for an eating disorder, studies have shown that as many as 20% of adolescent girls engage in subthreshold levels of disordered eating behaviors (Felts, Parrillo, Chenier, & Dunn, 1996). Behaviors such as dieting, bingeing, purging, and excessive exercise are not uncommon even among preadolescent and early adolescent girls. At all levels, these behaviors are associated with serious emotional and physical health consequences and for some girls, they represent the early stages of a chronic and even life-threatening eating disorder (Fisher, Schneider, Pegler, & Napolitano, 1991; French, Perry, Leon, & Fulkerson, 1995).

Although the majority of studies on the etiology of the eating disorders have tended to focus on internal biological and psychological factors (Crandall, 1988), recent studies have begun to consider the role of the support system in shaping patterns of disordered eating in preadolescent and adolescent girls. These studies, however, have tended to focus on the negative effects of the support system, exploring characteristics that contribute to the disordered behaviors rather than considering the protective or mediating role of social support.

Studies that have investigated the role of the family have generally shown that characteristics of the family unit as a whole, as well as the behaviors of individual family members play an important role in the development of adolescent eating problems, particularly for girls. Disturbances in general family functioning that are characteristic of the families of women with diagnosable eating disorders, have also been evidenced in the families of adolescents with subthreshold eating disordered behaviors (Graber, Brooks-Gunn, Paikoff, & Warren, 1994; Pike & Rodin, 1991). Although family characteristics such as disorganization, lack of cohesion, and high conflict have been consistently linked with disordered eating attitudes and behaviors, the mechanism to explain why these general patterns of interaction within a family lead to specific constellations of disordered eating behaviors and attitudes remain unclear. Other studies have shown that maternal attitudes and behaviors—both general and weight specific—relate to their daughters' disordered eating (Rieves & Cash, 1996). For example, Pike and Rodin (1991) found that mothers of eating disordered daughters were more dissatisfied with their general family functioning (themselves starting to diet at an early age), had more disordered eating behaviors, and were more critical of their daughter's appearance. Other researchers have shown that teasing by siblings, particularly brothers, contributes to high level of body dissatisfaction and disturbed body image in adolescent and young adults females (Cash, 1995).

Relatively few researchers have investigated the role of friends and peer networks in the development of disordered eating behaviors. Studies have shown that middle-school girls who talk with their friends about body weight and shape concerns have higher levels of body dissatisfaction and disordered eating behaviors (Levine, Smolak, & Hayden, 1994). Gibbs (1986) found that dieting behaviors of friends were not predictive of eating disordered attitudes and behaviors in a sample of high school-aged adolescents. However, in a longitudinal study of new members of a college sorority, Crandall (1988) found that through their first year of membership, the new members increased their level of binge eating to be consistent with the level that was considered normative in the group. Other researchers have shown that teasing about body weight and appearance by peers has a strong negative effect on body image and satisfaction (Levine, Smolak, & Harden, 1994).

The attitudes and behavior of peers and family influence eating behaviors of adolescent girls through various means including: (1) active processes such as direct criticism and disapproval, (2) more passive processes such as modeling disordered eating behaviors and attitudes, and (3) creating an environment in which body weight and shape are highly salient (Pike & Rodin, 1991). It is likely that these interpersonal processes heighten the importance of body weight and shape as an important source of self-definition and contribute to the formation of related body weight self-schema and possible selves that subsequently motivate disordered patterns of eating and weight control.

In a study of middle adolescent girls, Stein and Hedger (1997) found that the content of body weight and shape self-schema predicted emotional well-being and patterns of eating behaviors. Girls who defined themselves as currently "fat and out-of-shape" endorsed significantly thinner possible selves in both the eighth and ninth grades. Furthermore, they reported significantly lower levels of global self-esteem, appearance, and athletic competence, and higher depression and dieting behavior scores than girls who defined themselves as "slim and athletic." These findings provide evidence to suggest that the body weight and shape self-schema and possible selves play an important role in regulating emotional well-being and eating behaviors in nonclinical samples of adolescent girls. As such, social support systems that increase the salience and importance of body weight and contribute to the formation of conceptions of the self as "fat" play a central role in the formation of disordered patterns of eating and weight control.

As described, the protective effects of social support in the development of disordered eating in adolescent girls has not been systematically addressed.

In an 8-year longitudinal study of eating problems, however, Graber, Brooks-Gunn, Paikoff, and Warren (1994) found that girls who consistently showed no evidence of problem eating behaviors reported higher levels of family cohesion and lower levels of conflict. The investigators suggested that a cohesive and harmonious family may serve as a protective factor by mediating the effects of other sources of pressure regarding body weight and appearance. Although speculative, it is possible that strong, cohesive families provide the resources and supports necessary to the development of an array of positive identities such as soccer player, good student, cello player, healthy teenager, and good friend, while ignoring or otherwise downplaying the sources of self-definition that put one at risk for disordered eating. Additional studies in which the relationship between characteristics of the family environment, adolescent identity formation, and body weight self-definition are explored are needed to increase the understanding of the interaction between social support, self-definition, and disordered eating in adolescent girls.

SOCIAL SUPPORT AND THE SELF-SYSTEM: IMPLICATIONS FOR HEALTH-RELATED INTERVENTIONS

To date, no studies using self-concept or self-schema as a basis for interventions to promote healthy behaviors and decrease risky behaviors have appeared in the adolescent literature. However, among adults, Shadel, Mermelstein, and Borrelli (1996) explored domain-specific self-concepts in relation to success in smoking cessation. They assessed the smoker self-concept (smoking is part of my image, smoking is part of "who I am," etc.) and the abstainer self-concept (I am able to see myself as a nonsmoker, I am comfortable with the idea of being a nonsmoker, etc.) of European-Americans and African Americans prior to, immediately following, and 3 months after a smoking cessation program. The 7-week smoking cessation program consisted of a variety of strategies including self-monitoring, nicotine fading, stimulus control, and building self-management and coping skills. Prior to intervention, the smoker and abstainer self-concepts did not differ for persons who abstained and persons who resumed smoking after the intervention. Interestingly, the smoker self-concept scores of abstainers decreased significantly immediately after and 3 months posttreatment, whereas the scores for continuing smokers decreased significantly from baseline to immediately posttreatment but increased at 3 months to baseline levels. The abstainer self-concept scores of those who abstained increased significantly across each time point while these scores of smokers did not change significantly between any time points. Both smoker self-concept and abstainer self-concept appeared to change as a function of exposure to the traditional cognitive-behavioral cessation program even though they were not the specific targets of intervention. These results suggest that directly targeting domain specific self-schemas and possible selves may be a promising intervention strategy to prevent initiation of smoking and other risky behaviors as well as an approach to promoting healthy behaviors. The role of the self-system in behavior change among adolescents needs rigorous study.

Since intervention studies incorporating social support and self-system constructs have not yet been conducted with adolescents, these authors offer preliminary recommendations for approaches to intervention that could potentially lead to enhanced development of positive self-schemas, self-competence, and well-being among adolescents. Our recommendations are derived from our theoretical analysis and review of the descriptive research and focus on three possible forms of intervention. The three forms of interventions and examples include:

1.   Interventions to promote communication, involvement, and support among family members and within peer groups as a means of promoting the development of group-valued domains of positive self-definition. Examples include: (a) involve entire families in activities that help youth to develop skills in community action, volunteer services and social support giving such as, house builds, health fairs, elder assistance programs, (b) involve families in academic and school-related activities to create shared valuing, positive thoughts and feelings as part of the student self-schema, (c) strengthen family relationships and communication so that adolescents feel comfortable asking for support and help with relational and situational dilemmas that they confront during their adolescent years, and (d) involve peer groups of adolescents in meaningful activities that build emotional connection and caring self-schemas in a given domain such as conflict resolution, community clean-up, child care, educational television programming and filming.

2.   Interventions to directly promote involvement in health behaviors and activities that can lead to the elaboration of positive self-schemas and possible selves. Examples include: (a) focus on targeted skills training such as making healthy food choices, learning relaxation techniques, or gaining expertise with creative hobbies, (b) assist youths in developing

problem-solving and decision-making skills in desired behavioral domains such as sexuality or substance use, (c) assist youths to experience success in behavioral areas important to them such as music, athletics, computers, and (d) help adolescents to incorporate positive feeling states into various self-schemas such as connecting happiness, enjoyment, and feeling good with physical activity, eating healthily, or social interactions.

3. Interventions to provide role models and opportunities to observe others to promote the formation of positive desired possible selves. Examples include: (a) facilitate exposure to multiple positive adult role models with healthy lifestyles as a basis for envisioning positive health related possible selves, (b) assist youth to establish relationships with peer groups that value and enact healthy lifestyles and exhibit concern for self and others through service-learning projects, and (c) provide role models in the media that depict valuing and enjoyment of healthy lifestyles.

Readers are cautioned that these recommendations are based on theoretical analysis and on descriptive studies that are largely correlational in nature rather than on studies in which theoretically-based interventions have been systematically tested. Intervention studies remain to be conducted.

DIRECTIONS FOR ADOLESCENT RESEARCH IN SOCIAL SUPPORT, THE SELF-SYSTEM, AND HEALTH BEHAVIORS

Few studies to date provide direct evidence about the effects of social support on development of the self-system and emergence of resilience and health-related behaviors among adolescents in varying sociocultural contexts. Thus, much research is needed to develop effective interventions for increasing healthy behaviors and decreasing risky behaviors in adolescent populations. Tailoring health-promoting and preventive interventions to developmental stage and to the multiple contexts in which adolescents live and function, is a major challenge facing adolescent researchers in the years ahead. Further, the usefulness of the schema model of the self-concept to understanding and modifying health behaviors must yet be determined. Areas for productive research include:

1. Explore the role of social support in development of current self-schemas and possible selves among adolescents

2. Assess the self-concept of adolescents in the domains of social self-schema in terms of both *supported self* and *supportive self*
3. Develop valid and reliable measures of behavior-specific social support and health-relevant self-schema for adolescents from varying cultural backgrounds
4. Identify the mechanisms through which social support creates or activates resilience in vulnerable youth
5. Explore the extent to which self-schema mediate the effects of social support on adolescent health and health behaviors
6. Test interventions that enhance health relevant self-schema to promote the adoption and maintenance of healthy behaviors and the avoidance of risky behaviors
7. Test multilevel strategies of social support for their confluence in fostering healthy self-schemas and healthy lifestyles among adolescents

With the many health challenges that face youth during the adolescent years, an increased understanding of the specific ways in which social support impacts resilience, well-being, and health related lifestyles is critical. The schemas model of the self-system offers one potentially productive paradigm for achieving a better understanding of how social support influences health and health behaviors.

REFERENCES

Allender, M. E. (1998). Adolescent. In C. L. Edelman & C. L. Mandle (Eds.), *Health promotion throughout the lifespan* (4th ed., pp. 553–581). St. Louis: Mosby.
Barbaran, O. A. (1993). Coping and resilience: Exploring the inner lives of African-American children. *Journal of Black Psychology, 19*(4), 478–492.
Barrera, M., & Prelow, H. (2000). Interventions to promote social support in children and adolescents. In D. Cicchetti (Ed.), *The promotion of wellness in children and adolescents* (pp. 309–339). Washington, DC: Child Welfare League of America.
Berndt, T. J. (1996). Transition in friendship and friends' influence. In J. A. Graber, J. A. Brooks-Gunn, & A. C. Petersen (Eds.), *Transitions through adolescence: Interpersonal domains and context* (pp. 57–84). Mahwah, NJ: Erlbaum.
Brown, B. B., & Mounts, N. S. (1989). Peer group structures in single versus multi-ethnic high schools. Paper presented at the Biennial Meeting of the Society for Research in Child Development, Kansas City, MO.
Bukowski, W. M., Hoza, B., & Boivin, M. (1994). Measuring friendship quality during pre- and early adolescence: The development and psychometric properties of the

Friendship Qualities Scale. *Journal of Social and Personal Relationships, 11,* 471–484.

Bullerdick, S. K. (2000). Social connectedness and the relationship to emotional well-being among urban American Indian youth. *Dissertation Abstracts International, 60*(12-A), UMI No. 4603.

Cairns, R. B., & Cairns, B. (1995). *Lifelines and risks: Pathways of youth in our time.* New York: Cambridge University Press.

Camarena, P. M., Sarigiani, P. A., & Petersen, A. C. (1990). Gender-specific pathways to intimacy in early adolescence. *Journal of Youth and Adolescence, 19,* 19–32.

Cantor, N., & Kihlstrom, J. (1987). *Personality and social intelligence.* Englewood Cliffs, NJ: Prentice-Hall.

Cantor, N. (1990). From thought to behavior: "Having" and "Doing" in the study of personality and cognition. *American Psychologist, 45,* 735–750.

Cash, T. (1995). Developmental teasing about physical appearance: Retrospective descriptions and relationships with body image. *Social Behavior and Personality, 23,* 123–130.

Cauce, A. M., Hannan, K., & Sargeant, M. (1992). Life stress, social support, and locus of control during early adolescence: Interactive effects. *American Journal of Community Psychology, 20*(6), 787–798.

Cheever, K. H., & Hardin, S. B. (1999). Effects of traumatic events, social support, and self-efficacy on adolescents' self-health assessments. *Western Journal of Nursing Research, 21*(5), 673–684.

Colarossi, L. G. (2000). Gender differences in social support from parents, teachers, and peers: Implications for adolescent development. *Dissertation Abstracts International, 61*(2-A), UMI No. 767.

Connell, J. P., Spencer, M. B., & Aber, J. L. (1994). Educational risk and resilience in African-American youth: Context, self, action and outcomes in school. *Child Development, 65,* 493–506.

Crandall, C. (1988). Social contagion of binge eating. *Journal of Personality and Social Psychology, 55,* 588–598.

Dolcini, M. M., & Adler, N. E. (1994). Perceived competencies, group affiliation, and risk behavior. *Health Psychology, 13*(6), 496–506.

Eccles, J. S., Early, D., Frasier, K., Belansky, E., & McCarthy, K. M. (1997). The relation of connection, regulation, and support for autonomy to adolescents' functioning. *Journal of Adolescent Research, 12*(2), 263–286.

Epstein, L. H., Paluch, R. A., Coleman, K. J., Vrro, D., & Anderson, K. (1996). Determinants of physical activity in obese children assessed by accelerometer and self-report. *Medicine and Science in Sports and Exercise, 28,* 1157–1164.

Felts, W., Parrillo, A., Chenier, T., & Dunn, P. (1996). Adolescents' perceptions of relative weight and self-reported weight-loss activities: Analysis of 1990 YRBS national data. *Journal of Adolescent Health, 18,* 20–26.

Fisher, M., Schneider, M., Pegler, C., & Napolitano, B. (1991). Eating attitudes, health-risk behaviors, self-esteem, and anxiety among adolescent females in a suburban high school. *Journal of Adolescent Health, 12,* 377–384.

French, S., Perry, C., Leon, G., & Fulkerson, J. (1995). Changes in psychological variables and health behaviors by dieting status over a three-year period in a cohort of adolescent females. *Journal of Adolescent Health, 16,* 438–447.

Frey, C. U., & Rothlisberger, C. (1996). Social support in healthy adolescents. *Journal of Youth and Adolescence, 25*(1), 17–31.

Froming, W., Nasby, W., & McManus, J. (1998). Prosocial self-schemas, self-awareness, and children's prosocial behavior. *Journal of Personality and Social Psychology, 75,* 766–777.

Garcia, A. W., Broda, M. A., Frenn, M., Coviak, C., Pender, N. J., & Ronis, D. L. (1995). Gender and developmental differences in exercise beliefs among youth and prediction of their exercise behavior. *Journal of School Health, 65*(6), 213–219.

Garcia, A. W., Pender, N. J., Antonakos, C. L., & Ronis, D. L. (1998). Changes in exercise beliefs and behaviors of adolescents across the elementary to junior high school transition. *Journal of Adolescent Health, 22,* 394–402.

Garcia, T., & Pintrich, P. (1994). Regulating motivation and cognition in the classroom: The role of self-schemas and self-regulatory strategies. In D. Schunk & Zimmerman (Eds.), *Self-regulation of learning and performance: Issues and educational applications* (pp. 127–153). Hillsdale, NJ: Erlbaum.

Garmezy, N. (1993). Children in poverty: Resilience despite risk. *Psychiatry, 56,* 127–136.

Gibbs, R. E. (1986). Social factors in exaggerated eating behavior among high school students. *International Journal of Eating Disorders, 5,* 1103–1107.

Gottlieb, B. H., & Sylvestre, J. C. (1994). Social support in the relationships between older adolescents and adults. In F. Nestman & K. Hurrelmann (Eds.), *Social networks and social support in childhood and adolescence* (pp. 53–73). New York: Walter deGruyter.

Graber, J., Brooks-Gunn, J., Paikoff, R., & Wareen, M. (1994). Prediction of eating problems: An 8-year study of adolescent girls. *Developmental Psychology, 30,* 823–834.

Harter, S. (1985). Manual for the self-perception profile for children. University of Denver. (Available from Susan Harter, Department of Psychology, University of Denver, University Park, Denver, CO 80208).

Harter, S. (1999). *The construction of the self: A developmental perspective.* New York: Guildford Press.

Hawkins, J. D., Catalano, R., & Miller, J. (1992). Risk and protective factors for alcohol and other drug problems in adolescence and early adulthood: Implications for substance abuse prevention. *Psychological Bulletin, 112,* 64–105.

Hirsch, B. J., & DuBois, D. L. (1992). The relation of peer social support and psychological symptomatology during the transition to junior high school: A two-year longitudinal analysis. *American Journal of Community Psychology, 20*(3), 333–347.

Kaltiala-Heino, R., Rimpelae, M., Rantanen, P, & Laippala, P. (2001). Adolescent depression: The role of discontinuities in life course and social support. *Journal of Affective Disorders, 64,*(2–3), 155–166.

Kendzierski, D. (1988). Self-schemata and exercise. *Basic and Applied Psychology, 9*(1), 45–59.

Kendzierski, D. (1990). Exercise self-schemata: Cognitive and behavioral correlates. *Health Psychology, 9*(1), 69–82.

Kendzierski, D., & Whitaker, D. (1997). The role of self-schema in linking intentions with behavior. *Personality and Social Psychology Bulletin, 23,* 139–147.

Levin, M., Smolak, L., & Hayden, H. (1994). The relation of sociocultural factors to eating attitudes and behaviors among middle school girls. *Journal of Early Adolescence, 14,* 471–490.

Markstrom, C. A, Marshall, S. K., & Tryon, R. J. (2000). Resiliency, social support and coping in rural low-income Appalachian adolescents from two racial groups. *Journal of Adolescence, 23*(6), 693–703.

Markus, H. (1977). Self-schemata and processing information about the self. *Journal of Personality and Social Psychology, 35*(2), 63–78.

Markus, H., Cross, S., & Wurf, E. (1990). The role of the self-system in competence. In R. J. Sternberg & J. Kolligian (Eds.), *Competence considered.* New Haven, CT: Yale University Press.

Markus, H., Hamill, R., & Sentis, K. (1987). Thinking fat: Self-schemas for body weight and the processing of weight relevant information. *Journal of Applied Social Psychology, 17,* 50–71.

Markus, H., & Nurius, P. (1986). Possible selves. *American Psychologist, 41*(9), 954–969.

Markus, H., & Ruvolo, A. (1989). Possible selves: Personalized representations of goals. In L. Pervin (Ed.), *Goal concepts and personality* (pp. 211–241). Mahwah, NJ: Erlbaum.

Markus, H., & Wurf, E. (1987). The dynamic self-concept: A social psychological perspective. In M. R. Rosenzweig & L. W. Porter (Eds.), *Annual Review of Psychology, 38,* 237–299.

Meeus, W., & Dekovic, M. (1995). Identity development, parental and peer support in adolescence: Results of a national Dutch survey. *Adolescence, 30,* 931–944.

Nettles, S. M., Mucherah, W., & Jones, D. S. (2000). Understanding resilience: The role of social resources, *Journal of Education for Students Placed at Risk, 5*(1, 2), 47–60.

Oyserman, D., & Markus, H. (1990). Possible selves and delinquency. *Journal of Personality and Social Psychology, 59,* 112–125.

Patten, C. A., Gillin, J. C., Farkas, A. J., Gilpen, E. A., Berry, C. C., & Pierce, J. P. (1997). Depression symptoms in California adolescents: Family structure and parental support. *Journal of Adolescent Health, 20,* 271–278.

Pender, N. J. (1998). Motivation for physical activity among children and adolescents. In J. J. Fitzpatrick (Ed.), *Annual Review of Nursing Research, 16* (pp. 139–172). New York: Springer.

Pender, N. J., Murdaugh, C. L., & Parsons, M. A. (2002). *Health promotion in nursing practice* (4th ed., pp. 237–255). Upper Saddle River, NJ: Prentice Hall.

Pierce, G. R., Lakey, B., Sarason, I. G., & Sarason, B. R. (Eds.). (1997). *Handbook of social support and personality* (pp. 187–214). New York: Plenum.

Pike, K., & Rodin, J. (1991). Mothers, daughters and disordered eating. *Journal of Abnormal Psychology, 100,* 198–204.

Raja, S. N., McGee, R., & Stanton, W. R. (1992). Perceived attachment to parents and peers and psychological well-being in adolescence. *Journal of Youth and Adolescence, 21,* 471–485.

Rieves, L., & Cash, T. (1996). Social developmental factors and women's body-image attitudes. *Journal of Social Behavior and Personality, 11*, 63–78.

Sallis, J. F., Prochaska, J. J., & Taylor, W. C. (2000). A review of correlates of physical activity of children and adolescents. *Medicine and Science in Sports and Exercise, 32*(5), 963–975.

Shadel, W. G., Mermelstein, R., & Borrelli, B. (1996). Self-concept changes over time in cognitive-behavioral treatment for smoking cessation. *Addictive Behaviors, 21*(5), 659–663.

Smokowski, P. R., Reynolds, A. J., & Bezruczko, N. (1999). Resilience and protective factors in adolescence: An autobiographical perspective from disadvantaged youth. *Journal of School Psychology, 37*(4), 425–448.

Stein, K. F. (1994). Complexity of the self-schema and responses to disconfirming feedback. *Cognitive Therapy and Research, 18*, 161–178.

Stein, K. F., & Hedger, K. (1997). Body weight and shape self-cognitions, emotional distress and disordered eating in middle adolescent girls. *Archives of Psychiatric Nursing, 11*, 264–275.

Stein, K. F., Markus, H. R., & Roeser, R. W. (1997). The consensual self and self-esteem in American adolescent girls and boys. (Unpublished manuscript.)

Stein, K. F., Roeser, R. W., & Markus, H. R. (1998). Self-schemas and possible selves as predictors and outcomes of risky behaviors in adolescents. *Nursing Research, 47*(2), 96–106.

Sussman, S., Dent, C. W., Stacy, A. W., Burciaga, C., Raynor, A., Tuerner, G. E., Charlin, V., Craig, S., Hansen, W. B., Burton, D., & Flay, B. R. (1990). Peer-group association and adolescent tobacco use. *Journal of Abnormal Psychology, 99*, 349–352.

Takanishi, R. (2000). Preparing adolescents for social change: Designing generic social interventions. In L. J. Crockett & R. K. Silberstein (Eds.), *Negotiating adolescence in times of social change* (pp. 284–293). New York: Cambridge University Press.

Taylor, R. D., & Roberts, D. (1995). Kinship support and maternal and adolescent well-being in economically disadvantaged African-American families. *Child Development, 66*, 1585–1597.

Underwood, P. (2000). Social support: The promise and the reality. In V. H. Rice (Ed.), *Handbook of stress, coping and health: Implications for nursing research, theory and practice* (pp. 367–391). Thousands Oaks, CA: Sage.

Urberg, K. A., Shiang-Jeou, S., & Liang, J. (1990). Peer influence in adolescent cigarette smoking. *Addictive Behaviors, 15*, 247–255.

Urberg, K. A., Degirmencioglu, S. M., Tolson, J. M., & Halliday-Scher, K. (1995). The structure of adolescent peer networks. *Developmental Psychology, 31*(4), 540–547.

Werner, E. E. (1992). The children of Kauai: Resiliency and recovery in adolescence and adulthood. *Journal of Adolescent Health, 13*, 262–268.

Winfield, L. F. (1995). The knowledge base on resilience in African-American adolescents. In L. J. Crockett & A. C. Crouter (Eds.), *Pathways through adolescence: Individual development in relation to social context* (pp. 87–118). Mahwah, NJ: Erlbaum.

Yarcheski, A., Mahon, N. E., & Yarcheski, T. J. (1997). Alternate models of positive health practices among adolescents. *Nursing Research, 46*(2), 85–92.

Yarcheski, A., Mahon, N. E., & Yarcheski, T. J. (2001). Social support and well-being in early adolescents: The role of mediating variables. *Clinical Nursing Research, 10*(2), 163–181.
Zakarian, J. M., Hovell, M. F., Hofstetter, C. R., Sallis, J. F., & Keating, K. J. (1994). Correlates of vigorous exercise in a predominantly low SES and minority high school population. *Preventive Medicine, 23,* 314–321.
Zimmerman, M. A., Salem, D. A., & Maton, K. I. (1995). Family structure and psychosocial correlates among urban African-American adolescent males. *Child Development, 66,* 1598–1613.

ACKNOWLEDGMENT

The assistance of Ms. Karen McIlroy, Administrative and Research Associate, Child and Adolescent Health Behavior Research Center, University of Michigan School of Nursing, is gratefully acknowledged. Her assistance with literature searches and manuscript preparation made the timely completion of this chapter possible.

PART 2

Health Promoting Behaviors

CHAPTER 3

Improving Diet and Nutrition in Children and Adolescents

**Andrew M. Tershakovec and
Linda Van Horn**

The bulk of preventive nutrition interventions for children and adolescents conducted to date have focused primarily on limiting risk factors for cardiovascular disease and preventing or treating childhood obesity, however, the total experience with preventive nutrition intervention in children is limited. This is due in part to the relatively recent documentation that the roots for nutrition related adult disease lie in childhood. In addition, others have questioned the effectiveness of nutrition intervention (Browner, Westenhouse, & Tice, 1991; Hunninghake et al., 1993) and the safety (with respect to supporting normal growth and development and providing a complete and balanced diet) of such interventions in children (Newman, Browner, & Hulley, 1990). Thus, dietary interventions must overcome the difficulties inherent in any behavioral modification effort and the skepticism and mixed information that are commonly publicized regarding nutrition and preventive health. This chapter provides an overview of the preventive health aspects of nutrition intervention in children, and questions and concerns surrounding these issues are addressed.

DIET AND HEALTH RISK

The first observations linking diet with atherosclerosis were made in 1908 (Committee on Diet and Health, Food and Nutrition Board, Commission on

Life Sciences, National Research Council, 1989). More recently, results from the Seven Countries study (Keys, 1970, 1980), the Framingham study (Castelli, Garrison, Wilson, et al., 1986), the MRFIT (Multiple Risk Factor Intervention Trial) (Neaton & Wentworth, 1992), and studies of groups migrating from one country to another, such as the Ni-Hon-San study (Nichaman et al., 1975), have solidified the evidence linking diet, blood cholesterol level, and risk of heart disease in adults. The link between diet and cholesterol levels has also been described in children. Shea and colleagues (1991) showed significant relationships between total fat and saturated fat intake and cholesterol levels in 4–5 year-old Hispanic children. Data from the Bogalusa Heart Study demonstrated a positive association between saturated fat intake and cholesterol level in 10-year-old children (Frank, Berenson, & Webber, 1978), and dietary cholesterol and cholesterol levels in 4- and 7-year-old children (Nicklas, 1988). Furthermore, blood lipid levels have been correlated with the presence of early atherosclerotic changes in children and young adults (McGill et al., 2000; Newman et al., 1986). Higher fat diets have also been associated with caloric excess and greater weight gain or attainment of greater body fat (Heitmann, Lissner, Sorensen, & Bengtsson, 1995; Prewitt et al., 1991; Sheppard, Kristal, & Kusha, 1991; Tucker & Kano, 1992). Most of these data are limited to adults, but evidence of similar associations in children is emerging (Gazzaniga & Burns, 1993; Tershakovec et al., 1997). In addition, children who are overweight have an increased risk of becoming obese adults, while older children and children with greater degrees of obesity also have greater chances of remaining obese (Charney, Goodman, McBride, Lyon, & Pratt, 1977; Garn & La Velle, 1985; Guo, Roche, Chumlea, Gardner, & Siervogel, 1994; Whitaker, Wright, Pepe, Seidel, & Deitz, 1997).

EPIDEMIOLOGY OF DIET, HYPERCHOLESTEROLEMIA, AND OBESITY

As we are aware of the links between diet, health, and disease, it is useful to evaluate the prevalence of dietary factors that may be associated with poor health outcomes. Nationwide surveys and other data from the 1970s and 1980s (Kimm, Gergen, Malloy, Dresser, & Carroll, 1990; McPherson, Nichaman, Kohl, Reed, & Labarthe, 1990; Nicklas, Webber, Srinivasan, & Berenson, 1993) revealed that children's fat intake was 35–36% of total calories, and 13–14% of total calories as saturated fat. National Health and Nutrition Examination Survey [NHANES] III data, collected between 1988 and 1991, demonstrated a slightly lower fat intake for children and adolescents (33–34% of calories as fat, and 12–13% of calories as saturated fat) than previously described (Lenfant & Ernst, 1994). An even lower fat intake (29–30% calories as fat) was reported in a suburban, largely White, middle-to-upper socioeconomic status group of 4–10 year-old children (Tershakovec et al., 1997). Though results from NHANES are similar across gender and racial subgroups, other researchers have reported that African American children and children of lower socioeconomic status are less adherent to dietary recommendations regarding fat and saturated fat intake (Thompson & Dennison, 1994).

Data suggest that the average fat intake among adults is decreasing (McDowell et al., 1994; Stephen & Wald, 1990). The decreasing mean blood cholesterol levels in adults is consistent with this dietary change (Johnson et al., 1993). Similarly, dietary intakes of 10-year-old children in Bogalusa, Louisiana from 1973 to 1988, showed decreasing trends for total fat, saturated fat, and cholesterol intake (Nicklas et al., 1993). NHANES III data for adolescents are consistent with Bogalusa observations; however mean intake levels remain above current dietary recommendations (McDowell et al., 1994). Data from NHANES III also suggest a concomitant trend toward lower blood cholesterol levels in adolescents (Hickman et al., 1998).

As the National Cholesterol Education Program defines children with LDL-cholesterol (LDL-C) levels above the 75th percentile as hypercholesterolemic, 25% of children are theoretically at risk and thus eligible for individualized dietary intervention. An evaluation of the recommended selective screening process for hypercholesterolemia in children (screening only children with a family history of hypercholesterolemia or premature heart disease) in a rural area suggested that 38% of the children would be recommended to complete cholesterol screening (Dennison, Jenkins, & Pearson, 1994). However, the limited utility of the selective screening process to actually identify hypercholesterolemic children has also been demonstrated (Dennison, Kikuchi, Srinivasan, Webber, & Berenson, 1989; Garcia & Moodie, 1989).

Despite the apparent decreases in fat intake in American children, the prevalence of obesity is increasing at an alarming rate. The prevalence of obesity among White and African American boys and girls generally increased 50–100% from 1963 to 1991 so that 20–30% of children are considered obese (Troiano, Flegal, Kuczmarski, Campbell, & Johnson, 1995). Longitudinal data from the Bogalusa Heart Study revealed a similar trend (Freedman, Srinivasan, Valdez, Williamson, & Berenson, 1997). Prevalence rates of obesity differ somewhat among ethnic and racial groups (Winkleby, Robinson, Sundquist, & Kraemer, 1999). For example, the prevalence of obesity has risen more rapidly among African American children than White children. African American girls are one of the highest risk groups for becoming obese adults and suffering the attendant medical complications (Kumanyika, 1987; Troiano et al., 1995; Winkleby et al., 1999). The 10-fold increase in the incidence of non-insulin dependent diabetes reported among adolescents in Cincinnati suggested one of the dramatic consequences of such escalating obesity prevalence (Pinhas-Hamiel et al., 1996). It is not clear how much overlap there is within children with hypercholesterolemia and obesity, but reviewing the prevalence data relating to hypercholesterolemia and obesity together, it is clear that at least 25% of American children would potentially benefit from therapeutic dietary intervention.

DIET RECOMMENDATIONS

Based upon these associations and trends, expert groups have formulated dietary recommendations for children. Most of these are associated with the prevention or treatment of premature cardiovascular disease. Nutrition recommendations for healthy children (above the age of 2 years) and adolescents have been developed to lower average population levels of blood cholesterol in children and adolescents, to reduce the incidence of adult coronary heart disease, and generally to improve health (Report of the Expert Panel on Blood Cholesterol Levels in Children and Adolescents, 1992, American Academy of Pediatrics [AAP] Committee on Nutrition, 1998). These dietary recommendations also represent the first line of therapy for hypercholesterolemic children. According to these guidelines, the child's diet should include a wide variety of foods, and provide adequate calories to support growth and development and reach and maintain a desirable body weight. Daily food intake should provide no > 30% (and no < 20%) of total calories from fat, < 10% calories from saturated fat, and < 300 mg cholesterol per day. (These dietary recommendations are also collectively referred to as the Step I Diet.)

For children with elevated cholesterol levels, the minimum goal for dietary intervention is to achieve an LDL-C level below 130 mg/dl (approximately the 95th percentile), though ideally the LDL-C level should be below 110 mg/dl. If these goals are not achieved despite repeated attempts and adherence to the Step 1 Diet, the Step 2 Diet (< 7% calories as saturated fat and < 200 mg cholesterol/day) should be considered. The timing required to observe the response to these dietary changes is somewhat flexible. The National Cholesterol Education Program (NCEP) recommends 6 weeks–3 months of dietary intervention before repeating lipid profile analysis. With good adherence, diet induced lipid responses can be detected after 3 weeks. In addition, due to the variability in lipid levels, at least two lipid evaluations should be considered before making therapeutic decisions.

In contrast to these specific dietary guidelines for hypercholesterolemic children, no specific recommendations currently exist for dietary intervention related to weight management in obese children. Weight management programs for children tend to be multifaceted, and include dietary change, exercise promotion, and behavior modification. Keys to effective dietary modification efforts for obese children include a simple program that can be understood by children and implemented by their parents, and that generally lowers calorie and fat intake. The Stoplight Diet (Epstein, Valoski, Wing, & McCurley, 1990) is one example of such a program (see Weight Management Programs for Children and Adolescents section below).

A risk of nutritional intervention in weight management efforts appears to be that parents and children sometimes focus exclusively on lowering dietary fat content but ignore total caloric intake. The high caloric content of some low-fat foods can make this problematic. This may also complicate the management of hyperlipidemia, as weight gain or a high sugar intake may increase blood lipid levels, especially triglyceride level. Furthermore, obese adolescents, on average, have been shown to underreport caloric intake by about 40% (Bandini, Schoeller, Cyr, & Dietz, 1990), making the assessment of response to dietary change in weight management especially difficult. Assessment of resting energy expenditure and comparison of measured energy expenditure with reported caloric intake may provide important diagnostic information in such cases, and may be helpful in counseling and behavioral modification.

The Third Report of the National Cholesterol Education Program Expert Panel on Detection, Evaluation, and Treatment of High Blood Cholesterol in Adults (Adult Treatment Panel III) was recently published (NCEP, 2001). Though this report pertains to adults, there are a few aspects that should be considered with respect to children. ATP III recommends a full lipid profile for all individuals above the age of 20 years. Though previous guidelines had defined 35 mg/dl as a low HDL-C level, ATP III has raised this to 40 mg/dl. ATP III also defines a high triglyceride level as > 200 mg/dl in adults.

Adult Treatment Panel III supports the implementation of the Therapeutic Lifestyle Changes Diet for hyperlipidemic individuals, which includes the following: < 7% calories as saturated fat, up to 10% calories as polyunsaturated fat, up to 20% calories as monounsaturated fat, 50–60% calories as carbohydrate, 20–30 g/day fiber, approximately 15% calories as protein, < 200 mg/day cholesterol, and total calories to maintain a desirable body weight. (Note that these dietary guidelines resemble the Step II Diet.) ATP III also emphasizes the connection between hyperlipidemia and obesity, and interventions to minimize the so-called metabolic syndrome. In general, ATP III addresses several issues relating to cardiovascular risk assessment and intervention in adults which have not been addressed in pediatric guidelines. Reevaluation of pediatric guidelines should be considered to assess new information and broader based issues and recommendations.

Special Considerations for Young Children

Children less than 2 years of age grow very rapidly, and thus need a large amount of energy. Due to the high caloric density of fat (9 calories/gram versus 4 calories/gram for carbohydrates and protein), children less than 2 years of age typically require higher fat intake owing to their limited volume of intake capacity and the high energy needed to sustain normal growth. The rapidly developing central nervous system of a young child also requires an adequate fatty acid intake (Hamosh, 1988). For these reasons, current recommendations do not limit fat intake of children less than 2 years old. However, data exist suggesting the safety of lower fat diets for younger children. The Special Turku Coronary Risk Factor Intervention Project (STRIP) described the safety and efficacy of a diet containing 26–31% calories from total fat in lowering blood lipid levels and supporting normal growth in children when initiated at 7 months of age (Niinikoski et al., 1997; Rask-Nissila et al., 2000; Niinikoski, Viikari, Ronnemaa, et al., 1997; Lagstrom et al., 1999). Despite these reports of apparent safety, any attempts to implement such a diet with young children should be closely monitored.

PEDIATRIC DIETARY INTERVENTIONS: LIMITATIONS OF EXISTING RESEARCH

Before reviewing the experience with preventive and therapeutic dietary intervention in children, a few qualifiers are necessary. Many of the existing studies on hypercholesterolemic individuals do not define the cause of the hyperlipidemia (e.g., familial hypercholesterolemia, familial combined hyperlipidemia). Because children with different etiologies of hypercholesterolemia may respond differently to dietary interventions, differences in responses may be observed. Many of the studies control for only one aspect of the diet, while other dietary factors vary, leaving it unclear which change stimulated the observed response. Other limitations include the lack of adequate nutrient analyses at baseline in both the intervention and control groups. To define the response to the diet, it is necessary to define dietary change. Since few intervention studies have been completed with children, some of the current recommendations are derived from observations in adults. Also, most of the completed studies involve a small sample size, thus limiting their generalizability. Finally, few of these studies utilize a random control group, suggesting that some of the observed response to diet is actually regression to the mean (Morrison et al., 1979).

Defining the specific influence of dietary intervention in weight management programs for children may even be harder. Few researchers have limited the variability between groups to dietary change only or to different types of dietary change. Thus it is hard to assign specific changes to specific aspects of the diets.

Pediatric Response to Dietary Change

Most of dietary intervention for children has sought to follow recommended dietary guidelines, such as the Step I Diet. For example, Cortner and colleagues (1987), evaluated the response of 54 children (mean age 9.2 years) with LDL-C greater than 90th percentile and a family history of premature heart disease who were advised to follow the Step I Diet. The average decrease in LDL-C was 12%. Response was independent of age, duration of therapy, and initial LDL-C level. The individual variability in LDL-C response to diet ranged from an increase of 24%, to a decrease of 34%. Similar results have been described elsewhere (Quiver et al., 1992).

When the children followed by Cortner and colleagues(1987) were divided into those with heterozygous familial hypercholesterolemia (FH) and those with familial combined hyperlipidemia (FCHL), a differential response was suggested. The FH children demonstrated a mean decrease in LDL-C of 8% (none was below the 90th percentile) while the FCHL children's mean level decreased 13% (45% were below the 90th percentile). Widhalm (1985) reported similar results when reviewing outpatient trials of dietary intervention for FH children, but significantly larger average responses (e.g., −24%) with trials completed with inpatients. Greater compliance and more controlled conditions may be responsible for this difference in observed response between the outpatient and inpatient setting.

Kwiterovich et al. (1985) varied the dietary goals somewhat and compared responses between children with isolated hypercholesterolemia and those with combined hypercholesterolemia and hypertriglyceridemia following a diet limiting cholesterol intake to < 300 mg per day and maintaining a polyunsaturated fat to saturated fat (P:S) ratio > 2. In addition to significant decreases in total cholesterol and LDL-C levels, a significant drop in HDL-cholesterol (HDL-C) was observed in both groups, as reported in other dietary trials with adults and children (Mata, Alvarez-Sala, Rubio, Nuno, & De Oya, 1992; Widhalm, 1985). Whether the positive health consequences of a substantial reduction in LDL-C are counterbalanced by a reduction in HDL-C among growing children requires further study.

The Diet Intervention Study in Children (DISC), (Obarzanek, Hunsberger, Van Horn, et al., 1997; Obarzanek, Kimm, Barton, et al., 2001) is the largest study in which questions of efficacy, safety, and feasibility of diet intervention in growing adolescent children with elevated LDL-cholesterol were addressed. Six centers and a total of 663 children were enrolled in this controlled clinical trial. Children were randomly assigned to a Step II Diet for 3 years. Mean level of total fat intake in the intervention group was 28.6% at three years versus 33.0% in the usual care group. The mean net LDL-C difference between groups was −0.08 mmol/L (−3.23 mg/dl) with no apparent differences in any of the growth or psychosocial parameters measured. DISC excluded children at baseline who were diagnosed with familial hypercholesterolemia as well as children who were 30% above ideal body weight. Thus, DISC demonstrated that dietary intervention patterned on the Step II Diet can be safely implemented.

Response to Different Types of Fat

Varying responses to the ingestion of different types of fat have been reported. Two studies of boys in boarding schools in Massachusetts (13–18 years old) and South Africa (ages 12–18 years old) demonstrated the lipid lowering effect of a higher P:S ratio diet (McGancy, Hall, Ford, & Stare, 1972; Stein et al., 1975). In both studies, a differential response to the diet based on initial cholesterol level was observed (e.g. a greater lowering in cholesterol level was noted for boys whose initial total cholesterol was greater than 200 mg/dl, compared to those whose initial levels were less than 200 mg/dl). The difference in results related to initial cholesterol level between these authors and Cortner et al. (1987) may be due to specific clinical conditions. These boarding school students were not pre-selected and thus probably had a high incidence of environmental and polygenic hypercholesterolemia, while Cortner specifically selected children with familial forms of hyperlipidemia. Stein et al. (1982) observed a similar effect of a high P:S ratio. Studying 11 children and one adult with heterozygous FH, and 11 unaffected controls, the researchers suggested that a high P:S ratio had a lipid lowering effect, even with a higher total fat and cholesterol intake, while a high fat and cholesterol, and low P:S ratio diet had a significant deleterious effect, even on the unaffected siblings.

The potential positive health benefits of the high monounsaturated fat Mediterranean-type diet (high in olive oil, grains, fruits, and vegetables, with moderate fish and relatively limited red meat intake) have led to investigation of the effect of monounsaturated fat on lipid levels. Many of the older studies focused on P:S ratios; no reports of monounsaturated fat content were included. Investigators of adults suggested that a diet high in monounsaturated fat has a neutral or a slight lowering effect on LDL-C levels, but the more important effect may be associated with preserving HDL-C levels. Diets high in polyunsaturated fatty acids reportedly reduce both LDL-C and HDL-C levels. High monounsaturated fat-containing diets, on the other hand, seem to preserve or even raise HDL-C levels, while lowering or not raising LDL-C levels (Colquhoun, Moores, Somerset, & Humphries, 1992; Denke & Grundy, 1991; Mata et al., 1992; Mattson & Grundy, 1985; Mensink & Katan, 1989; Sirtori et al., 1992), though evidence supporting or contradicting these effects in children is lacking. In addition, there is concern that diets too high in polyunsaturated fat in adults may be related to increased cancer risk (Committee on Diet and Health, 1989).

There is increasing evidence that categorizing fatty acids and their effects on lipid levels into monounsaturated, polyunsaturated and saturated is overly simplistic. For example, the saturated fat, stearic acid, does not seem to raise LDL-C levels as seen with other saturated fats (Denke & Grundy, 1991; Derr, Kris-Etherton, Pearson, & Seligson, 1993; Kris-Etherton et al., 1993; Kris-Etherton, Mustad, & Derr, 1993). On the other hand, trans fatty acids (partially hydrogenated unsaturated fatty acids) have been shown to raise total cholesterol and LDL-C levels and lower HDL-C levels in adults (Troisi, Willett, & Weiss, 1992; Willett & Ascherio, 1994; Zock & Katan, 1992). The potential public health impact of the intake of trans fatty acids is widespread due to the frequent usage in processed foods, including foods which are considered to be "healthier" (Litin & Sacks, 1993; Willett & Ascherio, 1994). Because they are not quantified on the food label and because the nutrient database for trans fatty acids is incomplete, it is difficult or impossible for either the lay person or the nutrition community to gauge the actual content in foods. In an editorial, Willett and Ascherio (1994) estimated that 30,000 deaths occur yearly in the United States due to medical conditions exacerbated by the consumption of trans fatty acids. Further research is needed to document the exact impact, but avoidance of concentrated sources of trans fatty acids, such as hydrogenated shortenings, offers a practical approach. No data specifically relating to trans fatty acid intake and health impact in children exist.

Fiber

Dietary fiber, especially soluble fiber (such as oat bran), has been shown to have a moderate cholesterol lowering effect in hypercholesterolemic adults (Anderson et al., 1984; Anderson et al., 1991; Anderson, Riddell-Mason, Gustafson, Smith, & Mackey, 1992; Bell, Hectorn, Reynolds, & Hunninghake, 1990; Denmark-Wahnefried, Bowering, & Cohen, 1990; Jenkins et al., 1993; Kashtan et al., 1992; Kestin, Moss, Clifton, & Nestel, 1990; Kirby et al., 1981; Lampe et al., 1991; McIntosh, Whyte, Mcarthur, & Nestel, 1991; Ripsin et al., 1992; Van Horn et al., 1986). Several potential mechanisms have been proposed. Soluble fiber may bind with bile salts, causing greater bile excretion in the stool, however, observations are not all consistent with this hypothesis (Kirby et al., 1981; Kritchevsky, 1988; Lampe et al., 1991; Pilch, 1987). The most extensive intervention experience has been with oat fiber, rich in beta glucan (Ripsin et al., 1992). Studies with other sources of soluble fiber, such as sugar beets (Lampe et al., 1991), rice (Kestin et al., 1990), psyllium (Anderson et al., 1992), prunes (Tinker, Schneeman, Davis, Gallagher, & Waggoner, 1991) and barley (McIntosh et al., 1991), have had potentially favorable lipid-lowering results. The more modest lowering of lipid levels observed with insoluble fiber, such as wheat bran, may be due to replacement of low fiber, higher fat foods with lower fat, high fiber foods.

Experience with fiber supplementation in children is much more limited (Davidson et al., 1992; Dennison & Levine, 1993; Glassman et al., 1990) and the results somewhat mixed. Concern remains about the safety of such supplements in children. Very high fiber diets may limit caloric density and/ or impair micronutrient absorption (Sanders & Reddy, 1994). Though long-term experience is limited, children treated for encopresis (severe constipation) with a high fiber diet, laxatives and mineral oil did not suffer from nutritional inadequacies when followed over a six month period (McClung et al., 1993). To potentially aid in the prevention of cardiovascular disease, some cancers, adult-onset diabetes and to promote normal laxation, a fiber intake (in grams) of five plus the child's age (in years) has been recommended for children older than two years of age (Williams, Bollella, & Wynder, 1995). Higher fiber diets, with lower caloric densities, would also be recommended in weight management.

Vegetarian Diets

The efficacy of a vegetarian diet in lowering cholesterol levels in children has been demonstrated (Fernandes, Dijkhuis-Stoffelsma, Groot, Grose, & Ambagtsheer, 1981; Gaddi et al., 1987; Widhalm, Brazda, Schneider, & Kohl, 1993).The low cholesterol, low fat, high P:S, high fiber, and high micronutrient content may each have positive health effects by lowering cholesterol levels and by other mechanisms (Anderson, Smith & Gustafson, 1994; Fraser, 1994). The low caloric density and high bulk of the diet, phytate content, and other factors limiting micronutrient absorption, and the potential for vitamin B12 deficiency among pure vegans, has caused concerns (Sanders & Reddy, 1994). Well-controlled studies have shown that children following appropriate vegetarian diets can grow and develop normally despite being leaner than their meat-eating counterparts (Sabate, Lindsted, Harris, & Johnston, 1990). The therapeutic potential of a vegetarian diet in weight management has not been evaluated.

Soy protein has been shown to decrease total cholesterol, LDL-C, and triglyceride levels, while not lowering HDL-C levels (AHA Dietary Guidelines Committee, 2000; Anderson, Johnstone, & Cook-Newell, 1995; Baum, Teng, Erdman, et al., 1998; Crouse, Morgan, Terry, et al., 1999; Teixeira, Potter, Weigel, et al., 2000). This effect may be partially dependent on the isoflavone content of the soy protein; isoflavones have weak estrogenic activity. It should be noted that some processed soy food products lose much of the isoflavone content during production. The evidence supporting the positive effects of soy protein on blood lipid levels is so strong that the Food and Drug Administration has approved food label claims for reduced cardiovascular disease risk for food containing ≥ 6.25 grams of soy protein per serving (FDA Talk Paper T99–48). Though limited data exist regarding soy protein intake and children, incorporation of soy protein into a complete and balanced diet would be appropriate for children.

Miscellaneous Dietary Interventions

Data suggest that fish oil, antioxidants, and folic acid supplements may reduce the risk of coronary heart disease in adults by mechanisms largely independent of lowering blood lipid levels (Boushey, Beresford, Omenn, & Motulsky, 1995; Gey et al., 1993; Kinsella, Lokesh, & Stone, 1990; Renaud et al., 1995; Rimm et al., 1993; Stampfer et al., 1993). (Note that fish oil supplements have also been utilized to lower triglyceride levels in hypertriglyceridemic adult patients.) The potentially therapeutic effects of fish oil and antioxidants have been generally demonstrated with doses much greater than can practically be provided in a child's diet. Thus, without more safety information concerning the ingestion of such large, therapeutic amounts of these substances in children (e.g., fish oil or vitamin pills), the use of such potentially therapeutic food supplements should be discouraged in favor of optimized dietary patterns. Diets with larger numbers of servings of fruits and vegetables will optimize natural sources of antioxidants. This, combined with regular intake of fish and olive oil as seen with the Mediterranean diet, can safely be recommended for children and adolescents as part of an overall balanced diet.

Plant sterols are ingested in a regular diet. However, food products enriched with plant sterols have demonstrated a cholesterol lowering effect (Jones & Raeini-Sarjaz, 2000; Nguyen, 1999; Tammi et al., 2000; Miettinen, Pekka, Gylling, Vanhanen, & Vartiainen, 1995; Hallikainen, 2000). The mechanism of action is not fully understood, but it seems the plant sterol interferes with cholesterol-micelle interaction and subsequent cholesterol absorption. However, as one study suggested a lower serum beta carotene level associated with the use of a plant stanol ester margarine in 6 year old children (Miettinen, Pekka, Gylling, Vanhanen, & Vartiainen, 1995), such products should be carefully utilized in children.

WEIGHT MANAGEMENT PROGRAMS FOR CHILDREN AND ADOLESCENTS

Though few dietary intervention programs for hypercholesterolemic children have been completed, relative to the number completed for adults, even fewer dietary interventions have been completed for obese children. Epstein and colleagues (Epstein et al., 1980, 1990), have conducted the most comprehensive and well documented long-term weight management programs for children. In this program, 6–12 year old children were enrolled into group therapy in which diet, exercise, and behavior management information was provided. In general, dietary modification in weight management programs has included easy-to-follow dietary programs. The Traffic Light diet utilized in Epstein's programs is an example of such a program. Foods were designated as green, yellow, or red light foods, based upon their caloric density. Children were then given guidelines concerning caloric intake, and limits pertaining to the number of red light foods they were allowed to eat per week. An accompanying behavioral modification program encouraged compliance with all aspects of the program via contracting and self-monitoring. Parents and children paid a certain amount of money at the beginning of the program, and then received refunds in exchange for successful weight loss, self-monitoring of dietary intake, meeting red food intake limitations, and other desirable behaviors. Families were asked to reinforce the desired behavioral changes and to act as role models. Efforts focusing the program on children versus combined approaches with children and their parents were compared. Though the children in the child-focus group demonstrated the greatest initial weight loss (at 8 months), the child-parent focus group showed the best long-term outcome. At 10 years, the child-parent group had decreased their percent overweight by 7%, while the child-focus group had increased their percent overweight by 4.7% As the researchers enrolled a relatively select group of children (only 76 children were accepted into the trial from the 185 families who applied to participate), the efficacy of Epstein's program in the general population is not known.

Wadden and colleagues (1990), implemented a weight management program for obese African American adolescent girls with similar components as described above in Epstein's program. Participants were randomly assigned to one of three groups—child alone, child and mother together, and child and mother separately. In the child alone group, the girls attended the sessions alone, while in the child and mother together group, the mothers and daughters attended the sessions together. In the child and mother separately group, the mothers and daughters attended separate sessions. Though there were no significant differences between groups, a trend suggested the child alone group lost less weight (1.6 kg) than the other two groups (3.7 kg and 3.1 kg). It was also found that daughters of mothers who demonstrated good program attendance lost more weight (4.9 kg) than daughters of mothers with poor (1.9 kg) or no attendance (1.6 kg). After 6 months, the daughters in the child and mother together group gained less weight (1.7 kg) than the daughters in the child alone (3.0 kg) and the child and mother separately (3.5 kg) groups. Thus, these programs seem to demonstrate the importance of familial involvement in pediatric weight loss programs.

A recent meta-analysis of treatment for child and adolescent obesity sought to evaluate the utility of different components of the programs (Haddock, Shadish, Klesges, & Stein, 1994). The researchers demonstrated that programs that were comprehensive in nature (e.g., included behavior modification procedures, dietary change, and exercise) produced better results, and that inclusion of behavior modification techniques in particular was important. In this analysis, the components of the dietary modification were separately evaluated. Surprisingly, programs that included the recommended components of dietary modification (diet easily understood by the child, caloric intake tailored to the child's needs, diet focused on decreasing fat and caloric intake, dietary component supervised by a dietary expert) were less or no more effective than programs without these components. In addition, the efficacy of parental involvement was not confirmed in this analysis. The reasons for the lack of improved outcome when the programs included the recommended dietary components or when parents participated, given the previously described results supporting the importance of parental involvement, are unknown and should be studied more fully. The overall results also suggest that weight loss programs for obese children have produced modest results.

A protein-modified-fast has also been utilized to induce a relatively rapid weight loss in severely obese individuals. Though the experience is relatively limited in children, one study involving twelve obese adolescents who followed a diet providing 880 kcal/day and 2.5 g protein per kg ideal body weight has been reported. These participants decreased their percent overweight from 54% to 25% over 3 months, and were able to maintain their relative weight over the next nine months (Stallings, Archibald, Pencharz, Harrison, & Bell, 1988). Such programs must be instituted with careful supervision to ensure the participants are ingesting a complete and appropriately balanced diet, and to monitor for possible complications. For example, persons undergoing such rapid weight loss may be at risk for cholelithiasis (Thomas, 1995). Though it seems immediate weight loss can be induced with such programs, anecdotal reports of poor long-term weight maintenance after the transition to a regular diet are common.

There has been much recent interest in the use of low carbohydrate diets in weight management. It has been proposed that high glycemic index diets promote overeating and increased weight gain and worsening of blood lipid levels (Morris & Zemel, 1999; Ludwig, Majzoub, Al-Zahrani, Dallal, Blanco, & Roberts, 1999). This is consistent with the recently described association between consumption of sugar-sweetened drinks and obesity and excess weight gain in children (Ludwig, Peterson, & Gortmaker, 2001). Preliminary data also suggest that a ketogenic diet or a low glycemic index can induce greater weight loss over 3–4 months, for obese adolescents (Spieth et al., 2000; Ludwig, Peterson, & Gortmaker, 2001; Sondike, Jacobson, & Cooperman, 2000). However, the longer term efficacy and safety of such diets has not been studied in children or adults.

DIET MODIFICATION, NUTRIENT ADEQUACY AND FAILURE-TO-THRIVE

One of the major concerns relating to dietary intervention in children is whether such an altered diet can supply a complete and balanced diet, and support normal growth and development. In addressing these issues, it is useful to begin by evaluating the changes in nutrient intake associated with such dietary modification. The major sources of fat in children's diets are whole milk and other dairy products, and meats. The major sources of cholesterol are eggs and whole milk (Sigman-Grant, Zimmerman, & Kris-Etherton, 1993; Thompson & Dennison, 1994). These observations suggest that relatively narrow and focused dietary modifications may have significant impact on the fat and cholesterol content of children's diets. Sigman-Grant et al. (1993) investigated this potential and evaluated the impact of different strategies commonly used to meet dietary recommendations on the nutrient intake of young (2–5 year-old) children. Various strategies were implemented, including replacing high fat meats with low fat meats, high fat milk with skim milk, and high fat meat with medium fat meat, and using fat modified products, low fat preparation techniques and limiting added fat. They found it was more difficult to meet the recommendations for the 2 and 3 year-old children while providing a complete and balanced diet utilizing these strategies. For the 4–5 year olds, simply switching to skim milk brought the diet into the recommended range. Though other tested strategies also were successful, multiple combined strategies resulted in some very low fat diets (e.g., a diet including lean meats, low fat cheeses, egg substitutes, fat modified products, and skim milk provided 17% calories as fat to the 4–5 year old children) that may not provide adequate calories for some children.

In real life settings, lower fat diets were shown to be potentially less complete. In the Bogalusa Heart Study, an observational, epidemiological study, Nicklas, Webber, Koschak, and Berenson (1992) evaluated the diets of ten year old children who reported eating a diet containing less than 30% calories as fat. Compared to the high fat diet group (greater than 40% calories as fat), the children in the low fat group were at greater risk for not meeting the recommended daily allowance for vitamins B_6, B_{12}, and E, thiamine, riboflavin, and niacin.

These findings raised concerns about the potential negative impact of dietary intervention on the nutrient content of children's food. Two groups of researchers, however, have demonstrated that children and families, provided with appropriate guidance, can safely lower the fat content of children's diet. DISC assessed the relationship between energy intake from fat and anthropometric, biochemical, and dietary measures of nutritional adequacy and safety (Obarzanek et al., 1997; Obarzanek et al., 2001). Lower fat intake was not related to anthropometric measures or to serum zinc, retinol, albumin, B-carotene or vitamin E levels. Lower fat intake in DISC participants was related to higher levels of red blood cell folate, and hemoglobin, with a trend toward higher serum ferritin. Higher intakes of folate, vitamin C, and vitamin A were also associated with lower fat intakes with a trend toward higher iron intake as well. Those children who consumed less fat also consumed less calcium, zinc, magnesium, phosphorus, vitamin B_{12}, thiamin, niacin, and riboflavin. Risks of not meeting two thirds of the recommended daily allowances were evident only in zinc and vitamin E, and inconsistently for calcium.

In the second study, hypercholesterolemic 4–10 year old children received traditional dietary counseling with a registered dietitian or an innovative, home-based nutrition intervention program (Shannon, Tershakovec, & Martel, 1994; Shannon et al., 1991; Tershakovec et al., 1998). This parent-child autotutorial program utilized story books with accompanying audio cassette tapes, children's games and activities and a parents' manual to serve as a model for a nutrition intervention that could be prescribed for children. Children who completed standard nutrition counseling and children who completed the innovative home-based program decreased their fat and saturated fat intake without negatively impacting their micronutrient intake (McKenzie et al., 1996).

However, inappropriately applied dietary restrictions can negatively impact the growth of children. Lifshitz and Moses (1989) reported that of 40 children referred to a nutrition center for management of hypercholesterolemia, growth failure was noted in 8. There was inadequate caloric intake in the children with growth failure related to dietary modification instituted by the family *without appropriate medical and nutritional supervision.* In addition, Hansen, Michaelson, and Skovby (1992) reported that 13 children with familial hypercholesterolemia who were treated with a diet which approximated the prudent diet, showed decreased growth over an average of 8.5 years of follow-up. At the follow-up evaluation, growth was still within the normal range, as compared to WHO standards.

In other settings, normal growth has been observed despite significant dietary variation. Shea et al. (1993) evaluated the diet and growth of 215 3 to 4 year old children and found no difference in stature or growth over one year between children in the lowest quintile for total fat intake (27% calories as fat) as compared to those in the highest quintile for fat intake (38% calories as fat). Reviewing these publications together, it is evident that in most cases in which adverse effects were reported, low energy intake rather than low fat intake was the primary cause of growth failure, underscoring the need for comprehensive dietary management.

Evaluating the growth of vegetarian children, who generally eat a lower fat diet, adds further evidence supporting the potential for adequate growth while ingesting a lower fat diet. A survey of Seventh Day Adventist children, many of whom adhere to a lacto-ovo vegetarian diet, showed that, compared to public school children, Seventh Day Adventist boys were slightly taller, while no difference in the girls' heights was noted (Sabate et al., 1990). In a similar survey, O'Connell and colleagues (1989) evaluated the growth of vegetarian children in a collective community in Tennessee. The largest deviation from growth norms occurred between one and three years of age. By 10 years of age, the mean height of the study children was 0.7 centimeters less than the norm. In an effort to investigate the potential impact on growth of a vegetarian diet more closely, Kaplan and Toshima (1992) reviewed studies of growth in vegetarian children, and reported a similar trend of slightly delayed growth for the younger children. The transition from a high fat breast milk or formula-based diet to the lower fat vegetarian diet may account for this discrepancy in toddlers. The minimal or nonexistent growth differences seen in the older children suggest this difference is temporary and reversible.

Less information is available concerning the growth of children in dietary intervention. In the DISC study (1995), growth was a primary safety outcome measure. After 3 years on the DISC diet there was no significant difference between the groups in adjusted mean height, serum ferritin or other safety outcome measures. Mean body weight was not significantly different between groups at the end of three years. DISC researchers concluded that, despite adherence to a low fat, low cholesterol diet over three years, adolescents maintained adequate growth, iron stores, and nutritional adequacy during this critical period. These observations and confirmation of the safety of a low fat diet for child has recently been extended up to an observation period of seven years, when the children were 15–17 years old (Obarzanek et al., 2001).

Despite the previously noted concerns about dietary fat restrictions for children under the age of 2 years, there are suggestions that lower fat diets can support normal growth, even for such young children. Though such a diet in not recommended in the United States for children under the age of 2, Niinikoski and colleagues randomized 7-month-old Finnish infants into an intervention group which ingested 26–31% calories as fat and observed no change in the growth of children in the intervention group over the next 5 years, as compared to a control group, or when compared to standard measures for Finnish infants growth (Lagstrom et al., 1999; Niinikoski et al., 1997; Rask-Nissila et al., 2000).

Less concerns have been raised about the growth of overweight children entering weight management. This may be due to the fact that most obese prepubertal children are tall for their age (Vignolo et al., 1988). Obese children can maintain normal growth even when decreasing their relative weight or actually losing weight (Epstein, McCurley, Valoski, & Wing, 1990; Peipert, Stallings, Berry, & Henstenburg, 1992).

FOLLOWING THE RECOMMENDATIONS: IMPLEMENTING SAFE DIETARY INTERVENTION

Due to the potential for inadequate or inappropriate dietary restrictions provided by well meaning, but uninformed caretakers, dietary modification in children must be undertaken with care. At a minimum, growth and development should be monitored and dietary intake should be periodically assessed to prevent subtle inadequacies from progressing. As most physicians rate themselves as unable to provide effective dietary counseling (Kimm, Payne, Lakatos, Darby, & Sparrow, 1990; Nader, Taras, Sallis, & Patterson, 1987), making referral to qualified pediatric dietitians is a useful strategy. Unfortunately, few such dietitians are available outside of tertiary care pediatric medical centers and even then, their availability is limited by inadequate support of third party payers for dietitian's services.

Pediatric preventive health initiatives utilizing the population and individualized high-risk approaches have been recommended (Report of the Expert Panel on Blood Cholesterol Levels in Children and Adolescents, 1992). Most of the studies on pediatric nutrition interventions have been school-based, utilizing the population approach. The easy access to children, the presence of trained staff, a structure well suited for education and behavior modification, and common provision of at least one meal per day make the schools uniquely suited as a site for such population-wide interventions. The most comprehensive of these, The Child and Adolescent Trial for Cardiovascular

Health, was developed to lower the fat intake and increase the moderate-to-vigorous physical activity of third through fifth grade children by focusing on the school environment, classroom curricula, and home-based programs (Luepker et al., 1996). Schools in the intervention group lowered the fat content of the lunches they served, increased the intensity of physical activity provided in physical education classes, and the children in the intervention schools reported a lower fat intake and greater physical activity than schools and children in the control group, respectively. There were no differences in body size, blood pressure, or blood cholesterol levels between the groups. This contrasts with the results of a less comprehensive intervention, The Know Your Body curriculum, that demonstrated decreases in blood cholesterol level after 5 years (Walter, Hofman, Vaughan, & Wynder, 1989).

Two recent school-based studies aimed at reducing obesity have demonstrated the potential utility of alternative and broad-based approaches. Robinson implemented a 6-month curriculum that aimed to reduce television, videotape, and video game use in third and fourth grade children in an attempt to prevent obesity (Robinson, 1999). Children in the intervention group demonstrated a decrease in body mass index, triceps skinfold thickness, and waist circumference. Gortmaker and colleagues (1999) implemented a school-based interdisciplinary intervention for sixth through eighth grade children, which aimed to decrease obesity by decreasing television watching, and intake of high fat foods, and increasing fruit and vegetable intake, and moderate physical activity. A decrease in the prevalence of obesity was demonstrated in the girls, but not the boys. Similar to the results reported by Robinson, reductions in television viewing predicted obesity change. Though it seems reasonable that these interventions reduce obesity by increasing physical activity energy expenditure, and/or altering caloric intake, it is interesting that these results are more positive than for interventions which focus specifically on altering physical activity and caloric intake.

Access to families is sometimes difficult to attain with school-based programs. Though school-based programs allow relatively easy access to many children, a meta-analysis of treatment programs for childhood obesity showed that the school-based programs were similarly or less effective than non-school based programs (Haddock et al., 1994). Alternate approaches may include the use of multidisciplinary teams made up of physicians and other health care workers to provide population-wide and high-risk, individualized interventions for children and families through physicians' offices. Such approaches provide easy access to the family, as an adult must accompany the child to the physician's office. In addition, such programs could build upon the established relationship the family has with the health care provider. Furthermore, parents identify their child's primary care provider as a person they look to for nutrition and preventive health information. Considering physician's self-rated poor ability to provide effective pediatric nutrition intervention, this area of preventive health intervention is open for further development and innovation. As previously noted, an alternative, home-based dietary education program for 4–10 year old hypercholesterolemic children has been developed and has demonstrated efficacy in increasing knowledge, lowering fat and saturated fat content of the children's diet, and lowering LDL-C levels (Shannon et al., 1994; Tershakovec et al., 1998).

Going from this relatively limited research experience in pediatric nutrition intervention to practical, wide-scale implementation is problematic. Most health promotion behavior modification programs have produced modest changes in lifestyle (Winkleby, 1994). Though some may find this discouraging, part of the problem may lie in the extent of the intervention. Children with long term, chronic issues, such as hypercholesterolemia and obesity are provided with very limited attempts at intervention and behavioral modification. The task seems even more difficult when balanced against the secular changes directly competing with the goals of the dietary intervention and health promotions programs (e.g., easy access to high calorie, and high fat foods, increased availability of fun, sedentary activities [such as television, video games]) and due to financial constraints. As previously mentioned, most of the dietary intervention projects completed for children have been conducted in a school-setting. Unfortunately, few school districts have established such programs as a high enough priority to continue once outside funding ends. In clinical settings, interventions are limited as insurance reimbursement for assessment and management of hyperlipidemia or obesity in children is commonly limited (Tershakovec, Watson, Wenner, & Marx, 1999).

Despite these obstacles, efforts to provide comprehensive support for nutrition intervention/health promotion should be intensified, given the current epidemic of childhood and adult obesity. As previously noted, multidisciplinary interventions for obesity and hypercholesterolemia have been shown to be moderately effective. Primary care providers should be familiar with appropriate preventive health recommendations and approaches that have been effective, and actively work to provide nutrition-related anticipatory guidance to families. Physicians, nurse practitioners, and nurses should work together to provide a consistent and supportive message. Existing educational materials should be utilized; appropriate organizations should be encouraged to support the development of other needed materials. (It is important to remember that nutrition intervention materials and programs need to be ethnically and socioeconomically appropriate for the children and family.) Primary care providers should become familiar with the availability of resources in the community, including pediatric dietitians, child and pediatric exercise programs, pediatric and family counselors and psychologists, which can help in the multidisciplinary approach to these issues. Third party payers should be encouraged to support the provision of nutrition related preventive care to children and adolescents. However, it must be emphasized that providing information in itself is generally not enough. Behavior modification efforts should be based upon sound behavior modification and education theory and practice.

As part of anticipatory guidance, primary care providers should educate children and families about a healthy lifestyle and encourage them to adopt these guidelines into their everyday life. These influences begin early in life; dietary intake and physical activity of 3 year old children have been associated with potential risk factors for obesity (Johnson & Birch, 1994; Klesges, Klesges, Eck, & Shelton, 1995). The importance of parental influence on these behaviors should also be emphasized. For example, children whose mothers exert more control on their food intake seem to have less internal control on their own dietary intake (Johnson & Birch, 1994). In addition, parental physical activity is strongly associated with the physical activity of the child (Moore et al., 1991), and parental participation in weight management programs for children has been associated with improved outcome (Epstein, Valoski, Wing, & McCurley, 1994; Wadden et al., 1990). In fact, it has been demonstrated that a weight management program for 6–11 year old children was more effective when the program focused on parents as the agents of change, as opposed to the behavior modification program which focused on the children as the agents of change (Golan, Weizman, Apter, & Fainaru, 1998). Though parents may express limited interest in adopting a healthy lifestyle for themselves, in our experience, parents are more open to lifestyle changes if it will help their children.

If a child is identified as hypercholesterolemic, though the primary care provider may consider initiating dietary intervention; to provide more complete dietary recommendations, to assess compliance and to assure that the child is ingesting a complete and balanced diet, referral to a pediatric lipid referral center should be considered. If the child requires the Step II Diet, or is in the range where medications may be considered (for children greater than 10 years old who have a LDL-C greater than 160 mg/dl and have other risk factors for cardiovascular disease, or greater than 190mg/dl without other risk factors [Report of the Expert Panel on Blood Cholesterol Levels in Children and Adolescents, 1992]), such referral is essential. Similarly, as previously noted, primary care providers should promote a prudent diet and an active lifestyle to help prevent and overcome obesity. However, as the comprehensive and labor intensive treatments required for obesity are generally not practical for primary care providers, obese children should be referred to a specific pediatric obesity center. Unfortunately, the availability of such centers is limited.

DEFINING SUCCESS IN PEDIATRIC DIETARY INTERVENTION

As it is difficult to get some families interested in dietary modification, it is especially important to educate families about the expected response, as many families have unrealistic expectations regarding the response to the intervention. Children with elevated cholesterol levels can usually lower their LDL-C levels significantly with dietary modification, but patients should be forewarned that individual response to diet is variable. Reduction through diet is usually in the range of 10–15%. Families of hypercholesterolemic children often express frustration by the lack of response to dietary management. However, children referred for dietary intervention for hyperlipidemia and children from some subgroups (e.g., suburban, middle to upper socioeconomic status) may be already ingesting diets that meet NCEP recommendations (Kuehl et al., 1993; Tershakovec et al., 1997), thus further significant lowering of blood lipids levels due to dietary change would not be expected. This potential must be explained to families. As previously stated, managing expectations regarding magnitude of change in blood lipids is an important aspect of lipid management and long-term dietary adherence.

Unrealistic expectations for success create an even greater problem with respect to weight management. Even modest weight reduction in obese adults (5–10% of body weight) has demonstrated significant improvements in health measures, such as blood lipid levels and control of non-insulin dependent diabetes (Bosello, Armellini, Zamboni, & Fitchet, 1997; Van Gaal, Wauters, & De Leeuw, 1997). However, few persons participating in a weight loss program would be satisfied with such a response. These improvements in health measures with modest weight loss, and the improved measures of health with adults who are physically fit, (Blair et al., 1996) suggest the need to redefine the subjective evaluation of success in weight management.

Research to define the longer term health implications of relative weight loss in children and adolescents needs to be undertaken to help better define how we can help obese children grow to be healthier adults. The goals should be to help children become healthier, in the broadest sense of the word.

NUTRITION, PREVENTIVE HEALTH AND THE MEDIA

Despite the best efforts of health professionals, many of our efforts can be significantly undermined by the inappropriate or inaccurate reporting of nutrition related news. People are commonly confused by the conflicting results reported by the press. Judging by the number of nutrition related stories that are regularly reported, nutrition seems to be a topic of special interest to the public. However, much active misinformation concerning nutrition and preventive health exists. Promoters of food supplements, freed from the regulations that apply to medications, commonly make unsubstantiated health claims. It is the responsibility of the health professional to try to refute such unsubstantiated claims. In addition, health professionals have some responsibility to advise patients and their families about emerging medical data and the state of current health care knowledge.

PUTTING PEDIATRIC DIETARY INTERVENTION INTO PERSPECTIVE

With the wide availability of healthy, affordable food in developed countries, eating a broad-based diet that helps keep a child happy and healthy is possible and not cumbersome. Both parents and children reported that following the DISC diet was not a major problem (Reimers et al., 1998). Parents viewed DISC as being good for their child and the family as a whole. The greatest difficulty encountered was eating out, but nutritionists provided children with numerous alternatives.

In addition to such practical factors, it is important to present the dietary recommendations in perspective to the child and family. If a child is found to have an elevated cholesterol level, it should be emphasized that hypercholesterolemia is one of several risk factors for premature heart disease which will have little immediate effect on a child's health. It is important to avoid negative psychosocial aspects of labeling, as has been noted with other medical conditions (MacDonald, Sackett, Haynes, & Taylor, 1984). Obese children, on the other hand, commonly endure significant teasing and may suffer from low self-esteem and other psychosocial problems (Baum & Forehand, 1984; Ilade, 1973; Monello & Mayer, 1963; Strauss, Smith, Frame, & Forehand, 1985). The potential for a child or adolescent developing an eating disorder while pursuing an active weight loss program, must also be considered. These psychosocial components must be included when addressing the total therapeutic plan for an obese child. In any dietary intervention for children, the goal is to make gradual changes with which the child and family can comply, to help the child develop a lifelong habit of a happy and healthy lifestyle in which food and eating provide appropriate physiologic and psychological support and fulfillment.

REFERENCES

American Academy of Pediatrics Committee on Nutrition. (1998). Cholesterol in children. *Pediatrics, 101,* 141–147.

Anderson, J. W., Gilinsky, N. H., Deakins, A., Smith, S. F., O'Neal, D. S., Dillon, D. W., & Oeltgen, P. R. (1991). Lipid responses of hypercholesterolemic men to oat-bran and wheat-bran intake. *American Journal of Clinical Nutrition, 54,* 678–683.

Anderson, J. W., Johnstone, B. M., & Cook-Newell, M. D. (1995). Meta-analysis of the effects of soy protein intake on serum lipids. *New England Journal of Medicine, 333,* 276–282.

Anderson, J. W., Riddell-Mason, S., Gustafson, N. J., Smith, S. F., & Mackey, M. (1992). Cholesterol-lowering effects of psyllium-enriched cereal as an adjunct to a prudent diet in the treatment of mild to moderate hypercholesterolemia. *American Journal of Clinical Nutrition, 56,* 93–98.

Anderson, J. W., Smith, B. M., & Gustafson, N. J. (1994). Health benefits and practical aspects of high-fiber diets. *American Journal of Clinical Nutrition, 59*(Suppl.), 1242–1247.

Anderson, J. W., Story, L., Sieling, B., Chen, W-J., Petro, M. S., & Story, J. (1984). Hypocholesterolemic effects of oat-bran intake for hypercholesterolemic men. *American Journal of Clinical Nutrition, 40,* 1146–1155.

Bandini, L. G., Schoeller, D. A., Cyr, H. N., & Dietz, W. H. (1990). Validity of reported energy intake in obese and nonobese adolescents. *American Journal of Clinical Nutrition, 52,* 421–425.

Baum, C. G., & Forehand, R. (1984). Social factors associated with adolescent obesity. *Journal of Pediatric Psychology, 9,* 293–302.

Baum, J. A., Teng, H., Erdman, J. W., et al. (1998). Long-term intake of soy protein improves blood lipid profiles and increases mononuclear cell low-density-lipoprotein receptor messenger RNA in hypercholesterolemic, post-menopausal women. *American Journal of Clinical Nutrition, 68,* 545–551.

Bell, L. P., Hectorn, K. J., Reynolds, H., & Hunninghake, D. B. (1990). Cholesterol-lowering effects of soluble-fiber cereals as part of a prudent diet for patients with mild to moderate hypercholesterolemia. *American Journal of Clinical Nutrition, 52,* 1020–1026.

Blair, S. N., Kampert, J. B., Kohl, H. W., Barlow, C. E., Macera, C. A., Paffenbarger, R. S., & Gibbons, L. W. (1996). Influences of cardiorespiratory fitness and other precursors on cardiovascular disease and all-cause mortality in men and women. *Journal of the American Medical Association, 276,* 205–210.

Bosello, O., Armellini, F., Zamboni, M., & Fitchet, M. (1997). The benefits of modest weight loss in type II diabetes. *International Journal of Obesity, 21*(Suppl.), 10–13.

Boushey, C. J., Beresford, S. A., Omenn, G. S., & Motulsky, A. G. (1995). A quantitative assessment of plasma homocysteine as a risk factor for vascular disease: Probable benefits of increasing folic acid intakes. *Journal of the American Medical Association, 274,* 1049–1057.

Browner, W. S., Westenhouse, J., & Tice, J. A. (1991). What if Americans ate less fat? A quantitative estimate of the effect of mortality. *Journal of the American Medical Association, 265,* 3285–3291.

Castelli, W. P., Garrison, R. J., Wilson, P. W., et al. (1986). Incidence of coronary heart disease and lipoprotein cholesterol levels. The Framingham Study. *Journal of the American Medical Association, 256,* 2835–2838.

Charney, E., Goodman, H. C., McBride, M., Lyon, B., & Pratt, R. (1976). Childhood antecedents of adult obesity: Do chubby infants become obese adults? *New England Journal of Medicine, 295,* 6–9.

Colquhoun, D. M., Moores, D., Somerset, S. M., & Humphries, J. A. (1992). Comparison of the effects on lipoproteins and apolipoproteins of a diet high in monounsaturated fatty acids, enriched with avocado, and a high-carbohydrate diet. *American Journal of Clinical Nutrition, 56,* 671–677.

Committee on Diet and Health, Food and Nutrition Board, Commission on Life Sciences, National Research Council. (1989). Evidence associating dietary fats and other lipids with chronic diseases. In *Diet and Health* (3rd ed., pp. 159–258). Washington, DC: National Academy Press.

Cortner, J. A., Coates, P. M., Cryer, D. R., Faulkner, A., Sasanow, S. R., & Warman, N. (1987). Reduction of low-density lipoprotein cholesterol by dietary intervention in children at high risk for premature coronary artery disease. In L. Gallo (Ed.), *Cardiovascular disease* (pp. 515–520). New York: Plenum.

Crouse, J. R., Morgan, T., Terry, J. G., et al. (1999). A randomized trial comparing the effect of casein with that of soy protein containing varying amounts of isoflavones on plasma concentrations of lipids and lipoproteins. *Archives of Internal Medicine, 159,* 2070–2076.

Davidson, M. H., Dugan, L. D., Burns, J. H., Story, K., Bova, J., & Drennan, K. B. (1992). A psyllium-containing cereal for the treatment of hypercholesterolemia in children. *Clinical Research, 40,* 625.

Denke, M. A., & Grundy, S. M. (1991). Effects of fats high in stearic acid on lipid and lipoprotein concentrations in men. *American Journal of Clinical Nutrition, 54,* 1036–1040.

Denmark-Wahnefried, W., Bowering, J., & Cohen, P. S. (1990). Reduced serum cholesterol with dietary change using fat-modified and oat bran supplemented diets. *Journal of the American Dietary Association, 90,* 223–229.

Dennison, B. A., Jenkins, P. L., & Pearson, T. A. (1994). Challenges to implementing the current pediatric cholesterol screening guidelines into practice. *Pediatrics, 94*(3), 296–302.

Dennison, B. A., Kikuchi, D. A., Srinivasan, S. R., Webber, L. S., & Berenson, G. S. (1989). Parental history of cardiovascular disease as an indication for screening for lipoprotein abnormalities in children. *Journal of Pediatrics, 115,* 186–194.

Dennison, B. A., & Levine, D. M. (1993). Randomized, double-blind, placebo-controlled, two-period crossover clinical trial of psyllium fiber in children with hypercholesterolemia. *Journal of Pediatrics, 123,* 24–29.

Derr, J., Kris-Etherton, P. M., Pearson, T. A., & Seligson, F. H. (1993). The role of fatty acid saturation on plasma lipids, lipoproteins, and apolipoproteins: II. The plasma total and low-density lipoprotein cholesterol response of individual fatty acids. *Metabolism, 42,* 130–134.

The Dietary Intervention Study in Children (DISC). (1995). The Writing Group for the DISC Collaborative Research Group Efficacy and safety of lowering dietary intake of fat and cholesterol in children with elevated low-density lipoprotein cholesterol. *Journal of the American Medical Association, 273,* 1429–1435.

Epstein, L. H., McCurley, J., Valoski, A., & Wing, R. R. (1990). Growth in obese children treated for obesity. *American Journal of Diseases of Children, 144,* 1360–1364.

Epstein, L. H., Valoski, A., Wing, R. R., & McCurley, M. A. (1990). Ten-year follow-up of behavioral, family-based treatment for obese children. *JAMA, 264,* 2519–2523.

Epstein, L. H., Valoski, A., Wing, R. R., & McCurley, J. (1994). Ten-year outcomes of behavioral family-based treatment for childhood obesity. *Health Psychology, 13,* 373–383.

Epstein, L. K. H., Wing, R. R., Steranchak, L., Dickson, B., & Michelson, J. (1980). Comparison of family-based behavioral modification and nutrition education for childhood obesity. *Journal of Pediatric Psychology, 5,* 25–36.

Fernandes, J., Dijkhuis-Stoffelsma, R., Groot, P. H. E., Grose, W. F. A., & Ambagtsheer, J. J. (1981). The effect of a virtually cholesterol-free, high linoleic-acid vegetarian diet on serum lipoproteins of children with familial hypercholesterolemia (type II-A). *Acta Paediatrica Scandinavica, 70,* 677–682.

Food and Drug Administration. FDA Talk Paper T99-48, October 20, 1999, http://www.fda.gov/bbs/topics/ANSWSERS/ANS00980.html

Frank, G. C., Berenson, G. S., & Webber, L. S. (1978). Dietary studies and the relationship of diet to cardiovascular disease risk factor variables in 10-year-old children. The Bogalusa Heart Study. *American Journal of Clinical Nutrition, 31,* 328–340.

Fraser, G. E. (1994). Diet and coronary heart disease: Beyond dietary fats and low-density-lipoprotein cholesterol. *American Journal of Clinical Nutrition, 59*(Suppl.), 1117–1123.

Freedman, D. S., Srinivasan, S. R., Valdez, R. A., Williamson, D. F., & Berenson, G. S. (1997). Secular increases in relation to weight and adiposity among children over two decades: The Bogalusa Heart Study. *Pediatrics, 99,* 420–426.

Gaddi, A., Descovich, G. C., Noseda, G., Fragiacomo, C., Nicolini, A., Montanari, G., Vanetti, G., Sortori, M., Gatti, E., & Sirtori, C. R. (1987). Hypercholesterolemia treated by soybean protein diet. *Archives of Diseases of Children, 62,* 274–278.

Garcia, R. E., & Moodie, D. S. (1989). Routine cholesterol surveillance in childhood. *Pediatrics, 84,* 751–755.

Garn, S. M., & LaVelle, M. (1985). Two-decade follow-up of fatness in early childhood. *American Journal of Diseases of Children, 139,* 81–185.

Gazzaniga, J. M., & Burns, T. L. (1993). Relationship between diet composition and body fatness, with adjustment for resting energy expenditure and physical activity. *American Journal of Clinical Nutrition, 3,* 21–28.

Gey, K. F., Moser, U. K., Jordan, P., Stahelin, H. B., Eichholzer, M., & Ludin, E. (1993). Increased risk of cardiovascular diseases at suboptimal plasma concentrations of essential antioxidants: An epidemiological update with special attention to carotene and vitamin C. *American Journal of Clinical Nutrition, 56*(Suppl.), 787–797.

Glassman, M., Spark, A., Berezin, S., Schwarz, S., Medow, M., & Newman, L. J. (1990). Treatment of type IIa hyperlipidemia in childhood by a simplified American Heart Association diet and fiber supplementation. *American Journal of Diseases of Children, 144,* 973–976.

Golan, M., Weizman, A., Apter, A., & Fainaru, M. (1998). Parents as the exclusive agents of change in the treatment of childhood obesity. *American Journal of Clinical Nutrition, 67,* 1130–1135.

Gortmaker, S. L., Cheung, L. W., Peterson, K. E., Chomitz, G., Cradle, J. H., Dart, H., & Fox, M. E., et al. (1999). Impact of a school-based interdisciplinary intervention on diet and physical activity among urban primary school children: Eat well and keep moving. *Archives of Pediatric and Adolescent Medicine, 153*(9), 975–983.

Guo, S. S., Roche, A. F., Chumlea, W. C., Gardner, J. D., & Siervogel, R. M. (1994). The predictive value of childhood body mass index values for overweight at age 35 y. *American Journal of Clinical Nutrition, 59,* 810–819.

Haddock, C. K., Shadish, W. R., Klesges, R. C., & Stein, R. J. (1994). Treatments for childhood and adolescent obesity. *Annals of Behavioral Medicine, 16,* 235–244.

Hallikainen, M. A., Sarkkinen, E. S., & Uusitupa, M. I. J. (2000). Plant stanol esters affect serum cholesterol concentrations of hypercholesterolemic men and women in a dose-dependent manner. *Journal of Nutrition, 130,* 767–776.

Hamosh, M. (1988). Fat needs for term and preterm infants. In R. Tsang & B. Nichols (Eds.), *Nutrition during pregnancy* (pp. 107–123). Philadelphia: Hanley & Belfus, Inc.

Hansen, D., Michaelsen, K. F., & Skovby, F. (1992). Growth during treatment of familial hypercholesterolemia. *Acta Paediatrica, 81,*1023–1025.

Heitmann, B. L., Lissner, L., Sorensen, T. I., & Bengtsson, C. (1995). Dietary fat intake and weight gain in women genetically predisposed for obesity. *American Journal of Clinical Nutrition, 61,* 1213–1217.

Hickman, T. B., Briefel, R. R., Carroll, M. D., Rifkind, B. M., Cleeman, J. I., Maurer, K. R., & Johnson, C. L. (1998). Distributions and trends of serum lipid levels among United States children and adolescents ages 4–19 years: Data from the Third National Health and Nutrition Examination Survey. *Preventive Medicine, 27,* 879–890.

Hunninghake, D. B., Stein, E. A., Dujovne, C. A., Harris, W. S., Feldman, E. B., Miller, V. T., Tobert, J. A., Laskarzewski, P. M., Quiter, E., Held, J., Taylor, A. M., Hopper, S., Leonard, S. B., & Brewer, B. K. (1993). The efficacy of intensive dietary therapy alone or combined with lovastatin in outpatients with hypercholesterolemia. *New England Journal of Medicine, 328,* 1213–1219.

Jenkins, D. J., Wolever, T. M., Rao, A. V., Hegele, R. A., Mitchell, S. J., Ransom, T. P., Boctor, D. L., Spadafora, P. J., Jenkins, A. L., Mehling, C., Relle, L. K., Connelly, P. W., Story, J. A., Furumoto, E. J., Corey, P., & Wursch, P. (1993). Effect on blood lipids on very high intakes of fiber in diets low in saturated fat and cholesterol. *New England Journal of Medicine, 329,* 21–26.

Johnson, C. L., Rifkind, B. M., Sempos, C. T., Carroll, M. D., Bachorik, P. S., Briefel, R. R., Gordon, D. J., Burt, V. L., Brown, C. D., Lippel, K., & Cleeman, J. I. (1993). Declining serum total cholesterol levels among US adults. *Journal of the American Medical Association, 269,* 3002–3008.

Johnson, S. L., & Birch, L. L. (1994). Parent's and children's adiposity and eating style. *Pediatrics, 94,* 642–661.

Jones, P. J., & Raeini-Sarjaz, M. (2001). Plant sterols and their derivatives: The current spread of results. *Nutrition Reviews, 59*(1), 21–24.

Kaplan, R. M., & Toshima, M. T. (1992). Does a reduced fat diet cause retardation in child growth? *Preventive Medicine, 21,* 33–52.

Kashtan, H., Stern, H. S., Jenkins, D. J. A., Jenkins, A. L., Hay, K., Marcon, N., Minkin, S., & Bruce, W. R. (1992). Wheat-bran and oat-bran supplements' effects on blood lipids and lipoproteins. *American Journal of Clinical Nutrition, 55,* 976–980.

Kestin, M., Moss, R., Clifton, P. M., & Nestel, P. J. (1990). Comparative effects of three cereal brans on plasma lipids, blood pressure, and glucose metabolism in mildly hypercholesterolemic men. *American Journal of Clinical Nutrition, 52,* 661–666.

Keys, A. (1970). Coronary heart disease in seven countries. *Circulation, 41*(Suppl.), 11–1211.

Keys, A. (1980). *Seven countries: A multivariate analysis of death and coronary heart disease.* Cambridge, MA: Harvard University Press.

Kimm, S. Y. S., Gergen, P. J., Malloy, M., Dresser, C., & Carroll, M. (1990). Dietary patterns of U.S. children: Implications for disease prevention. *Preventive Medicine, 19,* 432–442.

Kimm, S. Y. S., Payne, G. H., Lakatos, E., Darby, C., & Sparrow, A. (1990). Management of cardiovascular disease risk factors in children. *American Journal of Diseases of Children, 144,* 967–972.

Kinsella, J. E., Lokesh, B., & Stone, R. A. (1990). Dietary n-3 polyunsaturated fatty acids and amelioration of cardiovascular disease: possible mechanisms. *American Journal of Clinical Nutrition, 52,* 1–28.

Kirby, R. W., Anderson, J. W., Sieling, B., Rees, E. D., Chen, W. J. L., Miller, R. E., & Kay, R. M. (1981). Oat-bran intake selectively lowers serum low-density lipoprotein cholesterol concentrations of hypercholesterolemic men. *American Journal of Clinical Nutrition, 34,* 824–829.

Klesges, R. C., Klesges, L. M., Eck, L. H., & Shelton, M. L. (1995). A longitudinal analysis of accelerated weight gain in preschool children. *Pediatrics, 95,* 126–130.

Kris-Etherton, P. M., Derr, J., Mitchell, D. C., Mustad, V. A., Russel, M. E., McDonnell, E. T., Salabsky, D., & Pearson, T. A. (1993). The role of fatty acid saturation on plasma lipids, lipoproteins, and apolipoproteins: I. Effects of whole food diets high in cocoa butter, olive oil, soybean oil, dairy butter, and milk chocolate on the plasma lipids of young men. *Metabolism, 42,* 121–129.

Kris-Etherton, P. M., Mustad, V., & Derr, J. A. (1993, May/June). Effects of dietary stearic acid on plasma lipids and thrombosis. *Nutrition Today, 30,* 30–38.

Kritchevsky, D. (1988). Dietary fiber. *Annual Review of Nutrition, 8,* 301–328.

Kuehl, K. S., Cockerham, J. T., Hitchings, M., Slater, D., Nixon, G., & Rifai, N. (1993). Effective control of hypercholesterolemia in children with dietary interventions based in pediatric practice. *Preventive Medicine, 22,* 154–166.

Kumanyika, S. (1987). Obesity in black women. *Epidemiology Review, 9,* 31–50.

Kwiterovich, P. O., Bachorik, P. S., Franklin, F. A., Margolis, S., Georgopoulos, L., Teng, B., & Sniderman, A. D. (1985). Effect of dietary treatment on the plasma levels of lipids, lipoprotein cholesterol and LDL B protein in children with type II hyperlipoproteinemia. *Progress in Clinical and Biological Research, 188,* 123–137.

Lagstrom, H., Seppanen, R., Jokinen, E., Niinikoski, H., Ronnemaa, T., Viikari, J., & Simell, O. (1999). Influence of dietary fat on the nutrient intake and growth of children from 1 to 5 y of age: The Special Turku Coronary Risk Factor Intervention Project. *American Journal of Clinical Nutrition, 69*(3), 516–523.

Lampe, J. W., Slavin, J. L., Baglien, K. S., Thompson, W. O., Duane, W. C., & Zavoral, J. H. (1991). Serum lipid and fecal bile acid changes with cereal, vegetable, and sugar-beet fiber feeding. *American Journal of Clinical Nutrition, 53,* 1235–1241.

Lenfant, C., & Ernst, N. (1994). Daily dietary fat and total food-energy intakes. Third National Health and Nutrition Examination Survey, Phase 1, 1988–91. *MMWR, Morbidity and Mortality Weekly Report, 43,* 116.

Lifshitz, F., & Moses, N. (1989). Growth failure. A complication of dietary treatment of hypercholesterolemia. *American Journal of Diseases of Children, 143,* 537–542.

Litin, L., & Sacks, F. (1993). Trans-fatty-acid content of common foods. [Letter to the editor]. *New England Journal Medicine, 329,* 1969–1970.

Llade, J. (1973). A comparison of the psychological adjustment of obese vs. non-obese children. *Journal of Psychosomatic Research, 17,* 89–96.

Ludwig, D. S., Majzoub, J. A., Al-Zahrani, A., Dallal, G. E., Blanco, I., & Roberts, S. B. (1999). High glycemic index foods, overeating, and obesity. *Pediatrics, 103*(3), 1–6.

Ludwig, D. S., Peterson, K. E., & Gortmaker, S. L. (2001). Relation between consumption of sugar-sweetened drinks and childhood obesity: a prospective, observational analysis. *Lancet, 357,* 490–491.

Luepker, R. V., Perry, C. L., McKinlay, S. M., Nader, P. R., Parcel, G. S., Stone, E. J., Webber, L. S., Elder, J. P., Feldman, H. A., Johnson, C. C., Kelder, S. H., & Wu, M. (for the CATCH Collaborative Group). (1996). Outcomes of a field trial to improve children's dietary patterns and physical activity. *Journal of the American Medical Association, 275,* 768–776.

MacDonald, L. A., Sackett, L., Haynes, R. B., & Taylor, D. W. (1984). Labelling in hypertension: A review of the behavioural and psychological consequences. *Journal of Chronic Diseases, 37,* 933–942.

Mata, P., Alvarez-Sala, L. A., Rubio, M. J., Nuno, J., & De Oya, M. (1992). Effects of long-term monounsaturated- vs polyunsaturated-enriched diets on lipoproteins in healthy men and women. *American Journal of Clinical Nutrition, 55,* 846–850.

Mattson, F. H., & Grundy, S. M. (1985). Comparison of effects of dietary saturated, monounsaturated, and polyunsaturated fatty acids on plasma lipids and lipoproteins in man. *Journal of Lipid Research, 26,* 194–202.

McClung, H. J., Boyne, L. J., Linsheid, T., Heitlinger, L. A., Murray, R. D., Fyda, J., & Li, B. U. K. (1993). Is combination therapy for encopresis nutritionally safe? *Pediatrics, 91,* 591–594.

McDowell, M. A., Briefel, R. R., Alaimo, K., Bischof, A. M., Caughman, C. R., & Carroll, M. D. (1994). Energy and macronutrient intakes of persons ages 2 months and over in the United States: Third National Health and Nutrition Examination Survey, Phase 1, 1988–1991. Advance Data from Vital and Health Statistics, No. 255. Hyattsville, MD: National Center for Health Statistics.

McGancy, R. B., Hall, B., Ford, C., & Stare, F. J. (1972). Dietary regulation of blood cholesterol in adolescent males: A pilot study. *American Journal of Clinical Nutrition, 25,* 61–66.

McGill, H. C., Herderick, E. E., Tracy, R. E., Malcom, G. T., Zieske, A. W., & Strong, J. P. (2000). Effects of coronary heart disease risk factors on atherosclerosis of selected regions of the aorta and right coronary artery. PDAY Research Group. Pathobiological Determinants of Atherosclerosis in Youth. *Arteriosclerosis, Thrombosis & Vascular Biology, 20*(3), 836–845.

McIntosh, G. H., Whyte, J., Mcarthur, R., & Nestel, P. J. (1991). Barley and wheat foods: Influence on plasma cholesterol concentrations in hypercholesterolemic men. *American Journal of Clinical Nutrition, 53,* 1205–1209.

McKenzie, J., Dixon, L. B., Smiciklas-Wright, H., Mitchell, D., Shannon, B. M., & Tershakovec, A. M. (1996). Change in nutrient intakes, numbers of servings, and contributions of total fat from food groups in 4- to 10-year-old children enrolled in a nutrition education study. *Journal of the American Dietary Association, 96,* 865–873.

McPherson, R. S., Nichaman, M. Z., Kohl, H. W., Reed, D. B., & Labarthe, D. R. (1990). Intake and food sources of dietary fat among schoolchildren in the Woodlands, Texas. *Pediatrics, 86,* 520–526.

Mensink, R. P., & Katan, M. B. (1989). Effect of a diet enriched with monounsaturated or polyunsaturated fatty acids on levels of low-density and high-density lipoprotein cholesterol in healthy women and men. *New England Journal of Medicine, 321,* 436–441.

Miettinen, T. A., Puska, P., Gylling, H., Vanhanen, H., & Vartiainen, E. (1995). Reduction of serum cholesterol with sitostanol-ester margarine in a mildly hypercholesterolemic population. *New England Journal of Medicine, 333,* 1308–1312.

Monello, L. F., & Mayer, J. (1963). Obese adolescent girls. An unrecognized minority group? *American Journal of Clinical Nutrition, 13,* 35–39.

Moore, L. L., Lombardi, D. A., White, M. J., Campbell, J. L., Oliveria, S. A., & Ellison, R. C. (1991). Influence of parents' physical activity levels on activity levels of young children. *Journal of Pediatrics, 118,* 215–219.

Morris, K. L., & Zemel, B. M. (1999). Glycemic index, cardiovascular disease, and obesity. *Nutrition Reviews, 57*(9), 273–276.

Morrison, J. A., Laskarzewski, P., deGroot, I., Kelly, K. A., Mellies, M. J., Khoury, P., & Glueck, C. J. (1979). Diagnostic ramifications of repeated plasma cholesterol and triglyceride measurements in children: Regression toward the mean in a pediatric population. *Pediatrics, 64,* 197–201.

Nader, P. R., Taras, H. L., Sallis, J. F., & Patterson, T. L. (1987). Adult heart disease prevention in childhood: A national survey of pediatricians' practices and attitudes. *Pediatrics, 79,* 843–850.

National Center for Health Statistics. (1984). *Health, United States.* (DHHS Publication No. PHS 85-1232). Washington, DC: Public Health Service.

National Cholesterol Education Program. Report of the Expert Panel on Blood Cholesterol Levels in Children and Adolescents. (1992). *Pediatrics, 89*(Suppl.), 525–584.

National Cholesterol Education Program. Executive Summary of the Third Report of the NCEP Expert Panel on Detection, Evaluation and Treatment of High Blood Cholesterol in Adults (Adult Treatment Panel III) (2001). *Journal of the American Medical Association, 285*(19), 2486–2497.

Neaton, J. D., & Wentworth, D. (1992). Serum cholesterol, blood pressure, cigarette smoking, and death from coronary heart disease. *Archives of Internal Medicine, 152,* 56–64.

Newman, T. B., Browner, W. S., & Hulley, S. B. (1990). The case against childhood cholesterol screening. *Journal of the American Medical Association, 264,* 3039–3043.

Newman, W. P., Freedman, D. S., Voors, A. W., et al. (1986). Relation of serum lipoprotein levels and systolic blood pressure to early atherosclerosis: The Bogalusa Heart Study. *New England Journal of Medicine, 314,* 138–144.

Nguyen, T. T. (1999). The cholesterol-lowering action of plant stanol esters. *Journal of Nutrition, 129,* 2109–2112.

Nichaman, M. Z., Hamilton, H. B., Kagan, A., Grier, T., Sacks, T., & Syme, S. L. (1975). Epidemiologic studies of coronary heart disease and stroke in Japanese men living in Japan, Hawaii and California: Distribution of biochemical risk factors. *American Journal of Epidemiology, 102,* 491–501.

Nicklas, T. A., Farris, R. P., Smoak, C. G., Frank, G. C., Srinivasan, S. R., Webber, L. S., & Berenson, G. S. (1988). Dietary factors relate to cardiovascular risk factors in early life. Bogalusa Heart Study. *Arteriosclerosis, 8,* 193–199.

Nicklas, T. A., Webber, L. S., Koschak, M., & Berenson, G. S. (1992). Nutrient adequacy of low fat intakes for children: The Bogalusa Heart Study. *Pediatrics, 89,* 221–228.

Nicklas, T. A., Webber, L. S., Srinivasan, S. R., & Berenson, G. S. (1993). Secular trends in dietary intake and cardiovascular risk factors of 10-y-old children: The Bogalusa Heart Study (1973–1988). *American Journal of Clinical Nutrition, 57,* 930–937.

Niinikoski, H., Lapinleimu, H., Viikari, J., Ronnemaa, T., Jokinen, E., Seppanen, R., Terho, P., Tuominen, J., Valimaki, I., & Simell, O. (1997). Growth until 3 years of age in a prospective, randomized trial of a diet with reduced saturated fat and cholesterol. *Pediatrics, 99,* 687–694.

Niinikoski, H., Viikari, J., Ronnemaa, T., Helenius, H., Jokinen, E., Lapinleimu, H., Routi, T., Lagstrom, H., Seppanen, R., Valimaki, I., Simell, O. (1997). Regulation of growth of 7- to 36-month-old children by energy and fat intake in the prospective, randomized STRIP baby trial. *Pediatrics, 100*(5), 810–816.

Obarzanek, E. O., Hunsberger, S. A., Van Horn, L. V., Hartmuller, V. V., Barton, B. A., Stevens, V. J., Kwiterovich, P. O., Franklin, F. A., Kimm, S. Y. S., Lasser, N. L., Simons-Morton, D. G., & Lauer, R. M. (1997). Safety of a fat-reduced diet: The Dietary Intervention Study in Children (DISC). *Pediatrics, 100,* 51–59.

Obarzanek, E. O., Kimm, S. Y., Barton, B. A., Van Horn, L. L., Kwiterovick, P. O., Simons-Morton, D. G., Hunsberger, S. A., Lasser, N. L., Robson, A. M., Franklin, F. A., Lauer, R. M., Stevens, V. J., Friedman, L. A., Dorgan, J. F., Greenlick, M. R., DISC Collaborative Research Group. (2001). Long-term safety and efficacy of a cholesterol-lowering diet in children with elevated low-density lipoprotein cholesterol: seven-year results of the Dietary Intervention Study in Children (DISC). *Pediatrics, 107*(2), 256–264.

O'Connell, J. M., Dibley, M. J., Sierra, J., Wallace, B., Marks, J. S., & Yip, R. (1989). Growth of vegetarian children: The Farm Study. *Pediatrics, 84,* 475–481.

Peipert, J. M., Stallings, V. A., Berry, G. T., & Henstenburg, J. A. (1992). Infant obesity, weight reduction with normal increase in linear growth and fat-free body mass. *Pediatrics, 89,* 143–145.

Pilch, S. M. (Ed.). (1987). *Physiological effects and health consequences of dietary fiber.* Bethesda, MD: Life Sciences Research Office, Federation of American Societies for Experimental Biology.

Pinhas-Hamiel, O., Dolan, L. M., Daniels, S. R., Standiford, D., Khoury, P. R., & Zeitler, P. (1996). Increased incidence of non-insulin-dependent diabetes mellitus among adolescents. *Journal of Pediatrics, 128,* 608–615.

Prewitt, T. E., Schmeisser, D., Bowen, P. E., Aye, P., Dolecek, T. A., Langenberg, P., Cole, T., & Brace, L. (1991). Changes in body weight, body composition, and energy intake in women fed high- and low-fat diets. *American Journal of Clinical Nutrition, 54,* 304–310.

Quivers, E. S., Driscoll, D. J., Garvey, C. D., Harrist, A. M., Harrison, J., Huse, D. M., Murtaugh, P., & Weidman, W. H. (1992). Variability in response to a low-fat, low-cholesterol diet in children with elevated low-density lipoprotein cholesterol levels. *Pediatrics, 89,* 925–929.

Rask-Nissila, L., Jokinen, E., Ronnemaa, T., Viikari, J., Tammi, A., Niinikoski, H., & Seppanen, R., et al. (2000). Prospective, randomized, infancy-onset trial of the effects of a low-saturated-fat, low-cholesterol diet on serum lipids and lipoproteins before school-age: The Special Turku Coronary Risk Factor Intervention Project (STRIP). *Circulation, 102*(13), 1477–1483.

Reimers, T. M., Brown, K. M., Van Horn, L., Stevens, V., Obarzanek, E., Hartmuller, G., Snetselaar, L., von Almen, T. K., & Chiostri, J. (1998). Maternal acceptability of a dietary intervention designed to lower children's intake of saturated fat and cholesterol: The Dietary Intervention Study in Children (DISC). *Journal of the American Dietetic Association, 98*(1), 31–34.

Renaud, S., de Lorgeril, M., Delaye, J., Guidollet, J., Jacquard, F., Mamelle, N., Martin, J-L., Monjaud, I., Salen, P., & Toubol, P. (1995). Cretan Mediterranean diet for prevention of coronary heart disease. *American Journal of Clinical Nutrition, 61*(Suppl.), 1360–1367.

Rimm, E. B., Stampfer, M. J., Ascherio, A., Giovannucci, E., Colditz, G. A., & Willett, W. C. (1993). Vitamin E consumption and the risk of coronary heart disease in men. *New England Journal of Medicine, 328,* 1450–1456.

Ripsin, C. M., Keenan, J. M., Jacobs, D. R., Elmer, P. J., Welch, R. R., Van Horn, L., Liu, K., Turnbull, W. H., Thye, F. W. M., Kestin, M., Hegsted, M., Davidson, D. M., Davidson, M. H., Dugan, L. D., Denmark-Wahnefried, W., & Beling, S. (1992). Oat products and lipid lowering. *Journal of the American Medical Association, 267,* 3317–3325.

Robinson, T. N. (1999). Reducing children's television viewing to prevent obesity: A randomized controlled trial. *Journal of the American Medical Association, 282*(16), 1561–1567.

Sabate, J., Lindsted, K. D., Harris, R. D., & Johnston, P. K. (1990). Anthropometric parameters of schoolchildren with different life-styles. *American Journal of Diseases of Children, 144,* 1159–1163.

Sanders, T. A. B., & Reddy, S. (1994). Vegetarian diets and children. *American Journal of Clinical Nutrition, 59*(Suppl.), 1176–1181.

Serdula, M. K., Ivery, D., Coates, R. J., Freedman, D. S., Williamson, D. F., & Byers, T. (1993). Do obese children become obese adults? A review of the literature. *Preventive Medicine, 22,* 167–177.

Shannon, B., Greene, G., Stallings, V. A., Achterberg, C., Berman, M., Gregoire, J., Mareci, M., & Shallcross, U. (1991). A dietary education program for hypercholesterolemic children and their parents. *Journal of the American Dietary Association, 91,* 208–212.

Shannon, B. M., Tershakovec, A. M., & Martel, J. K. (et al). (1994). Reduction of elevated LDL-cholesterol levels of 4–10 year old children through home-based dietary education. *Pediatrics, 94,* 923–927.

Shea, S., Basch, C. E., Irigoyen, M., Zybert, P., Rips, J. L., Contento, I., & Gutin, B. (1991). Relationships of dietary fat consumption to serum total and low-density lipoprotein cholesterol in Hispanic preschool children. *Preventive Medicine, 20,* 237–249.

Shea, S., Basch, C. E., Stein, A. D., Contento, I. R., Irigoyen, M., & Zybert, P. (1993). Is there a relationship between dietary fat and stature or growth in children three to five years of age? *Pediatrics, 92,* 579–586.

Sheppard, L., Kristal, A. R., & Kusha, L. H. (1991). Weight loss in women participating in a randomized trial of low-fat diets. *American Journal of Clinical Nutrition, 54,* 821–828.

Sigman-Grant, M., Zimmerman, S., & Kris-Etherton, P. M. (1993). Dietary approaches for reducing fat intake of preschool-age children. *Pediatrics, 91,* 955–960.

Sirtori, C. R., Gatti, E., Tremoli, E., Galli, C., Gianfranceschi, G., Franceschini, G., Colli, S., Maderna, P., Marangoni, F., Perego, P., & Stragliotto, E. (1992). Olive oil, corn oil, and n-3 fatty acids differently affect lipids, lipoproteins, platelets, and superoxide formation in type II hypercholesterolemia. *American Journal of Clinical Nutrition, 56,* 113–122.

Sondike, S. S., Jacobson, M. S., & Cooperman, N. (2000). The ketogenic diet increases weight loss but not cardiovascular risk: A randomized controlled trial. *Journal of Adolescent Health Care, 26,* 91.

Spieth, L. E., Harnish, J. D., Lenders, C. M., Raezer, L. B., Pereira, M. A., Hangen, S. J., & Ludwig, D. S. (2000). A low-glycemic index diet in the treatment of pediatric obesity. *Archives of Pediatric Adolescent Medicine, 154,* 947–951.

Stallings, V. A., Archibald, E. H., Pencharz, P. B., Harrison, J. E., & Bell, L. E. (1988). One-year follow-up of weight, total body potassium, and total body nitrogen in obese adolescents treated with the protein-sparing modified fast. *American Journal of Clinical Nutrition, 48,* 91–94.

Stampfer, M. J., Hennekens, C. H., Mason, J. E., Colditz, G. A., Rosner, B., & Willett, W. C. (1993). Vitamin E consumption and the risk of coronary disease in women. *New England Journal of Medicine, 328,* 1444–1449.

Stein, E. A., Mendelsohn, D., Fleming, M., Barnard, G. D., Carter, K. J., du Toit, P. S., Hansen, D. L., & Bersohn, I. (1975). Lowering of plasma cholesterol levels in free-living adolescent males; use of natural and synthetic polyunsaturated foods to provide balanced fat diets. *American Journal of Clinical Nutrition, 28,* 1204–1216.

Stein, E. A., Shapero, J., McNerney, C., Glueck, C. J., Tracy, T., & Gartside, P. (1982). Changes in plasma lipid and lipoprotein fractions after alteration in dietary cholesterol, polyunsaturated, saturated, and total fat in free-living normal and hypercholesterolemic children. *American Journal of Clinical Nutrition, 35,* 1375–1390.

Stephen, A. M., & Wald, N. J. (1990). Trends in individual consumption of dietary fat in the United States, 1920–1984. *American Journal of Clinical Nutrition, 52,* 457–469.

Strauss, C. C., Smith, K., Frame, C., & Forehand, R. (1985). Personal and interpersonal characteristics associated with childhood obesity. *Journal of Pediatric Psychology, 10,* 337–343.

Tammi, A., Ronnemaa, T., Gylling, H., Risk-Nissila, L., Viikari, J., Tuominen, J., Pulkki, K., & Simell, O. (2000). Plant stanol ester margarine lowers serum total and low-density lipoprotein cholesterol concentrations of healthy children: The STRIP project. *Journal of Pediatrics, 136,* 503–510.

Tershakovec, A. M., Jawad, A. F., Stallings, V. A., Zemel, B. S., McKenzie, J. M., & Shannon, B. M. (1998). Growth of hypercholesterolemic children completing physician-initiated low-fat dietary intervention. *Journal of Pediatrics, 133,* 28–34.

Tershakovec, A. M., Mitchell, D. C., Smiciklas-Wright, H., Martel, J. K., McKenzie, M. J., & Shannon, B. M. (1997). Pediatric preventive health screening and dietary intake. *Nutrition Research, 17,* 1239–1247.

Tershakovec, A. M., Shannon, B. M., Achterberg, C. L., McKenzie, J. M., Martel, J. K., Smiciklas-Wright, H., Pammer, S. E., & Cortner, J. A. (1998). A one-year follow-up of nutrition education for hypercholesterolemic children. *American Journal of Public Health, 88*(2), 258–261.

Tershakovec, A. M., Watson, M. H., Wenner, W. J., & Marx, A. I. (1999). Insurance reimbursement for the treatment of obesity in children. *Journal of Pediatrics, 134,* 573–578.

Teixeira, S. R., Potter, S. M., Weigel, R., et al. (2000). Effects of feeding 4 levels of soy protein for 3 and 6 weeks on blood lipids and apolipoproteins in moderately hypercholesterolemic men. *American Journal of Clinical Nutrition, 71,* 1077–1084.

Thomas, P. R. (Ed.). (1995). *Weighing the Options—Criteria for Evaluating Weight-Management Programs* (pp. 102–117). Washington, DC: National Academy Press.

Thompson, F. E., & Dennison, B. A. (1994). Dietary sources of fats and cholesterol in US children aged 2 through 5 years. *American Journal of Public Health, 84,* 799–806.

Tinker, L. F., Schneeman, B. O., Davis, P. A., Gallagher, D. D., & Waggoner, C. R. (1991). Consumption of prunes as a source of dietary fiber in men with mild hypercholesterolemia. *American Journal of Clinical Nutrition, 53,* 1259–1265.

Troiano, R. P., Flegal, K. M., Kuczmarski, R. J., Campbell, S. M., & Johnson, C. L. (1995). Overweight prevalence and trends for children and adolescents: The National Health and Nutrition Examination Surveys, 1963–1991. *Archives of Pediatric & Adolescent Medicine, 149,* 1085–1091.

Troisi, R., Willett, W. C., & Weiss, S. T. (1992). Trans-fatty acid intake in relation to serum lipid concentrations in adult men. *American Journal of Clinical Nutrition, 56,* 1019–1024.

Tucker, L. A., & Kano, M. J. (1992). Dietary fat and body fat: A multivariate study of 205 adult females. *American Journal of Clinical Nutrition, 56,* 616–622.

Van Gaal, L. F., Wauters, M. A., & De Leeuw, I. H. (1997). The beneficial effects of modest weight loss on cardiovascular risk factors. *International Journal of Obesity, 21*(Suppl.), 5–9.

Van Horn, L. V., Liu, K., Parker, D., Emidy, L., Liao, Y., Pan, W. H., Giumetti, D., Hewitt, J., & Stamler, J. (1986). Serum lipid response to oat product intake with a fat-modified diet. *Journal of the American Dietary Association, 86,* 759–764.

Vignolo, M., Naselli, A., DiBattista, E., Mostert, M., & Aicardi, G. (1988). Growth and development in simple obesity. *European Journal of Pediatrics, 147*(3), 242–244.

Wadden, T. A., Stunkard, A. J., Rich, L., Rubin, C. J., Sweidel, G., & McKinney, S. (1990). Obesity in Black adolescent girls: A controlled clinical trial of treatment by diet, behavior modification, and parental support. *Pediatrics, 85,* 345–352.

Walter, H. J., Hofman, A., Vaughan, R. D., & Wynder, E. L. (1989). Modification of risk factors for coronary heat disease: Five-year results of a school-based intervention trial. *New England Journal of Medicine, 318,* 1093–1100.

Whitaker, R. C., Wright, J. A., Pepe, M. S., Seidel, K. D., & Deitz, W. H. (1997). Predicting obesity in young adulthood from childhood and parental obesity. *New England Journal of Medicine, 337,* 869–873.

Widhalm, K. (1985). Effect of diet on serum lipoproteins in children with various forms of hyperlipidemias. In *Detection and treatment of lipid and lipoprotein disorders of childhood* (pp. 145–159). New York: Alan R. Liss, Inc.

Widhalm, K., Brazda, G., Schneider, B., & Kohl, S. (1993). Effect of soy protein diet versus standard low fat, low cholesterol diet on lipid and lipoprotein levels in children with familial or polygenic hypercholesterolemia. *Journal of Pediatrics, 123,* 30–34.

Willett, W. C., & Ascherio, A. (1994). Trans fatty acids: Are the effects only marginal? *American Journal of Public Health, 84,* 722–724.

Williams, C. L., Bollella, M., & Wynder, E. L. (1995). A new recommendation for dietary fiber in childhood. *Pediatrics, 96,* 985–988.

Winkleby, M. A. (1994). The future of community-based cardiovascular disease intervention studies. *American Journal of Public Health, 84,* 1369–1372.

Winkleby, M. A., Robinson, T. N., Sundquist, J., & Kraemer, H. C. (1999). Ethnic variation in cardiovascular disease risk factors among children and young adults: Findings from the Third National Health and Nutrition Examination Survey, 1988–1994. *Journal of the American Medical Association, 281*(11), 1006–1013.

Zock, P. L., & Katan, M. B. (1992). Hydrogenation alternatives: Effects of trans fatty acids and stearic acid versus linoleic acid on serum lipids and lipoproteins in humans. *Journal of Lipid Research, 33*, 399–410.

CHAPTER 4

The Importance of Physical Activity in Childhood and Adolescence

Han C. G. Kemper

In 1994 an international consensus conference on physical activity developed guidelines for adolescents based on scientific evidence related to the amount of physical activity needed to affect selected health variables in adolescents (Sallis & Patrick, 1994). Nine review papers were used to examine the dose response relation between physical activity and health variables, and to identify a level or amount of physical activity that reliably improved health outcomes in adolescence.

The conference participants advanced two guidelines for recommendations for the general adolescent population (Sallis & Patrick, 1994):

1) All adolescents should be physically active daily, or nearly every day, as part of play, games, sports, work, transportation, recreation, physical education, or planned exercise, in the context of family, school, and community activities. The activities should be enjoyable, involve a variety of muscle groups, and include some weight bearing activities. The intensity or duration of the activity is probably less important than the fact the energy is expended and a habit of daily activity is established.

2) Adolescents should engage in three or more sessions per week of physical activities that last 20 minutes or more and require moderate to vigorous levels of exertion. Moderate to vigorous activities are those that require at-large muscle groups and least as much effort as more than 7 times their basal metabolic rate.

This chapter will include a review of the literature on the development of physical activity patterns during youth including the extent to which these patterns satisfy the above mentioned guidelines.

It has long been recognized that physical activity is an important consideration during children's growing years in order to maintain normal growth and development (Bar-Or, 1983). Children are generally thought to be naturally physically active, but in recent years their activity levels have been a subject of great concern to health officials (Kohl & Hobbs, 1998; Shephard, 1982). Until a generation ago, physical activity was a natural part of life for most children. This is no longer so, and professionals are asking whether children and adolescents now get the physical activity required for healthy development. Hypoactivity is a direct or indirect cause or result of many pediatric diseases, such as arthritis, cerebral palsy, cystic fibrosis, severe cyanotic heart disease, obesity, and scoliosis. Children with bronchial asthma, diabetes mellitus, epilepsy, noncyanotic heart disease, and hemophilia can be active, but often they are not. Restrictions reflect overprotection by the parents or an uneducated attitude of teachers and health practitioners, or both (Bar-Or, 1983).

Physical inactivity is also an important direct and indirect risk factor for adult diseases such as cardiovascular diseases, cancer, and other chronic diseases. Powell, Thompson, Caspersen, and Kendrick (1987) and Berlin and Colditz (1990) have summarized the epidemiological evidence for indirect and direct causal relationships between physical activity and morbidity and mortality of cardiovascular diseases (CHD). Although many industrialized countries have adopted prevention policies designed to reduce the prevalence of the three risk factors: high serum cholesterol, smoking, and high blood pressure, physical inactivity should be added as a fourth important risk factor for coronary heart disease. Prompted by data linking physical inactivity and CHD, the American Heart Association and other agencies in the United States have placed more emphasis on physical inactivity as a risk factor for CHD.

Several large scale epidemiological studies indicate that physical inactivity results in CHD indirectly through various physiologic mechanisms that relate partly to beneficial effects of physical activities on blood pressure and serum lipoprotein profiles (Berlin & Colditz, 1990; Powell et al., 1987). Most studies that have statistically adjusted for the confounding effects of traditional risk factors indicate that physical inactivity is also an independent and direct risk factor for CHD. Technological progress in industrialized countries has led to decreasing physical activity in most jobs. Therefore, public health attention often is focused on leisure time physical activity.

The burden of physical inactivity on public health can be estimated as relative risks for the four selected risk factors. This *population attributable risk* (PAR) offers a balanced view of the need to act on stronger risk factors that affect fewer people versus the need to act on weaker risk factors that are far more prevalent. This population attributable risk for physical activity on all causes of mortality and mortality due to CHD seems, in 43 studies reviewed by Paffenbarger and others (Paffenbarger, Hyde, Wing, & Hsieh, 1986), greater than the effect of hypertension, hypercholesterolemia, and smoking, mainly because of the large number of physically inactive people. The increase in relative risk (RR) for each of these four CHD risk factors is of a similar magnitude. The RR varies between 1.9 (physical inactivity) and 2.5 (cigarette smoking). With the prevalences of the three other CHD risk factors being relatively low, compared to the prevalence of those failing to perform regular exercise, the PAR of physical inactivity is the highest. Therefore, physical activity is a greater concern for its population impact than the other three CHD risk factors (Caspersen, 1989). Physical inactivity is clearly an important risk factor for CHD.

The mechanization and automation of work and leisure activities have greatly decreased the externally imposed need for physical activity. Physical activity levels are now largely dictated by internal factors, such as body build, physical fitness, and the availability of recreational and sport facilities. Physical inactivity is an important risk factor for many chronic diseases, such as obesity, diabetes mellitus, chronic obstructive pulmonary diseases (COPD), osteoporosis and CHD. Atherosclerotic processes begin early in life (McGill et al., 1997; Montoye, 1985; Wissler, 1991). Researchers have suggested that a sufficient amount and intensity of regular physical activity could decelerate this process (Powell et al., 1987). Research to document this process longitudinally is nonexistent: an epidemiological prospective study, comparing physically active children with a randomized group of less active children over a long period, has never been conducted, and apparently cannot be carried out (Mednick & Baert, 1981). There is no possibility of a double-blind study to measure the effects of physical activity. Alternatively, an appropriate methodology would be to measure the natural history of habitual physical activity in children longitudinally, and to group individuals later according to registered activity patterns (Mirwald, Bailey, Cameron, & Rasmussen, 1981; Rutenfranz, Berndt, & Knauth, 1974; Rutenfranz, Seliger, Andersen, 1975; Sprynarova, 1974). Another possibility is to set up an experimental longitudinal study, such as the Canadian Trois Rivières region study (Jéquier et al., 1977), in which the effects of additional physical education classes were compared with those of control classes over 2 school years.

In the course of body growth and development come critical periods that influence patterns of physical activity (Masironi & Denolin, 1985):

- From ages 4–12, most children begin formal schooling and normally lose a considerable amount of play time.
- At age 12 most children enter secondary school, with free time further restricted by homework.
- At age 15 or 16 many teenagers in European countries shift from bicycles to motorcycles, while teens in the U.S. shift from bicycles to automobiles.
- From age 18 still more young people shift to utilization of automobiles.

The consequences of such facts for the development of physical activity in children was illustrated by Rowland (1990), who showed the change in total daily energy expenditure (Figure 4.1). The total daily energy expenditure per kilogram of body weight (kcal/kg) diminishes rapidly between 6–14 years of age, by almost 50% in both boys and girls. Boys are more active than girls at all ages by about 10%. During these years, lifestyle changes considerably, as do perspectives on activity and health also change.

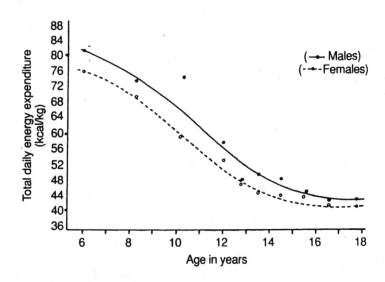

FIGURE 4.1   Total daily energy expenditure of boys and girls between ages 6 and 18 (Rowland, 1990).

Evaluating the natural history of physical activity in children and adolescents requires valid and accurate measurement methods. Daily physical activity, however, is a difficult lifestyle parameter to measure, because the measurement itself interferes with the normal physical activity pattern of the child. Also, children's activities change from day to day, week to week, and season to season.

Physical activity is related to multiple aspects of growth and health. From a physiological point of view, physical activity can be measured in terms of energy expenditure (in kilojoules) as the result of duration, intensity and frequency of the different physical activities. Both anaerobic and aerobic measures can be used to determine the total energy expenditure from oxygen uptake, heart rate, and other methods. Because the aerobic component is an important aspect of energy expenditure, this energetic physical activity has an effect on the body systems that take part in the oxygen delivering and transport systems of the body, such as ventilation (lungs), circulation (heart, vessels), and muscles (capillaries, mitochondria).

From a biomechanical point of view, physical activity causes stresses on the muscles and bones by muscle contractions and reaction forces from the body. These *peak strain* physical activities seem to be more important for their effects on the musculoskeletal system than the energetic component (Turner, 1998). These differential effects have to be taken into consideration when measuring daily physical activity (Kemper, Twisk, Koppes, Mechelen, & Post, 2001). Therefore, the gold standard of measurement of physical activity must include considerations of the mechanism of physical activities (Montoye, Kemper, Saris, & Washburn, 1996).

In summary the method that will be chosen for physical activity should meet at least the following four criteria:

1. socially acceptable and interfere minimally with normal daily activity;
2. applicable over at least 24 hr in order to include school and leisure activities;
3. valid with respect to the gold standard of physical activity measurement;
4. acceptable in financial cost.

DEVELOPMENTAL ASPECTS OF BEHAVIORAL HEALTH

Importance of Longitudinal Studies

Individual changes in growth, development, fitness and physical activity can only be studied if the same individuals are measured repeatedly over a period of time in longitudinal studies. Two types of longitudinal research can be distinguished.

1. In the nonintervention (observational) research, early characteristics are noted, and changes over time are analyzed on an individual basis. Most of this prospective longitudinal research is descriptive. From such nonintervention research no attempt can be made to establish causal relationships (Mednick & Baert, 1981).
2. If one is interested in the effects of physical activity in youth, one has to take on longitudinal research with an intervention component (experimental longitudinal research). Assuming that appropriate controls (e.g., no training) and research designs are used, certain causal statements could be made concerning the conclusions of such research.

There are several reasons that experimental longitudinal research in children and adolescents is needed.

1. Children and adolescents are in a phase of continuous growth and development. Their morphologic, physiological, and psychological characteristics are in flux, and these changes are similar to training effects.
2. Nonintervention comparisons of children who train against those who do not train cannot discern the effects of sports training over a period of time. Self-selection is a serious problem in comparing sporting with nonsporting groups (Cook & Campbell, 1979).

Only an intervention longitudinal study, in which the experimental and control group are randomly chosen and are compared over a period of time, could provide data necessary for solid conclusions about the effects of participation in sport and training.

Longitudinal Studies

The most common practical problems of longitudinal research include: long-term commitment of subjects, staff, financial and other resources; techniques that become obsolete; retention and adherence of subjects; and, final analysis and publication.

Children and adolescents vary in their rates of growth and development. Children who reach full biological maturity at an early chronological age are called *early maturers*, in contrast with *late maturers*, who reach full maturity at a later chronological age. Both types of subjects are included in longitudinal studies, therefore grouped data of children of the same chronological age include a mixture of subjects with different states of biological maturation. The effects of a training or sport program may be different depending on the level of maturation (Vrijens, 1978).

Changes that are related to biological development can be measured. In growth studies height and weight are measured at intervals of 2–6 months in order to calculate their velocities (for example height velocity in cm – year^{-1}). These velocities can be used as indicators for biological age. During puberty an increase in height occurs in both boys and girls, and the peak height velocity (PHV) correlates well with other parameters of biological maturation such as sexual maturation, axillary pubic hair development, and menarche and breast development in girls, and penis or testis development in boys (Faulkner & Tanner, 1978).

Using longitudinal data, the changes in dependent variables such as aerobic power or muscle power can be related not only to chronological age, but also to other age scales that may be more relevant to the effects of physical activity on the human body, such as age relative to PHV and skeletal age (Kemper, 1985) or peak muscle force velocity (Beunen & Malina, 1988). Evidence of these relationships is visible in Figures 4.2 and 4.3.

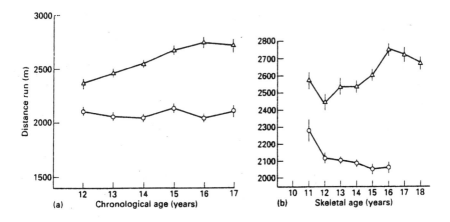

FIGURE 4.2 **Example of the aerobic endurance (12-min endurance run test) related to chronological age (a) and skeletal age (b) (Kemper, 1985).**

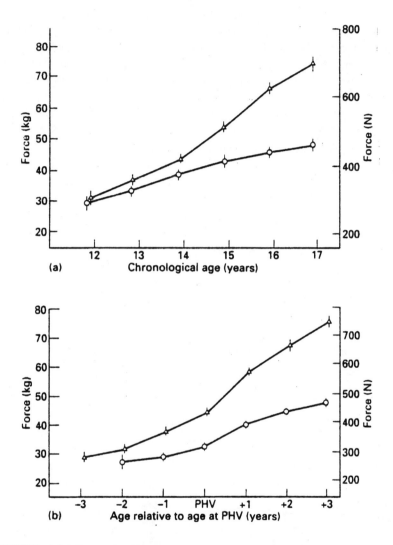

FIGURE 4.3   Example of static arm strength (arm pull test) related to chronological age (a) and peak height velocity (PHV) age (b) (Kemper, 1985).

Principles of Longitudinal Designs

In almost every study of growth, development and training, confounding effects will occur, no matter which design has been used. Three classical designs have been used most frequently: (1) the cross-sectional design; (2) the time-lag design; and (3) the longitudinal design. Each measurement taken on a subject at a particular point of time is influenced by three factors:

1. Chronological age of the subject, defined as the period that elapses between birth and time of measurement.
2. Birth cohort to which the subject belongs.
3. Time of measurement (i.e., the year in which the measurement is taken).

The three different designs are characterized in Figure 4.4. In a cross-sectional study the time of measurement is kept constant. Conversely, in a time-lag study, different groups of the same age are measured at different points of time, thus age is kept constant. In a longitudinal study information is gathered from one cohort sequentially (Schaie, 1965).

MULTIPLE LONGITUDINAL DESIGN: THE AMSTERDAM GROWTH AND HEALTH LONGITUDINAL STUDY

The research literature describes several designs that try to overcome the confounding effects (Kowalski & Prahl-Andersen, 1979; Rao & Rao, 1966; Tanner, 1962). The *multiple longitudinal* design uses repeated measurements on more than one cohort (Kemper & Van 't Hof, 1978), with overlapping ages during the study. This has the advantage of isolating the main effect, (e.g., the age effect) from interfering effects such as time of measurement and cohort (Van 't Hof, Kowalski, 1979).

Figure 4.5 shows an example of a multiple longitudinal design using three birth cohorts (1980, 1981, and 1982) that were measured during four consecutive years (1993–1996). Because there is an overlap in age, the cohorts can be compared at different ages (horizontal comparisons in Figure 4.5). A systematic difference between the cohorts at these ages is called a *cohort effect*. The factor of time of measurement can also be distinguished in a longitudinal study (Veling & Van 't Hof, 1980). If there are no cohort effects, the time of measurement is identified as a possible difference between the

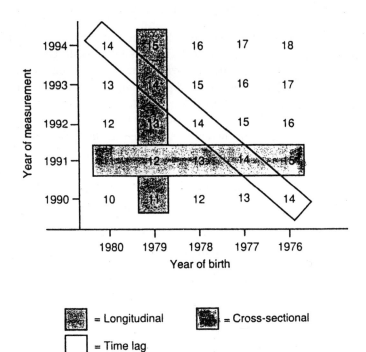

FIGURE 4.4   Graphical representation of the 3 classical study designs: cross sectional (vertical bar), time-lag (diagonal bar), and longitudinal (horizontal bar).

two groups. If it appears that there is no time of measurement effect and no cohort effect either, then the data of all cohorts at all points of time can be arranged in age groups, and a real developmental pattern can be discerned (Bell, 1954). This pattern is illustrated in Figure 4.6 with the data of maximal aerobic power (per kg body mass) from the Amsterdam Growth and Health Study (AGAHLS).

Testing or Learning Effects

Another problem with repeated measurements is a testing or learning effect. Many variables, physical as well as psychological, require a certain motivation

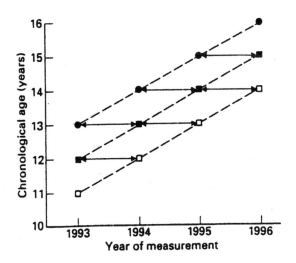

FIGURE 4.5 Example of a multiple longitudinal design, using three birth cohorts measured four consecutive years.

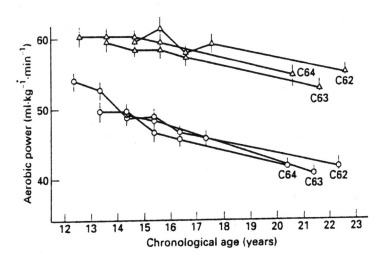

FIGURE 4.6 Maximal aerobic power (ml/kg.min) in males and females from three different birth cohorts (C_{62}, C_{63}, and C_{64}) related to chronological age.

or habituation of the subject while being measured. This introduces differences between periods of measurement that are solely due to the changes in attitude towards the measurement procedure itself. Such testing effects may be positive (i.e., when habituation or learning is important) or negative (i.e., when motivation decreases). Physical performance tests, where maximal motivation is needed, are particularly threatened by these effects. Repeated measurements may, therefore, have a disturbing influence on the quantity measured and diminish the external validity of the results. Systematic testing effects can be estimated if the design also includes a control group in which repeated measurements are not made (Figure 4.7).

Longitudinal Training Studies in the Child and Adolescent

Longitudinal studies in children that aim to analyze the effects of physical activity and training can be divided in two major types. In the first type, children are followed over a period of time. At the end of the study based on a retrospective determination, subgroups are made of children with differences in the observed or measured levels of physical activity. Children who

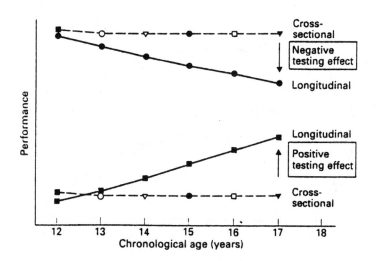

FIGURE 4.7 **Negative and/or positive testing effects of performance measurements: comparing longitudinal measurements with nonlongitudinal measurements in a comparable control group.**

showed a relatively high level of activity during the observation period are contrasted with children of the same sex, age, and other relevant characteristics who showed a relatively low level of activity during the same observation period. In four longitudinal studies (the Saskatchewan Growth and Development Study, Prague Growth Study, Bratislava Youth and Physical Activity, and AGAHLS), the following tracking procedure was taken: subjects were divided into high activity and low activity groups based on their longitudinally collected data (Kemper, 1986). In all these comparisons active children demonstrated higher physiological characteristics than the less active children. These results are not conclusive about the effects of physical activity, however, because the children made their own decisions about being active or not. Therefore, self-selection may have influenced the results (Kemper, 1995).

The second type of training studies utilizes the school environment: a change is initiated in the school curriculum by adding physical education (PE) lessons as extra or replacement for other school subjects. Comparisons are made before and after the change with control classes that did not have curriculum modifications. Kemper and colleagues (1976) reviewed these studies and found in general no effects before puberty. The main reasons are: (1) high training status of prepubertal children; (2) low intensity of PE classes; (3) small number of extra PE lessons; (4) nonhomogeneity of maturation between subjects; (5) low specificity of training stimulus: most of the PE lessons are devoted to motor coordinations improvement and less to endurance and resistance training. In most of the studies motor coordination increased significantly in the experimental groups compared to control groups but not maximal aerobic power (VO_{2max}) and maximal muscle force (F_{max}).

The only long-term intervention study (6 years) is the Trois Rivieres regional study in Canada (Shephard, 1982): Children enrolled in the experimental program received five PE lessons per week integrated into the normal primary school curriculum. Control subjects received the usual one lesson of PE per week. This study followed boys and girls from 6–12 years of age. VO_{2max} and other physical fitness characteristics increased significantly more in the experimental classes than in the control classes in the last 3 years, from age 8–11 years.

Aerobic Training

Several critical reviews (Rowland, 1985) have been written about aerobic training effects in children. Sady (1986) and Kemper and Van de Kop (1995) reviewed more than 20 training studies. Only those studies using a control group were included. The increase in $VO_{2max}.kg^{-1}$ body weight appeared to vary considerably, and there seemed to be no differences between pubescent and postpubescent children. The researchers showed that in training studies with a duration of between 4–15 weeks, effects varied from between −2% (in two studies detraining was measured) and +20% of baseline $VO_{2max}.kg^{-1}$ body weight. In training studies with a duration between 0.5–5 years the effects vary from −10 to +10% of baseline $VO_{2max}.kg^{-1}$ body weight. Training programs in children that fail to demonstrate a beneficial effect on aerobic fitness do not comply with adult standards formulated by the American College of Sports Medicine (1991). Both pre- and postpubertal children are physiologically adaptive to endurance exercise training, as demonstrated by statistically significant increases in $VO_{2max}.kg^{-1}$ body weight in the training groups compared to the nontraining groups (Pate & Ward, 1990). Although it is possible that a critical age exists before which the child is less trainable (before, at, or after PHV age) (Kobayashi et al., 1978; Mirwald & Bailey, 1985), other authors (Weber, Kartodihardjo, & Klissouras, 1976; Cunningham, Waterschoot, Paterson, Lefcoe, & Sangal, 1984; Froberg, Andersen, & Lammert, 1991) cast considerable doubt on that hypothesis.

The critical stage of maturity during which endurance training has its greatest influence on the cardiorespiratory system has yet to be determined (Vaccaro & Mahon, 1987). The degree of trainability seems to be dependent on motivation (prepubescents are less trainable) and from pretraining levels (children can be very active even when not taking part in programmed sports training). Although in some studies no training effect, or even a negative effect, was shown in $VO_{2max}.kg^{-1}$ body weight, performance measures such as running time are always improved. Possible explanations for this apparent discrepancy are that training induces a higher mechanical efficiency and that VO_{2max} does not reflect well the maximal aerobic performance of children (Bar-Or, 1989).

Strength Training

Fewer studies have been performed on the effect of strength training than on aerobic training in children. While some authors have reported a small degree of trainability before puberty (Vrijens, 1978), other studies (Weltman, 1984) demonstrated a significant increase in 6–11 year-old boys following a period of strength training. The discrepancy can be explained by the way the strength effects were evaluated: Vrijens used nonspecific testing by training with dynamic exercises and testing the effects isometrically. In contrast,

Weltman trained and tested the effects isokinetically. The results of Weltman and of others (Sewall & Micheli, 1984; Pfeiffer & Francis, 1986) confirmed that increases in muscle strength are possible before puberty in boys and girls, and are not related to maturity levels. Such increases are reached without the risk of musculoskeletal injuries. Anaerobic muscle performances, such as the Margaria stair/running test (Margaria et al., 1966) and the Wingate 30-cycle test (Bar-Or, 1987) can also be improved during childhood and adolescence regardless of maturation level.

METHODS OF TRAINING AND PHYSICAL ACTIVITY

Short-Term Demands of Exercise

For mechanical energy to be released at the muscle level, adenosine triphosphate (ATP) must be split. Because this high-energy compound is available only in small quantities, there is a need for reinforcement of ATP, supplied by anaerobic sources (creatine phosphate [CP] and lactic acid system) and aerobic sources (oxygen transport system). Muscle contractions cannot be sustained from anaerobic sources for longer than 1 minute. In contrast, muscle contractions utilizing aerobic sources can last minutes or even hours unless there is a shortage of substrate, particularly glycogen. Most physical activities utilize both aerobic and anaerobic sources, but are roughly subdivided into low power/long duration (aerobic) activities such as long distance running, swimming, skating, cycling, and skiing; and high power/short duration (anaerobic) activities such as sprinting, jumping, and throwing (Bar-Or, 1983). Short-term high power output, even when standardized for body size (body mass or active muscle mass), is distinctly lower in children than in young adults. There are no large differences in the level of ATP and CP, but a lower glycolytic rate is suggested by lower lactate concentrations in blood and muscle (Eriksson, 1972).

The most commonly used index of maximal aerobic power is the maximal oxygen intake (VO_{2max}), the highest volume of O_2 that can be consumed by the body per unit of time. Until the age of 12 years, VO_{2max} values increase equally in both genders. Although the VO_{2max} of boys keeps increasing until the age of about 18 years, there is little change in girls beyond the age of 14 years. If VO_{2max} is expressed per kg of body mass (VO_{2max}/body mass), there is hardly any age-dependent change in boys, but the relative VO_{2max} declines in girls, reflecting an increase in body fatness and a relative decrease of lean body mass.

An alternative and more theoretical approach is based on the scaling theory. It is assumed that body segments retain fairly constant proportions during childhood and adolescence. Linear dimensions are described by length (L), surfaces have areas that are described by L^2, and volumes by L^3. Maximal muscle force should be scaled to L^2 (because they are proportional to cross-sectional area). Maximal aerobic power (VO_{2max}) as a volume per time unit is also proportional to L^2. If VO_{2max} should be related to body height squared, values for children are lower than in healthy young adults. Longitudinal studies show in adolescents, however, height exponents that are higher or equal than expected: from 2.25–3.0 in boys and 2.0 in girls (Kemper & Verschuur, 1987). These exponents suggest that in girls the state of the aerobic system remains relatively constant, while in boys one sees an increase over and above that expected from increasing body size.

Long-Term Effects of Exercise

A child exercising systematically over weeks and months induces the morphologic and functional adaptation of training. Research on the effects of children's training faces many methodological problems. Changes due to growth, development, and maturation can also influence the results. Control groups must be included in the design, but subjects can very seldom be assigned randomly. Owing to the above constraints, most studies of training in childhood are correlative and not causative. Changes are specific to the training stimulus. Aerobic, endurancelike activities induce systemic effects (e.g., hypertrophy and dilatation of the right ventricle) and improvements of oxidative capacity in active muscles (including increases of aerobic enzymes and capillary density). Anaerobic, short-term high-power activities induce different effects, such as muscle hypertrophy (increases of myofibrils and connective, tendinous, and ligamentous tissue) and adaptations in the nervous system (e.g., recruitment patterns and synchronization of motor units) (Fox, Bowers, & Foss, 1993).

Training is based on two general principles: recognition of the major energy system used to perform a given activity and overload throughout training. All training programs must be specific to the energy system(s) predominantly used during (sports) performances.

The overload principle implies that the exercise resistance is near maximal and that the resistance is increased gradually as the child's performance capacity improves. The amount of training can be characterized by its intensity, duration, and frequency. The intensity of an activity is determined by the metabolic demands (VO_2), the strain on the cardiovascular system (heart rate), or in the case of strength training, by the weight lifted. Although intensity is often described in absolute terms, in children and adolescents it should be described in relation to the maximal capability of the individual. There is no training effect below a certain threshold. For young adults, the threshold of aerobic power is about 65% of VO_{2max} or 75% of maximal heart rate, while for strength training the threshold is about 70% of maximal voluntary isometric contraction (F_{max}). When dynamic tasks are involved, the maximal number of repetitions of muscle contractions can be used, the so-called repetition maximum (RM). If the RM of a dynamic task appears to be below 10, it can be assumed that this equals an isometric force of over 70% of F_{max}. To maintain overload, a program must be progressive. There is no optimal frequency of training because frequency interacts with the intensity and the duration of training sessions. In therapeutic and fitness programs it is generally recommended that children should not train more than 3 times a week.

The duration of training sessions for children should be at least 30 min but not longer than 1 hr. The minimal duration of 30 min allows a 10-min warm-up at the beginning and a 5-min cooldown at the end of the session. The maximum of 60 min avoids a middle part of the session when the training threshold must be exceeded by a child who is already fatigued and becoming inattentive.

Training Methods: Strength Versus Endurance

Muscular strength is the force or tension a muscle can exert against resistance during a single maximal effort. Because there are three basic kinds of muscle contractions: isometric, miometric (or concentric), and pliometric (or eccentric), there are also three types of muscle training. There is no simple, optimal program to develop strength. The most recently recommended method is isokinetic training. Here, a device that permits the development of maximal muscular tension is used throughout the full range of joint movement (while the speed is kept constant) unlike in dynamic weight training. Programs to improve strength consist primarily of high loads and low repetitions. In contrast, muscular endurance (the ability to perform repeated contractions over an extended period) is developed by frequent repetitions at low loads.

Much of the improvement in sports performances over the past century can be attributed not only to early selection and to increased participation rates, but also to the refinement of training methods. Apart from well-known continuous endurance training programs, different interval training programs have been introduced: interval sprint training, interval tempo training, and interval duration training (Fox, Bowers, & Fox, 1993).

The goal of interval sprint training is to increase the capacity of the phosphate battery and is characterized by a high intensity and a short duration. Interval duration training combines the longest loading periods with the lowest intensity in order to involve the oxygen transport system. The interval tempo training is specifically loading the lactic acid system, and has intermediate intensity and duration. The alternating periods of load and recovery of the interval training are more tailored to children's behavior than continuous loading.

Measurements of Physical Activity and Energy Expenditure

An important aspect of any assessment of habitual physical activity is the definition and interpretation of the term *physical activity*. Because the law of the conservation of energy also applies to humans—who must fuel all activity by extracting energy from food—measurements of physical activity are often expressed in terms of energy expenditure. Alternately, physical activity can be expressed as the amount of work performed (watts), as the duration of activity (hr, min), as units of movements (counts), or even as a numerical score derived from responses to a questionnaire. Any particular assessment technique, however, measures only one part of so-called *habitual physical activity* (Montoye et al., 1996).

The term *energy expenditure* is not synonymous with physical activity or exercise. A child may expend the same amount of energy in a short burst of strenuous exercise (sprint) as in less intense endurancetype activity (walk), but the health and physiological effects of the two could be different.

It is essential to remember that the intake or expenditure of joules is related to body size. A young child who is very active may spend a similar number of kilojoules in 24 hr as a large person who is sedentary. Therefore, if exercise is expressed as energy expenditure in joules, body size must be taken into account. To this end, energy expended or ingested is sometimes given as kilojoules per unit of body weight or, in the case of oxygen uptake, as millimeters of O_2 per kg of body weight. The use of METs (metabolic) is another approach to correcting for body weight. A MET score represents the ratio of energy expended for a specific activity in kilojoules, divided by resting energy expenditure in kilojoules, either measured or estimated from body size of the individual. In estimating resting (not basal) energy expenditure, a value of 4.2 kJ per kg of body weight per hr or 3.5 ml O_2 utilized per kg of body weight per min is an accepted estimate. A MET score indicates the energy expenditure of physical activity in multiples of the resting energy expenditure.

Energy is expended in three ways in warm-blooded humans and animals. A certain amount of energy is required to maintain body temperature and involuntary muscular contraction at rest for functions, including circulation and respiration. This energy level represents the resting metabolic rate. Some energy is required to digest and assimilate food. This process, referred to as *dietary induced thermogenesis* or *thermic effect of food*, adds about 10% to the resting metabolic rate. These two represent but a small part of the total energy expenditure and can be altered only very slightly in individuals. Finally, by far the most important source of variation between individuals in energy expenditure (when adjusted for body size) is muscular activity. The sources of this activity in children are playing (at home, at school, and on play grounds) and organized sport activities.

The physiological and biomechanical principles underlying physical activity are complex. Numerous difficulties are encountered in developing simple techniques for assessing habitual activity. For the most part, laboratory methods are not useful in the field for measuring activity and energy expenditure, and do not directly apply to epidemiological studies of assessing habitual physical activity.

The physiologic methods measuring energy expenditure in the laboratory can be divided into three groups:

- measurement of energy consumption (food intake), valid only if there is a state of energy balance (i.e., energy intake is equivalent to energy expenditure);
- direct measurement of energy expenditure from heat production in a sealed, insulated chamber (calorimetry);
- indirect measurement of energy expenditure from oxygen consumption in a respiration chamber, or using procedures with closed and open circuit methods using a hood, small face mask, or nose clip and mouthpiece.

The biomechanical methods measure muscular activity by displacements and acceleration of whole body or body segments in two ways:

- photographs with high-speed camera or video with subsequent very elaborate analysis, (automatic registration systems and computerized analysis have been recent improvements);
- force transducers positioned on the corners of a force plate.

Laboratory methods for measuring human energy expenditure are precise but very restrictive and thus limited to use over a short period of time. Field methods are less restrictive and usable over longer periods, but are more imprecise. In the section below six different categories of field methods are summarized and evaluated for their usage in measuring physical activity in children and adolescents.

The Doubly Labeled Water Method

A newer procedure, the *doubly labeled water method* (DLW), bridges the gap between precise laboratory measurements and field measurements (Schoeller, 1983). The method measures integral CO_2 production for up to 3 weeks from the difference in elimination rates of the stable isotopes deuterium and oxygen-18 from doubly labeled body water after ingestion of a quantity of water enriched with both isotopes. Validation against the precise and near continuous respiratory gas exchange method, such as in a respiration chamber, has demonstrated that the method is accurate (1–3%), and has a precision of 4%–7%, depending on isotope dose, length of elimination period, and frequency of sampling (2-point versus multipoint). The method is based on a number of assumptions that must be taken into account, depending on the application field. The DLW method is considered the gold standard for assessing energy expenditure. The method has several advantages over other techniques. It requires only periodic sampling of body fluids, it is nonrestrictive, and ideally suited for use with free-living subjects; and, it has the potential to serve as a criterion for validation (gold standard) of other field methods as mentioned below.

Observational Methods

Assessing physical activity by observation works particularly well with small children, when most other assessment methods are unsuitable. With training, observers can be quite accurate. Various forms are available to make recording more efficient. Also, devices are available, some of them computer compatible, that facilitate the observation approach of assessing physical activity (Van der Beek et al., 1992). Observation, however, is time-consuming and expensive, and thus not suitable for use in even moderately large groups. In addition, observations are time-limited, and may not reflect habitual physical activity.

The Diary Method

The diary method requires complete cooperation and precision from the subject, so the technique is not practical with some populations, such as young children. In some instances, it is not reasonable to expect subjects to interrupt their activities frequently to record intake and activity. Data collection is inexpensive because many subjects can be keeping diaries simultaneously and an observer is not required. The method is subject to considerable individual error although the accuracy is sufficient for group estimates (Bouchard et al., 1983).

Questionnaires and Interviews

The validity and test/retest reproducibility of questionnaires/interviews concerning physical activity have not been adequately studied. The use of questionnaires is the only feasible method for epidemiological investigations. Despite the limitations of the method, the results are often correlated with longevity and morbidity. Before selecting a particular questionnaire/interview, it is necessary to define the purposes of the study, time and financial constraints, and the gender, age, and socioeconomic characteristics of the population. Questionnaire methods are usually inappropriate for use in children under 10 to 12 years of age.

The questionnaire method will probably not provide accurate measures of energy expenditures, but it should be possible to group people into 3–5 categories on the basis of habitual physical activity. Strenuous physical activity appears to be recalled with greater accuracy than mild to moderate activity, and recall of recent activities is more accurate than those done at an earlier time. Weekends and weekdays should be assessed, as well as seasonal variations.

For young children, techniques other than questionnaires, such as observation, movement counters, and heart rate recording, are optimal. If interview and questionnaire are the only alternatives, the possible errors must be reduced. Questionnaires and interviews should focus on the daily routines, such as transportation to and from school and organized sports. Another approach is to ask a parent, teacher, or supervisor about a child's favorite play activities in order to rank children according to their habitual physical activity.

Because most energy-cost tables of physical activity are based on adult data, substantial errors in estimating energy cost are likely if these tables are used with children (or the elderly) (Sallis, Buono, & Freedson, 1991). The use of METs minimizes this error (Washburn & Montoye, 1986a).

Movement Assessment Devices

Pedometers, or stepcounters, are inexpensive, simple movement counters that can be used to estimate habitual physical activity over a relatively long period without interfering with, or requiring modifications of subjects' normal lifestyles. The measurement principle is based on the number of steps taken during locomotion. There are, however, serious problems with reliability and validity. Currently, available pedometers vary in deviations from the actual step rate, even among those of the same type. The following recommendations have been made regarding the use of pedometers.

- Each pedometer should be calibrated by adjusting the tension of the spring, and thereafter validating the pedometer score against the actual step rate at different walking and running speeds (Kemper & Verschuur, 1977).
- Pedometers offer a good estimate of physical activity *if* most body movements coincide with vertical displacements of the body—center of gravity—as happens in walking, jumping, running, and stepping. Activities without vertical displacements of the body (such as cycling, skating, and rowing) yield an underestimation of physical activity if the pedometer is utilized.
- Pedometers total the number of vertical displacements of the body and do not distinguish, for instance, between type of steps caused by a short period of high-intensity running and a long period of low-intensity walking. Because activities of high-intensity require more energy and are more important for physical fitness and health, in some situations it may be judicious to change the sensitivity so that only activities of a relatively high intensity are measured (for example, running with a speed of 6 km/hr). Moreover, such adjustments prevent registration of passive movements like driving in a car over a bumpy road and other vibrational artifacts that are not caused by physical activities.

There is a sound theoretical basis for attempting to estimate physical activity or energy expenditure using a portable accelerometer. The instrument must be waterproofed to register swimming movements, and during cycling it must be worn on a lower limb, not on the trunk. An accelerometer does not reflect the added energy expenditure when weight is lifted or carried. Pedometers and mechanical accelerometers (converted watches, for example) are difficult to standardize.

Portable, single plane (vertical) and triple plane accelerometers are designed to estimate physical activity or energy expenditure (Caltrac, Tritac, and CSA). The interinstrument variability of this instrument is low, and validity is good in walking or running under controlled laboratory conditions. In the field, however, if kilojoules or kilocalories of energy expenditure in usual activity in a particular season are to be estimated, at least 3 days, including a weekend day, should be averaged.

Estimation of Energy Expenditure from Physiologic Functions

A number of physiological functions reflect the rate of energy expenditure, but heart rate (HR) is the most practical response to measure in the field. There are now dependable, self-contained, portable HR recorders available at reasonable cost. The Sports Tester—a small transmitter around the chest in combination with a receiver/recorder as a wristwatch—is rated the best. In populations where day-to-day variation has been studied, 4–5 days of recording (including a weekend day) are usually necessary to obtain a HR index that is typical for an individual (Léger & Thivierge, 1988). To interpret HR as an index of physical activity or energy expenditure, it is imperative to employ individual VO_2–HR calibration curves, or to subtract the resting HR from recorded HR. The second method is simpler and probably almost as accurate (Washburn & Montoye, 1986b). Nevertheless, HR is affected by factors other than the intensity of the physical activity, the most significant being emotions, and thus leaves much to be desired as an index of physical activity or energy expenditure. It is probably most useful when other methods are not feasible, in young children for example, or in combination with another method.

If one is interested in the amount of moderate and intense physical activity, the estimation of energy expenditure above 50% of VO_{2max} is a reasonable alternative, however, the determination of each individual's VO_{2max} is necessary (Saris, 1989). The use of motion sensors in combination with HR recording seems to be a promising approach. Currently, multiple systems are in the developmental stage, so practical applications for those systems cannot be recommended.

Final Evaluation Summary

Table 4.1 summarizes the characteristics of field methods of assessing physical activity in children and adolescents. This is useful in selecting a method

TABLE 4.1 Summary Evaluation of Nine Field Methods of Assessing Habitual Physical Activity and/or Energy Expenditure in Children and Adolescents

	Job classification	Observation	Diary	Questionnaire/ interview	Pedometer	Electronic motion sensors	Accelerometers	Heart rate	Doubly labeled water
1. Age group (yr) appropriate									
Children (< 13 yr)	No	Yes	No	No	Yes	Yes	Yes	Yes	Yes
Adolescents (13–14 yr)	No	Yes	Yes	Yes	Yes	Yes	Yes	Yes	Yes
2. Validity	Poor	Good/fair	Poor/ good	Fair	Fair/poor	Fair	Fair/good	Fair/good	High/ poor
3. Reproducibility	Unknown	Good	Unknown	Fair to good	Fair	Fair	Fair	Fair	Unknown
4. Instrument reliability	Unknown	Good	Unknown	Unknown	Poor	Good	Good	Good	—
5. Size of population (Small: < 50; Large: 50+)	Small/large	Small	Small/ large	Small/large	Small/large	Small	Small/large	Small	Small
6. Cost	Low	High	Mod.	Low/Mod.	Mod.	Mod./High	Mod./High	High	High
7. Subject effort	None	None	Great	Mod.	Little	Little	Little	Little	None
8. Affects behavior	No	Yes	Yes	No	Possibly	Possibly	Possibly	Possibly	No
9. Subject acceptability	Yes	Yes	Yes/No	Yes	Yes	Yes	Yes	Yes/No	Yes

for particular needs; however, some of the techniques (movement recorders, for example) are in early stages of development and changes should be expected.

Montoye and colleagues (1996) outline several areas and research needs relevant to assessment and measurement of physical activity in children and adolescents (Montoye et al., 1996):

1. There is a need to improve the validity and reproducibility of questionnaires and interviews for children.
2. Methods to improve physical activity recall among children requires further investigation.
3. If data from collection devices (questionnaires/interviews, observations, diaries, etc.) are to be converted to estimates of energy expenditure, more research is needed on the energy cost of particular activities of children. Most energy-cost data are based on measurements of young, male adults.
4. More precise ways of using questionnaires and diaries to assess the strenuousness of activities are needed.
5. More accurate and less expensive instruments, such as portable accelerometers, that could be worn by the subject for estimating activity and energy expenditure need to be developed.
6. Research is needed on the validity of combining methods, such as heart rate and movement recording, or movement recording and questionnaire/interview.
7. Exercise often has an anaerobic component, particularly for children during leisure activity. Research is needed to assess the importance of the anaerobic component in children's activity.

PHYSICAL ACTIVITY IN THE AMSTERDAM GROWTH AND HEALTH LONGITUDINAL STUDY (AGAHLS)

Methods selected to measure physical activity should not interfere with a child's normal activity pattern and should obtain an estimate of the energy expenditure, which also reflects the intensity of the activity (Edholm, 1996; Seliger, 1966). In large group studies such as the AGAHLS, with more than 200 boys and girls, the methods must be simple, cheap, and time efficient. These requirements and the need to limit the extent of the activity measurements (because so many other variables were included) led to the selection of three methods:

1. the eight-level heart rate integrator (HRI), which has proved to be a reliable and simple method for recording heart rate (HR) (Saris, Snel, & Binkhorst, 1977; Verschuur & Kemper, 1985);
2. the pedometer, reduced in sensitivity (Verschuur & Kemper, 1980) in order to give a more reliable measurement of energy expenditure by only counting large vertical movements (such as running) rather than small movements (such as walking); and,
3. a questionnaire-interview developed for this study, that aimed to trace activities with a minimal energy expenditure of 4 times the basal metabolic rate (4 METs) for 3 months before the interview (Verschuur, 1987)

These three methods were applied during 4 successive years in all subjects in winter (January through March). Physical activities during 2 randomly selected weekdays (approximately 48 hr) were measured simultaneously, using the HRI and the pedometer. The pedometer was also used to measure weekend activities, from Friday afternoon until Monday morning just before school started. The activity questionnaire was given during interviews that took place in a mobile laboratory near the school.

Heart-Rate Integrator

The heart rate integrator (HRI) (Saris et al., 1977) is an electronic system about the size of a pack of cigarettes. Each R-R interval is measured by two chest electrodes, and analyzed and stored in one of the eight registers of the integrator, corresponding to 8 heart rate levels. In order to transfer HR into aerobic energy expenditure, the relationship between HR and oxygen uptake, which is linear between a HR of 110–120 and 170–180 beats/min (Åstrand & Rodahl, 1986), was determined from the subjects' submaximal treadmill tests. The HR and oxygen uptake in steady state during running (8 km/hr) was measured at slopes of 0, 2.5%, and 5%.

Pedometer

The pedometer measures vertical displacement. Attached to the body, it registers all movement of the center of gravity. Before application, we tested its accuracy (Kemper & Verschuur, 1977) and reduced its sensitivity so that it would start counting at a walking speed of 8 km/hr or more, a jogging pace (Verschuur & Kemper, 1980). The pedometer was worn in a leather cover and hung from the inside of the pupil's waistband. The activity score on the pedometer was the number of vertical displacements counted of 2 weekdays and 1 weekend.

The Activity Interview

The standardized activity interview covered the previous 3 months and was based on a questionnaire developed for this study. It was given by the same interviewer throughout the study. In order to classify the activities according to their energy cost, independent of body weight, we used the ratio between the work metabolic rate and the basal metabolic rate (1 MET) (Reiff, Montoye, Remington, Napier, Metzener & Epstein, 1967). The interview was limited to activities with a minimal intensity level of approximately 4 times the basal metabolic rate (≥ 4 METs), which equals walking at a speed of approximately 5 km/hr. The scored activities were subdivided into three levels of intensity (light, medium to heavy, and heavy) in accordance with the three highest activity levels used by the World Health Organization (Andersen, 1971). They correspond to a relative energy expenditure of 4–7 METs for light activity, 7–10 METs for medium to heavy intensity activity, and 10 or more METs for heavy activity. The classification of activities into the 3 intensity levels was based on data from the literature (Andersen, 1971; Bink, Bonjer, & Sluys, 1966; Durnin & Passmore, 1967; Hollmann & Hettinger, 1976; Reiff et al., 1967; Seliger, 1966). The interview gathered information on the average weekly time spent during the previous 3 months in each of the three activity categories, with a minimum of 5 minutes (Table 4.2). The scores for the three levels were added, yielding a total METs/week score, a weighted activity score combining duration and intensity.

Confounding Effects

Inspection of the data on the three physical activity measurements was conducted over the four measurement years between 1976–1980. The pedometer week score showed a significant time of measurement effect, although there was a general trend of lower mean week scores, with increasing age of the three longitudinal cohorts and the control groups. This is not the case in all groups during the second year of measurement (1978). A possible explanation is provided by climatic conditions during the winter of 1978. In that year there was a longer period of frozen waters, so these Dutch youngsters were able to spend more time at their national sport, ice-skating.

**TABLE 4.2   Classification of Sports and Leisure Activities into Four
Categories on the Basis of Average Intensity (Kemper, 1995)**

Intensity	Activity	
Very light ≤ 4 METs	Domestic:	Dish washing, dusting, floor sweeping
	Outdoor:	Sitting, standing, strolling
	Sport:	Billiards, bowling, bridge, checkers, chess, cricket, fishing, gliding, golf, sailing, shooting, skittle, t'ai chi ch'uan
Light 4–7 METs	Domestic:	Beating carpets, carrying groceries, hammering, polishing floors, sawing, scrubbing floors
	Outdoor:	Bicycling, canoeing, rowing, walking
	Sport:	Ballet, baseball, bodybuilding, dancing (ballroom, modern, folk), gymnastics (rhythmic, remedial), hiking, horseback riding, softball, table tennis, tug of war, volleyball, water-skiing, weightlifting
Medium to heavy 7–10 METs	Domestic:	Stair climbing
	Outdoor:	Basketball (dribbling, shooting), swimming
	Sport:	Badminton, fencing, gymnastics, mountaineering, scuba-diving, skating (figure, speed), skiing (alpine), tennis (outdoor or indoor) track and field (field event)
Heavy ≥ 10 METs	Outdoor:	Basketball (game), running, soccer (game)
	Sport:	Basketball, canoeing, conditioning exercises, cycling (race), handball (European, indoor or outdoor), hockey (field, indoor or outdoor, ice, roller), jogging, kick boxing, netball (indoor or outdoor), martial arts (judo, jujitsu, karate, aikido, kendo, kung fu, tae kwon do), rowing, rugby, skiing (cross-country), soccer (indoor or outdoor), squash, swimming, track and field (track event), trampolining, water polo, wrestling

Note. Outdoor = unorganized recreational activity; Sport = activity in sports clubs.

Source: HCG Kemper (Ed.). (1995). The Amsterdam Growth Study: A longitudinal analysis of health, fitness, and lifestyle. *HK Sport Science Monograph Series, Vol. 6, Human Kinetics*, pp. 42–44. Champaign, IL: Human Kinetics.

The total time spent on physical activity, measured by the interview, revealed both a testing and a dropout effect. A testing effect was seen upon comparison of the longitudinal boys' total activity time per week spent above an intensity of 4 METs with that of control school boys. At age 12–13 the scores of the control group equal those of the longitudinal group. Thereafter there was a slight increase in the former and decrease in the latter. In addition, it appeared that of girls the dropouts were significantly more active than the longitudinal group.

Results of Longitudinal Measured Physical Activity Measured by HRI and Pedometers

In both girls and boys daily physical activity decreases from 12–17 years of age. This is the case in daily energy expenditure calculated as kJ per kg body mass from HRI and calculated as week scores from pedometers. In girls, the decrease is 23% in HRI scores and 52% in pedometer scores; in boys, 17% and 44%, respectively. Boys are significantly more active than girls before puberty (ages 13 and 14), but after puberty the differences become smaller.

When one takes the peak energy expenditure from the HRI by calculating the energy expenditure above 50% of VO_{2max}, the rate of decrease with age is much faster and the differences between boys and girls post puberty is no longer significant.

Physical Activity Measured From Interview

Physical activities at school determine 50% of activity time in girls and 45% in boys, and these percentages do not change with age although total activity time decreases. Youngsters are physically active in going to and from school: at age 12–13, 70–80% go to school by bicycle and 10% by foot. A minority of boys and girls change to mopeds after age 16, 3% of girls and 15%–20% of the boys. Only 15%–20% of girls and boys' activities take place in sport clubs. A cross-sectional classification of sport participation in girls showed a decrease from 61% to 44% between ages 13–17. In boys, sport participation varied little over the same age period (55%–60%; Verschuur, 1987). These results are comparable with those of Backx, Erich, Kemper, and Verbeek (1989), who measured a rate of club membership/organized sport participation in Dutch 8–16 year-olds of between 59% and 75%.

The highest participation rate was at age 10 (75%) and the lowest at age 15 (59%). A longitudinal analysis during the school years was used to indicate the stability of participation in sports. Approximately 25% of the teenagers were never members of a sport club. Only 30% of the girls and 40% of the boys played sports in a club during all 4 years of the study. Soccer was the most popular sport (30–40%) in boys. Girls preferred dance and ballet (10–15%). Unorganized activities represent approximately 35% of girls' activities and 40% of boys'. In both girls and boys, the total time spent on unorganized outdoor activities decreased by 50% from 12–18 years. This decline, caused by a shift with age from playing games in the streets to shopping and dancing, is the most important change in these youngsters during their teens.

Subjects were given the activity interview four times between ages 13–17, and again at ages 21–27. In both females and males the same trend continued: from early teens to early twenties, subjects reduced their medium to heavy (7–10 METs) and heavy (≥ 10 METs) activities. Only light activities (4–7 METs) increase with age.

The total activity score measured as a weighted score of the duration and intensity of the activities, showed a rapid decrease between ages 13–17 in both boys and girls, and thereafter a gradual decline till age 21–27. At all ages females were less active than males, but in young adulthood the differences are smaller and not significant.

Interrelation Between the Three Activity Methods

The three activity instruments indicated without exception a gradual decrease in habitual physical activity between ages 13–17 in both boys and girls. The extent of the decrease, however, depended on the method used. The pedometer week scores showed the steepest decline (45%–15%), followed by the total time spent on activity per week as indicated by the interview (15%–20%). The daily energy expenditure (per kg body mass) from HRI decreased only slightly over the same age range (10–15%).

These differences can be better understood if one realizes that all three instruments measured physical activity at different levels of intensity: HRI measures all daily activities, including sleep. The interview disregards very light activities and starts at 4 METs (walking). The pedometer, on the other hand, records only running (≥ 8km/hr). Thus, the more the methods records the heavier forms of physical activity, the more pronounced the decrease in daily activity. Moreover, the information gathered from the three activity methods overlapped only in part: the HRI and pedometer methods measured the activities of each individual during a relative short period of time. This time (2–4 days) is supposed to be representative of the whole year's activity.

The activity interview is a 3-month retrospective, but is also more general, and the results are more dependent on the memory of the subject. Pearson correlation coefficients were calculated between the activity scores obtained from the same subjects by the three instruments. The correlations in boys and girls, averaged over the 4 school years, range between .16 and .20. These values are significant (p < 0.05) but explain only a small part of the total variation. These findings illustrate that it is not possible to use only one of the three methods and that a combination of measurement and observational methods are needed to obtain a valid picture of children's daily activity patterns.

The longitudinal approach revealed not only a gradual decline in physical activity but also that sport participation appears to be important at an early age to define an active lifestyle. The stability of the sports choices among long-term participants also seemed to indicate that many (30%) children make their choices early in their teens. This stresses the importance of introducing children to a variety of sports and other forms of movement to create opportunities for them to choose lifelong physical activity. Experimental studies of changes in physical activity reveal that effective strategies have in common a dimension of social reinforcement (Dishman, Sallis, & Orenstein, 1985). Schools could provide such reinforcement.

Relationship of Daily Physical Activity with Aerobic Fitness

To investigate the relationship between habitual physical activity (the independent variable) and VO_{2max} (the dependent variable), all girls and boys measured during the first 4 years of the AGAHLS were divided into active and inactive groups (Verschuur, 1987). The selection was made on the basis of three activity variables:

1. energy expenditure measured with HRI over 48 hr;
2. pedometer week scores;
3. total time spent in activity per week according to an activity interview.

Active individuals were those who scored above the median in at least 3 of 4 years. Inactive subjects were those who scored below the median in 2 of 4 years. Comparing active and inactive pupils over time, there were no differences in height, weight, or fat-free mass.

In contrast, parameters directly related to aerobic fitness were significantly related to the level of physical activity. Active girls and boys had significantly

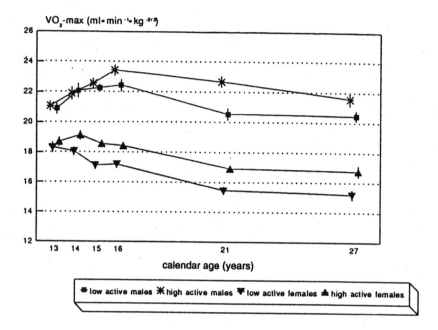

FIGURE 4.8   Changes in aerobic fitness (VO$_{2max}$/BM) in males and females, low activities and high activities, between ages 13–27 (Kemper, 1995; Kemper et al., 2001).

higher VO$_{2max}$/BM than inactive ones. Again, the differences are small, and inactive children had a reasonably high aerobic fitness: for inactive boys, 55 ml/kg; for inactive girls, from 40–47 ml/kg. Because the differences in VO$_{2max}$/BM between active and inactive youngsters already exist at age 13, self-selection rather than training may exert an influence here.

Because physical activity was measured in 1985 and in 1991 with the same activity interview as in previous years, the longitudinal group was divided into sport participants and non participants for the 15-year period between ages 13–27 (Kemper et al., 2001).

Figure 4.8 shows the maximal oxygen uptake per kg body mass for males and females who were relatively physically active (inactive during the 15 years of follow-up). Active males and females have significantly higher aerobic fitness than nonactives. The differences are 3–5 ml O$_2$ per kg body mass, and because they do not change systematically with age, these results support the hypothesis that youngsters are more active because they have high aerobic fitness rather than the reverse—that they have high aerobic fitness because they are active.

CHALLENGES FOR FUTURE RESEARCH

Longitudinal research measuring health and physical activity covering the whole period of puberty is relatively scarce. Comparison of the different longitudinal studies indicate the need for further standardization in sampling procedures, frequency of measurements, and methods of measuring physical activity. Most of the growth and training studies have used boys as subjects. Longitudinal growth and training studies have to be designed in which both genders are included. Much knowledge is still lacking about the trainability of children. To achieve a better understanding of trainability during growth and development the following research questions need to be resolved:

- What are evidence-based guidelines for healthy development of boys and girls?
- What are the best guidelines for adequate training stimuli in boys and girls?
- What is the impact of biological age on the training effects, and, is there any biological age where trainability is minimal or maximal?
- To what extent do physical activity behaviors track into adulthood; in other words are active children also active as adolescents?

REFERENCES

American College of Sports Medicine. (1991). *Guidelines for exercise testing and prescription* (4th ed.). Philadelphia: Lea & Febiger.
Andersen, K. L. (1971). *Fundamentals of exercise testing.* Geneva: World Health Organization.
Åstrand, P. O., & Rodahl, K. (1986). *Textbook of work physiology.* New York: McGraw-Hill.
Backx, F. J., Erich, W. B., Kemper, A. B., & Verbeek, A. L. (1989). Sports injuries in school-aged children: An epidemiologic study. *American Journal of Sports Medicine, 17*(2), 234–240.

Bar-Or, O. (1983). *Pediatric sports and medicine for the practitioner.* New York: Springer-Verlag.

Bar-Or, O. (1987). The Wingate anaerobic test. An update on methodology, reliability and validity. *Sports Medicine, 4,* 381–394.

Bar-Or, O. (1989). Trainability of the prepubescent child. *Physical Sports Medicine, 17*(5), 65–82.

Beek, A. J. van der, Gaalen, L. D. van, & Frings-Dresen, M. H. (1992). Working postures and activities of lorry drivers—A reliability study of on-site observation and recording on a pocket computer. *Applied Ergonomics, 23,* 331–336.

Bell, R. Q. (1954). An experimental test of the accelerated longitudinal approach. *Child Development, 25,* 281–286.

Berlin, J. A., & Colditz, G. A. (1990). A meta-analysis of physical activity in the prevention of coronary heart disease. *American Journal of Epidemiology, 132*(4), 612–620.

Beunen, G., & Malina, B. (1988). Growth and physical performance relative to the timing of the adolescent growth sport. *Exercise Sport Sciences Reviews, 16,* 503–541.

Bink, B., Bonjer, F. H., & Sluys, H. van der. (1966). Assessment of the energy expenditure by indirect time and motion study. In K. Evang & K. L. Andersen (Eds.), *Physical activity in health and disease* (pp. 207–215). Oslo, Norway: Scandinavian University Books.

Blair, S. N., Kohl, H. W. III, Paffenbarger, R. S., Clark, D. G., Cooper, K. H., & Gibbons, L. W. (1989). Physical fitness and all-cause mortality—A prospective study of healthy men and women. *Journal of the American Medical Association, 262*(17), 2395–2401.

Bouchard, C., Tremblay, A., Leblanc, C., Lortié, G., Savard, R., & Thériant, G. A. (1983). Method to assess energy expenditure in children and adults. *Journal of Clinical Nutrition, 37,* 461–467.

Caspersen, C. J. (1989). Physical activity epidemiology: Concepts, methods, and applications to exercise science. *Exercise and Sport Sciences Reviews, 17,* 423–473.

Cook, T. H., & Campbell, D. T. (1979). *Quasi Experimentation.* Chicago: Rand McNally.

Cunningham, D. A., Waterschoot, B. M. van, Paterson, D. H., Lefcoe, M., & Sangal, S. P. (1977). Reliability and reproducibility of maximal oxygen uptake measurement in children. *Medicine and Science in Sports and Exercise, 9,* 104–108.

Dishman, R. K., Sallis, J. F., & Orenstein, D. R. (1985). Determinants of physical activity and exercise. *Public Health Reports, 100*(2), 158–171.

Durnin, J. V. G. A., & Passmore, R. (1967). *Energy work and leisure.* London: Heinemann.

Edholm, O. G. (1966). The assessment of habitual activity. In K. Evang & K. L. Andersen (Eds.), *Physical activity in health and disease* (pp. 187–197). Oslo, Norway: Scandinavian University Books.

Eriksson, B. O. (1972). Physical training, oxygen supply and muscle metabolism in 11–15 year old boys. *Acta Physiologica Scandinavica, 384*(Suppl.), 1–48.

Faulkner, F., & Tanner, J. M. (Eds.). (1978). *Human Growth, Vol. 2. Postnatal Growth.* New York: Plenum.

Fox, E. L., Bowers, R. W., & Foss, M. L. (1993). *The physiological basis for exercise and sport.* Dubuque: Brown and Benckmark.

Froberg, K., Andersen, B., & Lammert, O. (1991). Maximal oxygen intake and respiratory functions during puberty in boy groups of different physical activity. In R. Frenkl &

I. Szmodis (Eds.), *Children and Exercise, Pediatric Work Physiology XV NEVI* (pp. 265–280). Budapest.

Gretebeck, R., & Montoye, H. J. (1992). Variability of some objective measures of physical activity. *Medicine and Science in Sports and Exercise, 24,* 1167–1172.

Hof, M. A. Van 't, & Kowalski, C. J. (1979). Analysis of mixed longitudinal data sets. In B. Prahl-Andersen, C. J. Kowalski, & P. Heydendael (Eds.), *A mixed-longitudinal, interdisciplinary study of growth and development.* San Francisco: Academic Press.

Hollmann, W., Hettinger, T., & Sportmedizin, Arbeits- und Trainung Grundlagen. (1976). [Sports medicine, occupational and training fundamentals]. Stuttgart: Schattauer Verlag.

Jéquier, J. C., Lavalée, H., Rajic, M., Beaucage, L., Shephard, R. J., & Labarre, R. (1977). The longitudinal examination of growth and development: History and protocol of the Trois Rivières regional study. In H. Lavallée & R. J. Shepard (Eds.), *Frontiers of activity and child health* (pp. 49–54). Ottawa, ON: Pelican.

Kemper. H. C. (Ed.). (1985). Growth, Health and Fitness of Teenagers: Longitudinal Research in International Perspective. *Medicine and Sport Sciences, 20.* Basel: Karger.

Kemper, H. C. (1986). Longitudinal studies on the development of health and fitness and the interaction with physical activity of teenagers. *Pediatrician, 13,* 52–59.

Kemper, H. C. (Ed.). (1995). The Amsterdam Growth Study, a longitudinal analysis of Health, Fitness and Lifestyle. *HKP Sport Science Monograph Series, 6.* Champaign, IL: Human Kinetics.

Kemper, H. C., & Hof, M. A. Van 't. (1978). Design of a multiple longitudinal study of growth and health in teenagers. *European Journal of Pediatrics, 129,* 147–155.

Kemper, H. C., & Kop, H. van der. (1995). Entrainement de la puissance maximale aerobic chez les enfants pre-pubères et pubères, une revue de la literature. *Science et Sports, 10*(1), 29–38.

Kemper, H. C., Twisk, J. W. R., Koppes, L. L. J. Mechelen, Van, W., & Post, G. B. (2001). A 15-year physical activity pattern is positively related to aerobic fitness in young males and females (13–27 years). *European Journal of Applied Physiology, 84,* 395–402.

Kemper, H. C., & Verschuur, R. (1977). Validity and reliability of pedometers in habitual activity research. *European Journal of Applied Physiology and Occupational Physiology, 37,* 71–82.

Kemper, H. C., & Verschuur, R. (1980). Measurement of aerobic power in teenagers. In K. Berg & B. Eriksson (Eds.), *Children and exercise: Vol. 10. International series on sport sciences* (pp. 55–63). Baltimore: University Park Press.

Kemper, H. C., & Verschuur, R. (1987). Longitudinal study of maximal aerobic power in teenagers. *Annals of Human Biology, 14*(5), 435–444.

Kemper, H. C., Verschuur, R., Ras, J. G., Snel, J., Splinter, P. G., & Tavecchio, L. W. (1976). Effect of 5 versus 3 lessons a week of physical education upon the physical development of 12 and 13 year old schoolboys. *The Journal of Sports Medicine and Physical Fitness, 16,* 319–326.

Kobayashi, K., Kitamure, K., Miura, M., et al. (1978). Aerobic power as related to body growth and training in Japanese boys: A longitudinal study. *Journal of Applied Physiology, 44,* 666–672.

Kohl, H. W., & Hobbs, K. E. (1998). Development of physical activity behaviors among children and adolescents. *Pediatrics, 101,* 549–554.

Kowalski, C. J., & Prahl-Andersen, B. (1979). *General considerations in the design of studies of growth and development.* In C. J. Kowalski, B. Prahl-Andersen, & P. Heyendael (Eds.), *A mixed longitudinal interdisciplinary study of growth and development* (pp. 3–13). New York: Academic Press.

Léger, L., & Thivierge, M. (1988). Heart rate monitors: Validity, stability, and functionality. *Physician and Sports Medicine, 16,* 143–151.

Margaria, R., Aghemo, P., & Rovelli, E. (1966). Measurement of muscular power (anaerobic) in man. *Journal of Applied Physiology, 21,* 1662–1663.

Masironi, R., & Denolin, H. (1985). *Physical activity in disease, prevention and treatment.* Padua, Italy: Piccin.

McGill, H. C., McMahan, C. A., & Malcom, G. T. for the PDAY Research group. (1997). Effects of serum lipoproteins and smoking on atherosclerosis in young men and women. *Arteriosclerosis, Thrombosis, and Vascular Biology, 17,* 95–106.

Mednick, J. A., & Baert, A. E. (Eds.). (1981). *Prospective Longitudinal Research: An Empirical Basis for the Primary Prevention of Psychosocial Disorders.* Oxford: Oxford University Press.

Mirwald, R. L., Bailey, D. A., Cameron, N., & Rasmussen, R. L. (1981). Longitudinal comparison of aerobic power in active and inactive boys aged 7.0 to 17.0 years. *Annals of Human Biology, 8*(5), 405–414.

Mirwald, R. L., & Bailey, D. A. (1985). *Longitudinal Analyses of Maximal Aerobic Power in Boys and Girls by Chronological Age, Maturity and Physical Activity.* Saskatoon: University of Saskatchewan.

Montoye, H. J. (1985). Risk indicators for cardiovascular disease in relation to physical activity in youth. In Binkhorst, Kemper, & Saris (Eds.), *Children and exercise, XI, Int. Series on Sport Sciences, 15* (pp. 3–26). Champaign, IL: Human Kinetics.

Montoye, H. J., Kemper, H. C., Saris, W. H., & Washburn, R. (1996). *Measuring physical activity and energy expenditure.* Champaign, IL: Human Kinetics.

Paffenbarger, R. S. Jr., Hyde, R. T., Wing, A. L., & Hsieh, C. C. (1986). Physical activity, all-cause mortality and longevity of college alumni. *New England Journal of Medicine, 314,* 605–613.

Pate, R. R., & Ward, D. S. (1990). Endurance exercise training ability in children and youth. In W. A. Grano, J. A. Lombardo, B. J. Sharkey, & J. A. Stone (Eds.), *Advances in sports medicine and fitness: Vol. 3* (pp. 37–55). Chicago: Year Book Medical Publishers.

Pfeiffer, R., & Francis, R. S. (1986). Effects of strength training on muscle development in prepubescent, pubescent and postpubescent males. *Phys Sports Med, 14,* 137–143.

Powell, K. E., Thompson, P. D., Caspersen, C. J., & Kendrick, J. S. (1987). Physical activity and the incidence of coronary heart disease. *Annual Review of Public Health, 8,* 253–258.

Rao, M. N., & Rao, C. R. (1966). Linked cross-sectional study for determining norms and growth rates—A pilot survey on Indian school-going boys. *Saykgya, 68,* 237–258.

Reiff, G. G., et al. (1967). Assessment of physical activity by questionnaire and interview. In M. J. Karvonen & A. J. Barry (Eds.), *Physical activity and the heart.* Springfield, IL: Charles C. Thomas.

Rowland, T. W. (1985). Aerobic response to endurance training in prepubescent children: A critical analysis. *Medicine and Science in Sports and Exercise, 17,* 493–497.

Rowland, T. W. (1990). *Exercise and children's health.* Champaign, IL: Human Kinetics.

Rutenfranz, J., Berndt, I., & Knauth, P. (1974). Daily physical activity investigated by time budget studies and physical performance capacity of schoolboys. In J. Borms & M. Hebbelink (Eds.), Children and exercise. *Acta Pediatrica Belgium, 28*(Suppl), 79–86.

Rutenfranz, J., Seliger, V., Andersen, K. L., et al. (1975). Differences in maximal aerobic power related to the daily physical activity in childhood. In G. Borg (Ed.), *Physical work and effort* (p. 279). London: Pergamon.

Sady, S. P. (1986). Cardiorespiratory exercise training in children. *Clinics in Sports Medicine, 5,* 493–514.

Sallis, J. F., Buono, M. J., & Freedson, P. S. (1991). Bias in estimating caloric expenditure from physical activity in children. Implications for epidemiological studies. *Sports Medicine, 11*(4), 203–209.

Sallis, J. F., & Patrick, K. (1994). Physical activity guidelines for adolescents. *Pediatric Exercise Science, 6*(4), 302–315.

Sallis, J. F., & Owen, N. (1999). *Physical activity and behavioral medicine.* Thousand Oaks, CA: Sage Publications.

Saris, W. H. (1982). *Aerobic power and daily physical activity in children with special reference to methods and cardiovascular risk indicators.* Thesis, Nijmegen University: Krips Repro Meppel.

Saris, W. H. (1989). Habitual physical activity in children: Methodology and findings in health and disease. *Medicine and Science in Sports and Exercise,, 18,* 253–263.

Saris, W. H., Snel, P., & Binkhorst, R. A. (1977). A portable heart rate distribution recorder for studying daily physical activity. *European Journal of Applied Physiology and Occupational Physiology, 37,* 19–25.

Schaie, K. W. (1965). A general model for the study of development problems. *Psychological Bulletin, 64,* 92–107.

Schoeller, D. A. (1983). Energy expenditure from doubly labeled water: Some fundamental considerations in humans. *American Journal of Clinical Nutrition, 38,* 999–1005.

Seliger, V. (1966). Circulatory responses to sports activities. In K. Evang & K. L. Andersen (Eds.), *Physical activity in health and disease* (pp. 198–206). Oslo, Norway: Scandinavian University Books.

Sewall, L., & Micheli, L. J. (1984). Strength training for children. *Journal of Pediatric Orthopedics, 6,* 143–146.

Shephard, K. (1982). *Physical activity and growth.* Chicago: Medical Publishers.

Sprynarova, S. (1974). Longitudinal study of the influence of different physical activity programs on functional capacity of boys from 11–18 years. *Acta Pediatrica Belgium, 28*(Suppl.), 204–213.

Stunkard, A. (1960). A method of studying physical activity in man. *American Journal of Clinical Nutrition, 8,* 595–561.

Tanner, J. M. (1962). *Growth at adolescence.* Oxford: Blackwell Scientific Publications.

Turner, C. H. (1998). Three rules for bone adaptation to mechanical stimuli. *Bone, 23,* 399–407.

Vaccaro, P., & Mahon, A. (1987). Cardiorespiratory response to endurance training in children. *Sports Medicine, 4,* 352–363.

Veling, S. H., & Hof, M. A. van 't. (1980). Data quality control methods in longitudinal studies. In M. Ostyn, G. Beunen, & J. Simons (Eds.), *Kinanthropometry II. International Series of Sports Science, 9* (pp. 436–442). Baltimore: University Park Press.

Verschuur, R. (1987). *Daily physical activity and health; Longitudinal changes during the teenage period. SO 12.* Haarlem, Netherlands: de Vrieseborch.

Verschuur, R., & Kemper, H. C. (1980). Adjustment of pedometers to make them more valid in assessing running. *International Journal of Sports Medicine, 1,* 87–89.

Verschuur, R., & Kemper, H. C. (1985). Habitual physical activity in Dutch teenagers measured by heart rate. In R. A. Binkhorst, H. C. G. Kemper, & W. H. M Saris (Eds.), *Children and exercise XI: Vol. 15. International series on sport sciences* (pp. 194–202). Champaign, IL: Human Kinetics.

Vrijens, J. (1978). Muscle strength development in the pre- and post pubescent ages. *Sports Medicine, 11,* 152–158.

Washburn, R. A., & Montoye, H. J. (1986a). The assessment of physical activity by questionnaire. *American Journal of Epidemiology, 123,* 563–570.

Washburn, R. A., & Montoye, H. J. (1986b). Validity of heart rate as a measure of mean daily energy expenditure. *Exercise Physiology, 2,* 161–172.

Weber, G., Kartodihardjo, W., & Klissouras, V. (1976). Growth and physical training with reference to heredity. *Journal of Applied Physiology, 40,* 211–215.

Weltman, A. (1984). Weight training in prepuberal children. Physiologic benefit and potential damage. In O. Bar-Or (Ed.), *Advances in pediatric sports sciences, 3.* Champaign, IL: Human Kinetics.

Wissler, R. W. (1991). USA multicenter study of the pathobiology of atherosclerosis in youth. *Annals of the New York Academy of Science, 623,* 26–39.

PART *3*

Preventable Conditions and the Impact of Behavior

CHAPTER *5*

Unintentional Injuries in Childhood and Adolescence

Kristi Alexander and Michael C. Roberts

> Safety first is an important rule
> At home, at play, and in your school!

Ⅰf only it were so easy! Despite the frequent warnings given to children and adolescents regarding their safety, unintentional injuries remain the single greatest threat to their health and well-being (Division of Injury Control, 1990; *Healthy People 2010*, 2000; Roberts & Brooks, 1987). Unintentional injuries (also referred to as nonintentional or inadvert injuries) are those unfortunate events that result in injuries to children that are *not* willfully precipitated by the actions of another person. Thus, a child who breaks an arm falling from a swing set is said to have sustained a nonintentional injury. In contrast, a similar injury, resulting from the actions of an angry parent is considered to be an instance of child abuse. This distinction, however, has been challenged by Peterson (1994) as imprecise, and possibly erroneous, in many instances.

Researchers in the field of childhood injuries have long rejected the term *accident* to describe unintentional injuries, as the former term implies an unavoidable, random event (Roberts, 1993; Rosen & Peterson, 1990). Indeed, injuries are perceived by most as resulting from behavioral and environmental factors that interact in such a way as to result in harm to an individual. Each year, countless young people experience trauma, disability, and death as the

145

result of an unintended injury. Despite the significant impact on the lives of children, adolescents, and their families, nonintentional injuries have remained the "neglected disease of modern society" (National Academy of Sciences, 1969 as cited in Rivara & Grossman, 1996).

As late as 1990, injury prevention and control were described as *"beginning* to receive a high priority" (Division of Injury Control, 1990, p. 627). Although there have been some notable exceptions (e.g., Pearn et al., 1979; Spiegel & Lindaman, 1977), attempts to reduce the high rates of unintentional injuries in childhood have been only moderately successful (Finney et al., 1993). Nonetheless, both researchers and parents agree that the vast majority of childhood unintentional injuries are preventable (Gullota & Finney, 2000; O'Shea, Collins, & Butler, 1982; Roberts, 1986; Roberts, Elkins, & Royal, 1984).

In order to develop effective prevention programs, a full understanding of the mechanisms that place children and their families at risk must be achieved. In this chapter, we will explore the many factors that affect children's injury rates, in the hopes of providing a summary of the body of empirical evidence that exists in this area. In the first section, we will report the current information regarding the prevalence and incidence of injuries to children and adolescents. Next, we will review the evidence for risk factors that emanate from children and their parents. Third, we will report the current efforts to increase children's safety by changing systems. Finally, we will discuss our thoughts about how the safety of children and adolescents may be improved.

PREVALENCE AND INCIDENCE

Among children 1–19 years old, injury is the leading cause of death (National Center for Injury Prevention and Control, 1996); accounting for more fatalities than the next six leading causes of death combined. For adolescents, the fatality rate from injuries is higher than in any other age group, except for the elderly (CDC, 2000). For children less than 15 years old, motor vehicle accidents, drownings, burns (and other fire-related injuries), and suffocations account for the majority of injury deaths. For adolescents, the causes of injury related deaths are somewhat different; motor vehicle collisions are the predominant event that results in teenage fatalities, closely followed by firearm injuries and drownings. Tragically, alcohol was associated with half of all automobile related fatalities involving teenagers (CDC, 2000). Although death in childhood is a relatively infrequent occurrence, it has been estimated that for every injury that results in death, there are 34 hospitalizations, and over 1200 emergency room visits (Gallagher, Finison, Guyer, & Goodenough, 1984). Furthermore, the difference between a fatal and nonfatal injury may be the result of a fortuitous circumstance. For example, the child who is hit by a car traveling at 25 instead of 45 mph, or the toddler who falls out of the first story window instead of a fifth floor window.

Injuries are costly for society, health care institutions, families, and victims. It was estimated that in 1990 the cost of childhood injuries was over $7.5 billion (Division of Injury Control, 1990); contributing to this sum were the nearly 16 million emergency room visits by children (Rodriguez, 1990). Furthermore, injuries are the most common condition attended to by school nurses (Nadar & Brink, 1981). Individual families also feel the financial burden of nonintentional injuries. Many families report substantial work and financial problems when their children receive even minor unintended injuries, and the financial impact increases exponentially when children and adolescents are seriously injured (Osberg, Kahn, Rowe, & Brooke, 1996; Wade et al., 2001).

CHILD RISK FACTORS

Although there is no empirical support for an injury prone child type, it does appear that some children are injured at a higher rate than others (Matheny, 1987). Furthermore, specific child characteristics, such as age and sex, appear to be related to a greater risk for injury (Rivara, 1982). In contrast to the gender and age differences, research exploring other psychosocial characteristics of children has been less conclusive (Horwitz, Morgenstern, DiPietro, & Morrison, 1988; Rivara, 1982; Rivara & Mueller, 1987). Variables such as temperament and activity level have not been consistently identified as predictors of children's risk for unintentional injuries (Horwitz et al., 1988; Rivara, 1982). In this section, we will summarize the epidemiological and behavioral evidence for factors that increase the risk of unintentional injury to children and adolescents.

Gender and Age

Several researchers have found that males have an overall higher rate of nonintentional injuries than do females beginning after 1 year of age and continuing into old age (Beautrais, Fergusson, & Shannon, 1982; Rivara, Bergman, LoGerfo, & Weiss, 1982; Rivara & Mueller, 1987). In a study of children between the ages of 1–4 years, male gender emerged as the only child variable associated with injury rates (Beautrais et al., 1982).

A sex difference has also been demonstrated for mild injuries and for close calls. Morrongiello (1997) found that with daily reporting over a 2-week period, boys presented significantly more injuries and potential injurious events than girls. Further, this researcher found that boys and girls were differentially affected by injury experiences. Boys who were injured during the 2-week period were more likely than girls to have previously engaged in the behavior that resulted in injury. In addition, boys were more likely than girls to state that they would repeat those behaviors in the future, despite the behavior having resulted in the present injury. Interestingly, despite similarities in the seriousness of the injuries sustained, boys were more likely than girls to rate their injuries as less severe. Morrongiello suggested that the sex differences in injury rates may be attributable, in part, to this discrepancy between experience and beliefs. That is, boys may be more likely to repeat risky behaviors that have resulted in injury because they rate their injuries as less critical than do girls.

Interestingly, this sex difference does not hold across injury types. In analyzing the data from nearly 200,000 injuries to children 18 years or younger, although Rivara et al. (1982) found that the overall rate for boys was higher than for girls, not all types of injuries showed this pattern. They found no sex difference for the rates of foreign body ingestions, poisonings, and burns. In contrast, lacerations and contusions were highly discrepant across sex, with boys sustaining significantly more cuts and head injuries than girls.

Some researchers have suggested that the sex difference in injury rates might be attributable to differences in exposure to risk (Manheimer & Mellinger, 1967). Rivara et al. (1982) explored this hypothesis by controlling for the differences in the amount of time children spent engaged in an activity. When controlling for children's exposure to risk, sex differences for bicycle injuries were eliminated. Rivara et al. (1982) concluded that boys had more injuries related to bicycles because they rode more. In contrast, the sex difference in playground slide injuries was not decreased when exposure was considered. Boys had more injuries involving the slide even though girls were more likely to play on the slide. They concluded that the differences in unintentional injury rates for boys and girls were not entirely due to differential exposure rates, but also appear to reflect behavioral differences.

Similarly, Routledge, Repetto-Wright, and Howrath (1974) found that despite spending equal amounts of time in road-crossing, boys had significantly higher injury rates.

In addition, the difference in nonintentional injury rates for boys and girls does not appear to be related to children's ability to assess the potential danger in a situation or to specify behaviors to reduce risk. Coppens (1985, 1986) has shown that no sex difference exists in the ability of children 3–8 to differentiate between safe and unsafe situations, or in their ability to verbalize appropriate prevention behaviors to avoid hazards depicted in pictures.

Age also contributes significantly to injury rates and is associated with both the type of injury children suffer and the resulting trauma (CDC, 2000; Matheny & Fisher, 1984; Rivara & Mueller, 1987). A developmental trend has been well documented for the types of injuries children sustain and appears to be related to the changing environments and behavior of the growing child. Toddlers, for example, are more likely to suffer falls and toxic ingestions (Matheny, 1986), while elementary school age children are more frequently involved in pedestrian accidents (Rivara et al., 1982). Adolescents between the ages of 13–19 are at highest risk for motor vehicle, firearms, sports, and drowning injuries (USDHH, 1987). Furthermore, teenage drivers are much more likely to be involved in automobile collisions in which a death occurs (Williams & Karpf, 1982). They are also 10 times more likely than younger children to be killed in a car collision (Division of Injury Control, 1990).

Age-related developmental considerations also impact child injuries. Younger children may be at greater risk for falls because of less well-developed motor skills (Angle, 1975). Likewise, the period of greatest risk for self-induced poisonings is relatively short, between the ages of 1–3 years (Flagler & Wright, 1987). Although older children may ingest toxic substances, toddlers are at greater risk because of both their newfound mobility and interest in orally exploring their environment (Baltimore & Meyer, 1968). Elementary school-age children may sustain more pedestrian injuries than adolescents because of their difficulty judging the distance and speed of oncoming cars (Malek, Guyer, & Lescohier, 1990; Phinney, Colker, & Cosgrove, 1985).

Behavioral Problems

The research exploring the relationship between nonintentional injuries and behavioral problems has often found contradictory results (Horwitz et al.,

1988; Rivara, 1982). Nonetheless, there does seem to be some relationship between behavioral problems in childhood and nonintentional injury. For example, Bijur, Golding, Haslum, and Kurzon (1988) found that overactivity and aggression partially predicted boys' injury rates. One study conducted with children from low socioeconomic backgrounds found that oppositional behavior as reported by parents predicted injury within a 1-year period, although aggression and hyperactivity did not (Jaquess & Finney, 1994). Matheny (1987) found that preschool children who had two or more nonintentional injuries were described by their mothers as more active and less adaptable than children who had not been injured.

Nyman (1987) found temperamental differences in children under 5 who had an injury-related hospitalization. Children who had been rated by their mothers at 6–8 months of age as having negative or difficult temperamental characteristics, such as negative mood and poor reactions to new situations, were more likely to have sustained a serious injury. Because this study investigated only hospitalized children, it is questionable if the relationship between temperament and injuries would hold with less severely impacted children.

Similarly, Cataldo and colleagues (1992) found significant differences between the behavior of injured and noninjured preschoolers in a simulated hazard situation. Children who had been previously injured were more disruptive in their play; they were observed to break objects, hit, and kick more than noninjured children. Further, previously injured children exhibited greater changes in activity and less appropriate play behaviors. Although this study did not examine the behavior of children in an actual injury event, the results appear to suggest that problem behaviors may contribute to children's injury risk.

The relationship between specific childhood disorders and injury risk is less clear. Gayton, Bailey, Wagner, and Hardesty (1986) found support for a relationship between hyperactivity and accident proneness for both boys and girls as reported by mothers on Achenbach's Child Behavior Checklist. In contrast, Davidson's (1987) extensive review of the literature on hyperactivity and childhood nonintentional injuries found equivocal support for a relation between the two.

Attentional Problems

The ability to attend appropriately to situations has been posited as a potential risk factor for unintended injury. In a study with adults, Hansen (1989) found that industrial workers who received many work related injuries also possessed high levels of distractibility. A similar relationship has been found for preschool children; those who had sustained two or more injuries were described by their mothers as less attentive than were children who had not been injured (Matheny, 1987).

Although an unequivocal relationship has not been established between attentional problems such as Attention Deficit Hyperactivity Disorder (ADHD) and nonintentional injuries, some evidence does exist that children with ADHD who are injured sustain more severe injuries than do children without ADHD (DiScala, Lescohier, Banthel, & Li, 1998). Components of ADHD such as impulsivity may increase children's risk for injury. In a study of child pedestrian injuries, the most frequently occurring injury was the result of the *midblock dart-out*. Midblock dart-out occurs when children run into the street, frequently from between parked cars, in the path of an oncoming vehicle. This behavior may occur when children are distracted by other children or an activity, and further supports the contention that impulsive responding to a situation may increase a child's risk for injury (Malek et al., 1990).

Risk-Taking

Several researchers (Jelalian et al., 1997; Potts, Martinez, & Dedmon, 1995) have found a positive relationship between self-reported risk taking in childhood and adolescence and nonintentional injury. Further, with the Injury Behavior Checklist (IBC; Speltz, Gonzales, Sulzbacher, & Quan, 1990), children's injuries were predicted accurately from parent-reported risk-taking. In contrast, Padilla, Rohsenow, and Bergman (1976) concluded that risk-taking behavior was *not* predictive of childhood nonintentional injuries.

Perception of risk may also influence unintentional injury rates, particularly with adolescents who may attribute less risk to their behavior. Indeed, Cohn, MacFarlane, Yanez, and Imani (1995) found that teenagers were more likely than their parents to regard behaviors such as not using seat belts as less harmful and less likely to result in injury. Similarly, surveys of parents and middle-school aged children found that "parents are largely ignorant of the extent to which their adolescents are involved in major risk behaviors" (Young & Zimmerman, 1998, p. 1137). In an interesting study, parents of 8–12 year-old boys were asked to predict their child's actual behavior if he found a gun (Jackman, Farah, Kellerman, & Simon, 2001). Contrary to parental predictions, close to three fourths of the boys handled a gun upon discovery (in a controlled situation) and some pulled the triggers hard enough to have caused it to fire. This study dramatically illustrated the discrepancy of parental perception and child risky behavior.

Previous Injuries

Several studies have found that previously injured children are more likely than their noninjured peers to sustain additional injuries. Bijur, Golding, and Haslum (1988) found that children who had one or two injuries during their first 5 years of life were twice as likely to be involved in multiple unintended injury events between the ages of 5–10 years. Furthermore, the best predictor of injuries for children in the 5–10 year old age group was the number of injuries reported at age 5. Similarly, Emission, Jones, and Goldacre (1986) found that preschool children who were hospitalized for a nonintentional injury were twice as likely to be hospitalized again, even when controlling for age and sex. For young, low-SES children attending a day camp, the best predictor of injury during the week long day camp was having received an injury in the past year (Jaquess & Finney, 1994). Furthermore, of the 10 children who had sustained an injury in the past year, 7 of these children were injured during the camp period. One study has examined the child factors that may be responsible for the high concordance between past and future injury rates. In a laboratory setting, it was found that previously injured children were more likely to touch simulated hazards than were children who had not been injured (Cataldo et al., 1992).

PARENTAL RISK FACTORS

Some parents appear to impose a greater injury liability on their children than others. In contrast to the literature examining children's risk factors, unintentional injury research has focused less on the actions of parents that may contribute to their progeny's injury rates (Peterson & Stern, 1997). That parents are responsible for the health and well-being of their children is, for the most part, an indisputable fact. It has been demonstrated that parents recognize that they hold the responsibility of preventing injury to their children (Peterson, Farmer, & Kashani, 1990) and in the case of young children, intervene most often in their child's activities to prevent injury (Gralinski & Kopp, 1993). Further, most parents believe that unintentional injury is avoidable and that more than half of serious injuries are preventable (Eichelberger,

Gotschall, Feely, Harstad, & Bowman, 1990). Nevertheless, despite the good intentions of parents, children continue to be injured.

Parental Age

Despite the comparatively fewer investigations of the characteristics of parents, there is support for some parental demographic variables as predictors of children's injury histories. One variable that has often been associated with children's injury risk is parental age. Taylor, Wadsworth, and Butler (1983) found that preschool children of teenage mothers had a greater number of hospital admissions for unintended injuries than did children of older parents. The authors found that injuries both in the home and outdoors occurred with significantly greater frequency among the children of adolescent mothers while those occurring in nursery schools or as a result of a traffic nonintentional injuries were not correlated with maternal age. Although the teenaged mothers' children were at greater risk for all types of injuries, they appeared particularly at risk for poisonings and burns and superficial injuries or lacerations. Expectant adolescent mothers, in a more recent study, were found to identify fewer potentially dangerous situations than were adult mothers (McClure-Martinez & Cohn, 1996).

Another study supporting a link between maternal age and unintentional injury examined household safety, a factor associated with nonintentional injuries. Alexander and Reeker (1997) found that younger mothers of preschool children (less than 30 years of age) had more potential hazards in their homes than did older mothers. Although household safety alone does not predict injuries, it does appear to pose an additional risk factor for children (Mori & Peterson, 1986; Scheidt, 1988).

Although research on demographic variables helps describe the parents and caregivers involved in children's unintended injuries, it contributes little to understanding of why injuries occur. Therefore, the need for information regarding parental *behavior* is essential for the development and implementation of injury prevention. Research has demonstrated that the experience of an unintended injury to one's child (Baker, 1980), the provision of safety devices (Dershewitz & Christophersen, 1984; Dershewitz & Williamson, 1977), or educational programs (Colver, Hutchinson, & Judson, 1982), are not sufficient to change the behavior of parents with respect to their children's safety. Other researchers have concluded that teaching parents or children safety behaviors is not enough; "we must investigate the beliefs, attitudes, and emotions that influence skills and the use of behavioral knowledge" (Peterson et al., 1990, p. 189).

Supervision

The ability of parents to provide appropriate supervision is a critical factor in children's injury rates (Garling & Garling, 1991; Peterson, Cook, Little, & Schick, 1991). One study found that the likelihood of children being injured by fireworks was more than 11 times greater if they were not supervised (McFarland, Harris, Kobayashi, & Dicker, 1984). Similarly, Morrongiello (1997) found that children were more likely to be injured not when supervised, but when they were with other children. This difference was particularly true for 8–10 year-old boys. It may be, however, that parents' supervision practices interact with children's behavior to result in injury. One study found that when parents were distracted, previously injured children exhibited more disruptive behavior (Cataldo et al., 1992). Interestingly, this study found no differences between the parents of injured and non injured children in the warnings they gave to their children to prevent potential injury.

Factors Decreasing Supervision

Research strongly suggests that any variable that reduces an adult's ability to supervise may increase children's risk for nonintentional injury (Rivara, 1982). Squires and Busuttil (1995) found that alcohol was involved in nearly a third of all child household fire fatalities during the past decade. In most of these cases, the parents were the ones who were intoxicated, although in others, grandparents, older siblings, and babysitters were the individuals who had used alcohol.

Similarly, other factors that may divert parents' attention may result in higher rates of unintended injury to their children. There is evidence that factors such as large families, poor urban neighborhoods, and frequent household moves increase children's risk for injury (Taylor et al., 1983). Abidin (1982) found that mothers who reported high and low levels of stress brought their children for medical care for injuries more often than mothers reporting moderate stress. Stress may affect an individual's ability to avoid injury to him or herself as well. The results of one study found that elite female gymnasts who reported greater stress were more likely to sustain an injury (Kerr & Minden, 1988).

Cognitive factors and beliefs may also affect parental supervision. The experience of injury to one's child would assumedly have the potential to impact a parent's beliefs about injury and safety. Glik, Kronfield, and Jackson (1991) found that parents of children injured in the past year were more likely to perceive potential risks as resulting in serious injury than were parents whose children had not been injured. Furthermore, this *perceived risk* was negatively associated the actual number of risk factors found in the home; the homes of injured children had fewer injury hazards than did the homes of noninjured children. In contrast, Langley and Silva (1982) found no differences among mothers with respect to their attitudes towards prevention, regardless of their children's unintentional injury histories. Because of the equivocal relationship found between parent's beliefs about accident prevention and their child's history of nonintentional injury, further investigations of the cognitive factors affecting parents' behavior are warranted (Peterson et al., 1990).

The problem in determining the relationship between beliefs and behaviors may be due, in part, to the competing demands experienced by parents. Caregivers struggle to raise healthy, autonomous individuals, but also must provide sufficient supervision to ensure their children's well-being. Squires and Busuttil (1995) contend that part of the difficulty may lie in the "poorly defined border between encouraging appropriate independence . . . and inadequate supervision" (p. 872). Evidence of this weak border is easily found. For example, a survey of parents of teenage drivers found that although parents supported a probationary license for 16–17 year olds, they rejected the idea of a restrictive license that would prohibit these young drivers from operating motor vehicle during a high-risk time period, between midnight and 6 a.m. (Plato & Rasp, 1983). Parents of teenagers attending drivers' education training reported that vehicle size and weight (i.e., crashworthiness) were not important features in choosing cars for the teens to drive, whereas gas mileage and other safety features that are considered less effective were higher priorities in selecting a car (Rivara, Rivara, & Bartol, 1998).

Fagot (1974) found that parents identified roughhouse play and aggressive behavior as appropriate for boys and therefore, may inadvertently encourage boys to participate in behaviors that have a higher risk for unintentional injury. Similarly, parents may not restrict the behavior of boys, even when they perceive the child's behavior to be risky (Block, 1983).

Parents' locus of control has also been suggested as a variable that may mediate the relationship between parental safety behavior and children's inadvertent injury rates (Coppens, 1985). Locus of control has been demonstrated to be related to overall parental functioning (Galejs & Pease, 1986; Swick & Graves, 1986), and parents' beliefs about the origin of their children's behavior problems (Harris & Nathan, 1973). With respect to injuries, one study found that mothers of previously injured children scored in the external direction on both Rotter's (1966) measure and on the Accident Locus of Control scale (Coppens, 1985), indicating that they believed they had less control over events in their lives. In contrast, like the high functioning parents described by Galejs and Pease (1986), the mothers of children who had not had an unintentional injury scored in the internal direction on both these measures (Alexander, 1992).

Safety Practices

Similar to supervision, parents' beliefs about the importance of safety practices may also affect children's risk for unintentional injury. Most parents report being aware of risk and dangers within the home and report taking action to decrease the household hazards (Thuen, 1992). However, many parents appear uninterested in learning specific ways to safeguard their children's environment (Eichelberger et al., 1990). O'Brien (1996) found that only 20% of parents of infants and toddlers reported needing household safety information, despite the high incidence of injuries stemming from household causes.

Despite the reported safety awareness of parents, household safety remains a serious problem in many homes. Furthermore, it has been found that mothers of preschoolers report more safety behavior (e.g., childproofing house, etc.) than was actually observed in their homes (Wortel & de Gues, 1993). In addition, considerable variability was found in safety behavior. For example, while 95% of mothers in this study stored medicines safely, nearly 30% did not take similar precautions with poisonous plants or cosmetics, both hazards for poisonings. Similar results were found within the burn-risk category. Although the vast majority of mothers kept coffee pots and matches out of children's reach, over 90% of mothers did not have a stove guard or safety mechanism on the oven doors (Wortel & de Gues, 1993). Interestingly, Langley and Silva (1982) found no difference between the safety practices of mothers whose children had sustained an injury and those mothers whose children had not been injured. This suggested that, for some individuals, the perception of risk may be unrelated to their personal experience. Supervisory style, in contrast, was strongly related to a reduction in household safety hazards (Glik, Greaves, Kronenfeld, & Jackson, 1993).

Educational level is another factor that may impact parental safety behavior. Glik et al. (1993) found that the homes of preschool children whose mothers had a high school education (or less) had more household hazards, notably accessible poisons. In contrast, Wortel and de Gues (1993) did not find that Dutch mothers with less than 9 years of education differed significantly from mothers with more education, in regard to their safety behavior. Farah, Simon, and Kellermann (1999) found that a little over half of parents who were firearms owners stored the guns loaded or unlocked (both unsafe practices) and underestimated the risk to their children.

In summary, supervision and safety practices have been shown to be important parent variables affecting children's injury rates. The factors that influence these behaviors, however, have yet to be clearly delineated (Gulotta & Finney, 2000). Much more work must be undertaken to develop the necessary understanding of these complex behaviors.

CHANGING SYSTEMS TO INCREASE SAFETY

Interventions to prevent injuries in childhood can focus on one of three overlapping mechanisms or targets of approach: (a) target caregivers to take preventive action on behalf of the child, (b) target children to take preventive action for themselves, and (c) target the environment and institutions (Roberts et al., 1984). This simple framework will organize the following sections as we discuss how systems can be changed to increase the safety of children and adolescents in the hazardous environments where they live, play, and learn.

Caregivers' Preventive Actions

Society assumes that parents and other caregivers (e.g., daycare providers) are responsible for arranging and maintaining the various situations in which children are placed (e.g., school, home, play areas). Consequently, over time, a great deal of expense and effort has been directed at providing information and motivation to influence parents and caregivers to improve, or childproof, environments. These efforts are based on three assumptions: (a) parents have the appropriate knowledge to make decisions about safe environments, (b) they are motivated to take action, and (c) they have effective control over their children's situations. Although these assumptions may not be true in all cases, much of the injury prevention effort has been directed at parents and caregivers to become safer.

General Health and Safety Information

The most frequent form of safety intervention is likely to be the provision of information to parents and other caregivers about potential hazards. As noted, the assumption of such education is that, once the appropriate information is available, parents will choose to take the necessary safety actions on behalf of their children. Most health information for parents is generally provided in brochures and handouts on a range of home safety situations such as household poisons, electrical hazards, or falls. Rarely have these types of informational interventions been evaluated for their efficacy. What evidence does exist regarding the effectiveness of these efforts is spotty at best (Pless & Arsenault, 1987). Nevertheless, they remain the most prevalent form of preventive interventions.

Success for parental health education programs was reported for increasing the use of child safety seats (Christophersen, Sosland-Edelman, & LeClaire, 1985), the acquisition of smoke detectors (Miller, Reisinger, Blatter, & Wucher, 1982), and home safety (Bass, Mehta, Otrovsky, & Halperin, 1985). In contrast, other early studies of health education found no change in caregivers' preventive behaviors such as poison control in the home (Lacouture, Minisci, Gouveia, & Lovejoy, 1978), buckling children in safety seats and seat belts before the advent of state laws (Roberts & Turner, 1984), and general home injury prevention (Dershewitz & Williamson, 1977; Schlesinger et al., 1966). In an evaluation of an intervention with day care center directors, information about playground safety was coupled with an expert's identification of hazards in the centers (Sacks, Brantley, Holmgreen, & Rochat, 1992). A return visit to check whether modifications had taken place to improve the centers' playgrounds revealed that the informational intervention was not effective. Despite the generally poor empirical evidence of their efficacy, informational campaigns directed at caregivers remain a popular form of injury prevention.

Instruction and Incentive Programs

When provided with relevant information and more importantly, also given a chance to practice and receive feedback about safety enhancing behaviors (often associated with incentives to perform them), parents do improve the safety of their children's environment. For example, one program successfully intervened with families whose hazardous homes posed risks to their children. The intervention involved the use of an assessment instrument coupled with comprehensive safety instructions (Barone, Greene, & Lutzker, 1986; Tertinger, Greene, & Lutzker, 1984). Similarly, rewarding parents for having their young children and infants riding in safety seats increased this safety behavior (Roberts & Turner, 1986). Nevertheless, these forms of intervention, despite demonstrated effectiveness, are infrequently employed because of the time, energy, and cost required.

Pediatrician-Provided Counseling and Information

Pediatricians are often the source of information about prevention of injuries. For example, physicians have been found to be the major providers of information about bicycle safety and helmet use by their patients (Ruch-Ross & O'Connor, 1993). A formal program was initiated by the American Academy of Pediatrics (AAP) entitled: The Injury Prevention Program—TIPP. The goal of this program was the provision of high-quality and accurate materials for assessment and information to pediatricians and parents. Regrettably, this program was not fully evaluated from its inception, some assessment of effects has been extrapolated from studies of injury prevention counseling during pediatric visits (Bass et al., 1993; Hansen, Wong, & Young, 1996; Miller & Galbraith, 1995).

Although not assessing TIPP, one intervention study found that when physicians counseled patients using an information pamphlet, there was no impact beyond a control condition in self-reported acquisition and use of children's bicycle helmets (Cushman, James, & Waclawik, 1991). This type of limitation on outcome led Runyan and Runyan (1991) to conclude: "very few successes have been reported in patient education about injury control" (p. 972). One moderate success was documented in teaching new parents about poisons and the need for having ipecac syrup in the house in case of ingestion of poisons by newborns and young children (Cooper, Widness, & O'Shea, 1988). Despite the limitations on effectiveness, pediatricians and health care personnel remain important sources of safety information for caregivers.

Community Efforts

In various communities, local agencies, institutions, and organizations combine efforts to target the adult caregivers to change unsafe situations or behavior in children and adolescents. These efforts can be associated with changes in laws (e.g., seat belt or bicycle helmet laws), or sometimes these activities are developed because of a perceived need to do something, but legislative action is not the goal. In some cases, community programs and public awareness campaigns are undertaken in order to avoid having to put legislation into effect. For example, some communities have developed giveaway or discount programs for smoke detectors (e.g., Gorman, Charney, Holtzman, & Roberts, 1985; Shaw, McCormick, Kustra, Ruddy, & Casey, 1988). In contrast, community organizations offering discount coupons and information about the need for bicycle helmets have had muted success (e.g., Bergman, Rivara, Richards, & Rogers, 1990; Cushman et al., 1991; DiGuiseppi, Rivara, Koepsell, & Polissar, 1989).

All too often, community interventions fail to empirically evaluate their effects or, when evaluations are conducted, fail to change as a result of any negative findings. For example, the DARE (Drug Abuse Resistance Education) program, the nationwide substance abuse intervention implemented by local police agencies and supported by federal funds, has been found to be ineffective (Ennett, Tobler, Ringwalt, & Flewelling, 1994). DARE, however, remained widely disseminated and considered a key part of the drug abuse prevention effort in America. It has been revamped recently, but the revised curriculum remains to be evaluated. In the case of prevention of sexual abuse, one survey of prevention materials found very little scientific base in their development (e.g., Roberts, Alexander, & Fanurik, 1990).

CHILD-ORIENTED PREVENTIVE ACTIONS

A second major approach to increasing children's safety is to target the children to take the necessary actions to protect themselves from harm. The rationale for this approach is that "training to assume responsibility for health behaviors early in life, may lead to lifelong positive habits. This involves both avoiding hazards and adopting positive behavior" (Roberts, 1986, p. 148). Often it is believed that targeting younger children to adopt safer behaviors will be more effective than waiting until risky behaviors become more prevalent, for example, in the adolescent years (Roberts, Maddux, & Wright, 1984). Programs to encourage children to take responsibility for safer behaviors, therefore, are oriented to improving the safety of the child at the time and also for the future.

Seatbelt Use

The reduction of fatalities and serious injuries by the use of seatbelts and child safety seats has been well-established (e.g., Osberg & Di Scala, 1992). Rates of seatbelt use are climbing as result of a number of factors, including laws in all 50 states mandating children's use of seat belts. The greater use, however, is a recent phenomenon. Previously, rates of safety belt use were extremely low. Consequently, behaviorally-oriented interventions directed to children to take responsibility for their own use of car safety devices were developed. In a series of studies at day care centers and elementary schools, Roberts and his colleagues demonstrated that rewarding the children directly could significantly increase their use of safety belts and seats (Roberts, Alexander, & Knapp, 1990; Roberts & Broadbent, 1989; Roberts & Fanurik, 1986; Roberts, Fanurik, & Layfield, 1987; Roberts, Fanurik, & Wilson, 1988, summarized in Roberts, Layfield, & Fanurik, 1991). The success of these interventions demonstrates that children's safety behavior may be changed, although not without significant effort.

Bicycle Helmet Use

Like seatbelts, the use of bicycle safety helmets has demonstrated value in reducing serious head injury and death (Thompson, Rivara, & Thompson, 1989). Nevertheless, most children do not wear these safety helmets; current usage rate estimates range from 15%–35% (Murray & Linscheid, 1991; Weiss, 1992). One student-oriented intervention program targeted children directly by offering safety information and incentives for helmet use. This study found an initial increase from 0% usage to 5% and a later rate of 17% (Murray & Linscheid, 1991). Another incentive program offering a popular collectible (i.e., POG disks) to children when wearing helmets found that use increased from 48% to 67% (Willis, 1997). These studies suggest that contingent reinforcement can be effective in increasing the use of bicycle helmets by children in much the same way as found by Roberts and colleagues for seat belt use.

Emergency Skills

Other child-oriented interventions have targeted children's behavior during emergencies (e.g., house fires) as one way to decrease the chances of injury or death. These programs, utilizing information, behavioral practice, and feedback, have taught children how to recognize an emergency situation and how to make emergency telephone calls, or how to exit a room or building in case of a fire (e.g., Hillman, Jones, & Farmer, 1986; Jones & Kazdin, 1980). These programs have demonstrated successful acquisition of safety response behaviors and their long-term retention for preschool and elementary school children, as well as children who are blind or mentally retarded.

Pedestrian Skills

Efforts to teach children safer ways to cross streets have shown some behavioral improvement and generalization beyond where the training took place (e.g., Yeaton & Bailey, 1978). A more recent pedestrian training intervention was conducted in a community-based program to teach school children (kindergarten through grade 4) street-crossing skills (Rivara, Booth, Bergman, Rogers, & Weiss, 1991). Although significant increases were observed in the children's safe behaviors, the overall effect was relatively modest, while the cost of the intervention was fairly expensive.

Other Safety Behaviors

Additional child-oriented preventive efforts have been evaluated for training children in home safety while alone (Peterson, 1989), spinal cord injury prevention through school-based curricula (Richards, Hendricks, & Roberts, 1991), and child self-protective behaviors for molestation and sexual abuse (Poche, Brouwer, & Swearingen, 1981; Wurtele & Miller-Perrin, 1992). These efforts typically rely on intensive, behaviorally-based interventions to achieve significant increases in the safety behavior. However, the most ubiquitous safety education program, driver's education in high school, does not appear to reduce motor vehicle crashes (Vernick et al., 1999). In fact, early licensure often associated with driver training may expose teenagers to higher risks for crashes.

Caveats About Child-Oriented Prevention

Several cautions regarding the child-oriented approach to improving children's safety must be considered. First, parents often assume that child is protected if he or she has been trained in an area (e.g., swimming lessons or "drown-proofing"). This parental perception might lead to decreased diligence of supervision (supervision being the key to injury prevention). Indeed, parents have been shown to hold beliefs about their children's safety behavior that are either not true or not safe enough (Eichelberger et al., 1990; Peterson, Farmer, & Kashani, 1991). Peterson (1989), for example, after designing a demonstrably successful program for home safety for children home alone after school, found that parents showed lessened supervision of their own. She expressed concern that these children's preparation for self-care was "overestimated, under rehearsed and unsafe" (p. 36). (A related issue was raised by Dershewitz, 1977, who found that there were no changes of improved safety after a health education program for parents, but the participants believed that their homes had fewer hazards afterwards.)

A second concern is that this approach assumes that children must be the responsible agents for safety when responsibility may more appropriately reside with the adults in the child's life, both proximal (parents/caregivers) and distal (legislators). Individual responsibility is an important American philosophy, but it may be inappropriately applied to children who have little control over their own environments (Finney et al., 1993; Roberts et al., 1984).

Third, child-oriented prevention assumes that children may have developmental skills that they do not have; for example, motoric or cognitive abilities characteristic of older children or adults (Finney et al., 1993; Maddux, Roberts, Sledden, & Wright, 1986). Placing responsibility on children for circumstances beyond their developmental understanding or ability to change is clearly inappropriate.

ENVIRONMENT AND PUBLIC POLICY

The third major approach to injury prevention/control is to change the environment, generally through public policy decision making. When advocating safer environments for children, injury preventionists frequently invoke the term passive prevention. This represents one end of a continuum of active to passive interventions (Finney et al., 1993). *Active injury* control strategies are those in which the individual must make repeated action each time in order to receive any protection from injury (e.g., putting on the seat belt each time for the car driver; wearing a safety helmet for the motorcyclist). *Passive interventions*, in contrast, are those in which there is limited or no individual action required; the injury control has been built-in so that it occurs regardless of the individual's behavior (e.g., safer road designs, air bags on car, childproof caps on medicines and poisons).

Passive prevention has also been called *environmental* or *structural intervention*. Of course, even in passive prevention, somebody has to take some action; first, to require some preventive improvement for the environment and second, to implement the changes necessary to gain safety benefit. Some public health advocates assert that passive prevention or environmental changes are best because protection is afforded everybody. Others acknowledge that passive prevention is often hard to implement given political realities, limitations on what structural change can be accomplished, and lack of consensus over what are the most appropriate changes. Additionally, active interventions may be most effective or necessary when the limits of passive efforts have been reached. The previous two sections dealt primarily with active interventions with individuals (caregivers, children) to improve their own safety behavior. In this section, we consider environmental or passive prevention measures. These include mandating structural changes to the child's environment through legislative acts and agency regulations to make it safer.

Consumer Product Safety Commission (CPSC)

A number of legislative acts to improve children's safety are now administered under the regulatory agency of the CPSC. These have restricted the ease of accessibility of poisons and drugs for infants and young children through the Poison Prevention Packaging Act of 1970 and later amendments. As a result, the number of inadvertent poisonings has declined significantly (Clarke & Walton, 1979; Smith & Falk, 1987; Walton, 1982). The Flammable Fabric Act of 1967 ensured that children's sleepwear is treated with flame retardants, resulting in fewer burns to children (McLoughlin, Clark, Stahl, & Crawford, 1977; Smith & Falk, 1987). The Refrigerator Safety Act of 1982 minimized the possibilities of entrapment of children in discarded refrigerators and freezers. Other regulations changed crib designs to prevent strangulation and suffocation by eliminating decorations and side slats.

A frequent safety intervention imposed by the CPSC has been the addition of warning labels about small parts in toys that might choke a younger child. These are not environmental interventions, but similar to health education for caregivers with similarly poor results. For example, research has demonstrated that some parents view age-appropriateness labels as indicating that the precocious younger child would be developmentally stimulated by an older-age toy, thus exposing the child to inappropriate hazards (Langlois et al., 1991).

Within their limited overview, the CPSC can require the recall of unsafe items, but more often it negotiates with manufacturers for voluntary action. Although much of the public believes that its safety is being protected through the review procedures and regulations of the CPSC, the reality is that very few of products on the market are actually covered (Christoffel & Christoffel, 1989). The CPSC has severely limited authority and insufficient staff to consider comprehensively the safety of all products for sale in the United States. For example, two major causes of death and injury, firearms and motor vehicles, are expressly stated as out of the CPSC jurisdiction. Many products, often used by or with children, remained in the marketplace for too long, despite being associated with high rates of injuries (e.g., eye-piercing projectiles, minibikes and all-terrain vehicles, thin plastic bags used by drycleaners, baby walkers, and fireworks). Thus, despite public perceptions, many products still contribute to a hazardous environment for children. Nonetheless, when imposed by regulations and policy, environmental changes can have significant effects.

Playground and Pedestrian Safety

Acknowledging the limitations of child training programs and children's ability to judge hazards, structural interventions have been proposed as the most effective for improving the safety of children at play or while walking close to traffic. Environmental designs are effective when barriers separate play and pedestrian areas from high volume, high speed traffic (Bergman & Rivara, 1991; Rivara, 1990).

Safety Seat and Safety Belt Laws

One legislative effort to improve children's safety has come through the enactment of state laws requiring the use of infant safety seats and seat belts for children in most states. This enhancement of car passenger safety was a long-term and often politically contentious effort (Roberts, 1994). Despite the fact that the state laws have numerous loopholes and variable enforcement, public health researchers have accumulated considerable evidence of the effectiveness of these laws in saving lives and controlling injury (Chorba, Reinfurt, & Hulka, 1988; Wagenaar, Maybee, & Sullivan, 1988).

Bicycle Helmet Laws

Legislation requiring bicycle riders to wear safety helmets has also had positive effects on children's usage. For example, in Australia, a mandatory helmet law resulted in an increase of use from 30–90% (Vulcan, Cameron, & Watson, 1992). In one county in Maryland, an increase from 4–47% resulted after passage of a law requiring helmets on county roads or bikepaths for children under 16 years of age (Dannenberg, Gielen, Beilenson, Wilson, & Joffe, 1993).

Gun Control Laws

Firearms are not under the legal purview of the CPSC and laws regulating firearms to reduce both intentional and unintentional death and injuries have been vehemently resisted by certain organizations such as the National Rifle Association. In states where children's access to guns is more restricted by law, there is increasing evidence of safety benefits in reduction of firearm deaths (Cummings, Grossman, Rivara, & Koepsell, 1997; Webster & Starnes, 2000).

Limitations on Regulations and Environmental Interventions

One important limitation on the CPSC and other public policy efforts toward greater safety through environmental changes has been the political sensitivity of the government at all levels in making regulations that affect business, cost money, and intrude into citizens' personal freedoms (Brooks & Roberts, 1990; Peterson & Roberts, 1992). The example of laws for the mandatory use of infant/child safety devices and seat belts for children and adults is particularly illustrative of a situation where such laws were resisted as intrusions in the private lives of citizens, but were eventually enacted in most states following over 20 years of political wrangling (Roberts, 1994). Thus, although usually quite effective, environmental changes are often the most difficult to enact.

CONCLUSIONS

As this review indicates, there does not seem to be one single target (caregiver, child, or environment) that allows for a complete and effective intervention to prevent injury to children. Multilevel, multitargeted, and multimethod approaches seem necessary.

In this chapter we have described the significance of children's injuries, how they occur, and how injuries might be prevented or controlled. In this description, we have relied on the scientific literature without discrimination as to the discipline or approach taken in the empirical study of injuries and their prevention. Some of the literature was derived from a public health perspective utilizing epidemiological techniques or health education programming. Some aspects have come from a pediatric or child health psychology orientation. Relatedly, traditions of medicine and nursing have made important contributions to understanding childhood injuries and their prevention or control. We find value in these various approaches both in explaining the circumstances of childhood injuries as well as in developing and evaluating effective intervention strategies. The debate over what is the most effective and appropriate approach to finding solutions to the injury has often been rancorous, sometimes obscuring the importance of the topic and its effects on the quality of life for children. Such methodological and philosophical antagonisms have diminished communication, such that Roberts (1987) called the clashes of orientation a "catfight." This manifested itself in professional iconoclasm and chauvinism, turf ownership, needless disparagement or put-down of alternative ideas in publications, and isolation of the professional fields. Although some amelioration of extreme positions has been made over time, there remain some significant differences in the approaches to injury prevention and control. These hinder development of effective solutions.

A multifaceted approach is necessary for greater progress in understanding the occurrence of injuries and their control. New approaches and methodologies are required in which methods are combined and new ones are developed. Thus, for example, there has been an increased consideration by public health epidemiologists in looking at more detailed or molecular examination of injury events and by behavioral psychologists in developing larger scale implications and data sets.

The comprehensive report, *Injury Prevention: Meeting the Challenge*, published in 1989 by the National Committee for Injury Prevention and Control, articulated the need for "thorough and systematic consideration of several basic questions" (pp. 35–36):

- Who is being injured?
- How are these people being injured?
- Where are these injuries taking place?
- What are the circumstances under which these injuries occur?
- How serious are these injuries?
- How many of these injuries have occurred, and over what period of time?
- Which of these injuries is most significant in its personal and social consequences?
- Is the local injury rate from a particular type of injury higher, or lower, than the national (or state) rate?
- What information will be needed to evaluate an intervention?

Answers to these questions will come not from a single discipline or a single methodological approach, but from a comprehensive view utilizing all sources of information. As *Injury Prevention: Meeting the Challenge* stated "it is rare that a single intervention will significantly reduce a complex injury problem" such that preventionists "should carefully consider a mix of legislation/enforcement/education/behavior change, and engineering/technology interventions that complement each other and increase the likelihood of success" (p. 72).

A developmental perspective is particularly important in the childhood injury area because children are developing organisms, ever changing in their abilities in reciprocal interactions with their environment (Maddux et al., 1986). Of course, these environments include not just the physical arrangements of their settings (e.g., home, school, play areas), but also the humans around them (e.g., parents/caregivers, other adults, siblings, peers). A developmental perspective helps determine when during the lifespan certain interventions and prevention efforts are most needed and for what kinds of problems and when the efforts should be offered to maximize efficacy and acceptance by a child or those responsible for the child (Roberts et al., 1984). The recognition of developmental aspects transcends discipline and methodological orientation. The interdisciplinary effort needed to control or prevent injuries in childhood will necessarily involve the contributions of numerous scientific disciplines in making all aspects of children's environments safer and conducive to health and development (*Healthy People 2010*, 2000).

REFERENCES

Abidin, R. R. (1982). Parenting stress and utilization of pediatric services. *Children's Health Care, 11,* 70–73.

Alexander, K. (1992). *Accidental injuries in childhood: Comparison of the contributions from parents and children.* Unpublished doctoral dissertation, University of Alabama, Tuscaloosa.

Alexander, K., & Reeker, J. (1997). Nonintentional injuries in preschool children: The relationship of maternal locus of control to household safety. Unpublished manuscript.

Angle, C. R. (1975). Locomotor skills and school accidents. *Pediatrics, 56,* 819–822.

Baltimore, C. L., & Meyer, R. J. (1968). A study of storage, child behavioral traits, and mother's knowledge of toxicology in 52 poisoned families and 52 comparison families. *Pediatrics, 42,* 312–317.

Baker, S. (1980). Prevention of childhood injuries. *The Medical Journal of Australia, 1,* 466–470.

Barone, V. J., Greene, B. F., & Lutzker, J. R. (1986). Home safety with families being treated with child abuse and neglect. *Behavior Modification, 10,* 93–114.

Bass, J. L., Christoffel, K. K., Widome, M., Boyle, W., Scheidt, P., Stanwick, R., & Roberts, K. (1993). Childhood injury prevention counseling in primary care settings: A critical review of the literature. *Pediatrics, 92,* 544–550.

Bass, J. L., Mehta, K. A., Otrovsky, M., & Halperin, S. F. (1985). Educating parents about injury prevention. *Pediatric Clinics of North America, 32,* 233–242.

Beautrais, A., Fergusson, D., & Shannon, F. (1982). Childhood accidents in a New Zealand birth cohort. *Australian Paediatric Journal, 18,* 238–242.

Bergman, A. B., & Rivara, F. P. (1991). Reducing childhood injuries in Sweden. *Pediatrics, 88,* 69–74.

Bergman, A. B., Rivara, F. P., Richards, D. D., & Rogers, L. W. (1990). The Seattle children's bicycle helmet campaign. *American Journal of Diseases of Children, 144,* 727–731.

Bijur, P., Golding, J., & Haslum, M. (1988). Persistence of occurrence of injury: Can injuries of preschool children predict injuries of school-aged children? *Pediatrics, 82,* 707–712.

Bijur, P., Golding, J., Haslum, M., & Kurzon, M. (1988). Behavioral predictors of injury in school-age children. *American Journal of Diseases of Children, 142,* 1307–1312.

Block, J. (1983). Differential premises arising from differential socialization of the sexes: Some conjectures. *Child Development, 54,* 1335–1354.

Brooks, P. H., & Roberts, M. C. (1990). Social science and the prevention of children's injuries. *Social Policy Report, 4* (Whole No. 1).

Cataldo, M. F., Finney, J. W., Richman, G. S., Riley, A. W., Hook, R. J., Brophy, C. J., & Nau, P. A. (1992). Behavior of injured and uninjured children and their parents in a simulated hazardous setting. *Journal of Pediatric Psychology, 17,* 73–80.

Centers for Disease Control and Prevention *Healthy People 2010.* (2000). Website: http://www.health.gov/healthypeople/document

Centers for Disease Control. (2000). Youth risk behavior surveillance—United States. 1999. *Morbidity and Mortality Weekly Report, 49,* 1–96.

Chorba, T. L., Reinfurt, D., & Hulka, B. S. (1988). Efficacy of mandatory seat-belt use legislation: The North Carolina experience from 1983 through 1987. *Journal of the American Medical Association, 260,* 3593–3597.

Christoffel, T., & Christoffel, K. K. (1989). The Consumer Product Safety Commission's opposition to consumer product safety: Lessons for public health advocates. *American Journal of Public Health, 79,* 336–339.

Christophersen, E. R., Sosland-Edelman, D., & LeClaire, S. (1985). Evaluation of two comprehensive infant car seat loan programs with 1-year follow-up. *Pediatrics, 76,* 36–42.

Clarke, A., & Walton, W. W. (1979). Effect of safety packaging on aspirin ingestion by children. *Pediatrics, 63,* 687–693.

Cohn, L., MacFarlane, S., Yanez, C., & Imani, W. (1995). Risk perception: Differences between adolescents and adults. *Health Psychology, 14,* 217–222.

Colver, A., Hutchison, P., & Judson, E. (1982). Promoting children's home safety. *British Medical Journal, 285,* 1177–1180.

Cooper, J. M., Widness, J. A., & O'Shea, J. S. (1988). Pilot study of instructing parents of newborns about poison prevention strategies. *American Journal of Diseases of Children, 142,* 627–629.

Coppens, N. M. (1985). Cognitive development and locus of control as predictors of preschoolers' understanding of safety and prevention. *Journal of Applied Developmental Psychology, 6,* 43–55.

Coppens, N. M. (1986). Cognitive characteristics as predictors of children's understanding of safety and prevention. *Journal of Pediatric Psychology, 11,* 189–202.

Cummings, P., Grossman, D. C., Rivara, F. P., & Koepsell, T. D. (1997). State gun safe storage laws and child mortality due to firearms. *Journal of the American Medical Association, 278,* 1084–1086.

Cushman, R., James, W., & Wacklawik, H. (1991). Physicians promoting bicycle helmets for children: A randomized trial. *American Journal of Public Health, 81,* 1044–1046.

Dannenberg, A. L., Gielen, A. C., Beilenson, P. L., Wilson, M. H., & Joffe, A. (1993). Bicycle helmet laws and education campaigns: An evaluation of strategies to increase children's helmet use. *American Journal of Public Health, 83,* 667–674.

Davidson, L. L. (1987). Hyperactivity, antisocial behavior, and childhood injury: A critical analysis of the literature. *Journal of Developmental and Behavioral Pediatrics, 8,* 335–340.

Dershewitz, R. A. (1977). Will mothers use free household safety devices? *American Journal of Diseases of Children, 133,* 61–64.

Dershewitz, R. A., & Christophersen, E. R. (1984). Childhood household safety: An overview. *American Journal of Diseases of Children, 138,* 85–88.

Dershewitz, R. A., & Williamson, J. W. (1977). Prevention of childhood household injuries: A controlled clinical trial. *American Journal of Public Health, 67,* 1148–1153.

DiGuiseppi, C. G., Rivara, F. P., Koepsell, T. D., & Polissar, L. (1989). Bicycle helmet use by children: Evaluation of a community-wide helmet campaign. *Journal of the American Medical Association, 262,* 2256–2261.

DiScala, C., Lescohier, I., Barthel, M., & Li, G. (1998). Injuries to children with attention deficit hyperactivity disorder. *Pediatrics, 102,* 1415–1421.

Division of Injury Control. (1990). Childhood injuries in the United States. *American Journal of Diseases of Children, 144,* 627–646.

Eichelberger, M. R., Gotschall, C. S., Feely, H. B., Harstad, P., & Bowman, L. M. (1990). Parental attitudes and beliefs of child safety: A national survey. *American Journal of Diseases of Children, 144,* 714–720.

Emission, C. J., Jones, H., & Goldacre, M. (1986). Repetition of accidents in young children. *Journal of Epidemiology and Community Health, 40,* 170–173.

Ennett, S. T., Tobler, N. S., Ringwalt, C. L., & Flewelling, R. L. (1994). How effective is drug abuse resistance education? A meta-analysis of Project DARE outcome evaluations. *American Journal of Public Health, 84,* 1394–1401.

Fagot, B. (1974). Sex differences in toddler's behavior and parental reaction. *Developmental Psychology, 10,* 554–558.

Farah, M. M., Simon, H. K., & Kellermann, A. L. (1999). Firearms in the home: Parental perceptions. *Pediatrics, 104,* 1059–1063.

Fergusson, D., Horwood, L., Beautrais, A., & Shannon, F. (1982). A controlled field trial of a poisoning prevention program. *Pediatrics, 69,* 515–520.

Finney, J. W., Christophersen, E. R., Friman, P. C., Kalnins, I. V., Maddux, J. E., Peterson, L., Roberts, M. C., & Wolraich, M. (1993). Society of Pediatric Psychology Task Force: Pediatric psychology and injury control. *Journal of Pediatric Psychology, 18,* 499–526.

Flagler, S. L., & Wright, L. (1987). Recurrent poisonings in children: A review. *Journal of Pediatric Psychology, 12,* 631–641.

Galejs, I., & Pease, D. (1986). Parenting beliefs and locus of control orientation. *The Journal of Psychology, 120,* 501–510.

Gallagher, S. S., Finison, K., Guyer, B., & Goodenough, S. (1984). The incidence of injuries among 87,000 Massachusetts children and adolescents: Results of the 1980–81 statewide childhood injury prevention program surveillance system. *American Journal of Public Health, 74,* 1340–1347.

Garling, A., & Garling, T. (1991). Mothers' supervision and perception of young children's risk of unintentional injury in the home. *Children's Environments Quarterly, 8,* 24–30.

Gayton, W. F., Bailey, C., Wagner, A., & Hardesty, V. A. (1986). Relationship between childhood hyperactivity and accident proneness. *Perceptual and Motor Skills, 63,* 801–802.

Glik, D. C., Greaves, P. E., Kronenfeld, J. J., & Jackson, K. L. (1993). Safety hazards in households with young children. *Journal of Pediatric Psychology, 18,* 115–131.

Glik, D., Kronenfeld, J., & Jackson, K. (1991). Predictors of risk perceptions of childhood injury among parents of preschoolers. *Health Education Quarterly, 18,* 285–301.

Gorman, R. L., Charney, E., Holtzman, N. A., & Roberts, K. B. (1985). A successful city-wide smoke detector give-away program. *Pediatrics, 75,* 14–18.

Gralinski, J. H., & Kopp, C. B. (1993). Everyday rules for behavior: Mothers' requests to young children. *Developmental Psychology, 29,* 573–584.

Gulotta, C. S., & Finney, J. W. (2000). Intervention models for mothers and children at risk for injuries. *Clinical Child and Family Psychology Review, 3,* 25–36.

Hansen, C. P. (1989). A causal model of the relationship among accidents, bio-data, personality, and cognitive factors. *Journal of Applied Psychology, 74,* 81–90.

Hansen, K., Wong, & Young, P. C. (1996). Do the Framingham safety surveys improve injury prevention counseling during pediatric health supervision visits? *Journal of Pediatrics, 129,* 494–498.

Harris, S. L., & Nathan, P. E. (1973). Parent's locus of control and perception of cause of children's problems. *Journal of Clinical Psychology, 29,* 182–184.

Hillman, H. S., Jones, R. T., & Farmer, L. (1986). The acquisition and maintenance of fire emergency skills: Effects of rationale and behavioral practice. *Journal of Pediatric Psychology, 11,* 247–258.

Horwitz, S. M., Morgenstern, H., DiPietro, L., & Morrison, C. L. (1988). Determinants of pediatric injuries. *American Journal of Diseases of Children, 142,* 605–611.

Husband, P., & Hinton, P. (1972). Families of children with repeated accidents. *Archives of Disease in Childhood, 47,* 396–400.

Jackman, G. A., Farah, M. M., Kellermann, A. L., & Simon, H. K. (2001). Seeing is believing: What do boys do when they find a real gun? *Pediatrics, 107,* 1247–1250.

Jacobi, A. (1983). Preschooler's discrimination of poisonous from nonpoisonous household items as identified by the Mr. Yuk poison prevention sticker. *Children's Health Care, 11,* 98–101.

Jaquess, D. L., & Finney, J. W. (1994). Previous injuries and behavior problems predict children's injuries. *Journal of Pediatric Psychology, 19,* 79–89.

Jelalian, E., Spirito, A., Rasile, D., Vinnick, L., Rohrbeck, C., & Arrigan, M. (1997). Risk taking, reported injury, and perception of future injury among adolescents. *Journal of Pediatric Psychology, 22,* 513–531.

Jones, R. T., & Kazdin, A. E. (1980). Teaching children how and when to make emergency telephone calls. *Behavior Therapy, 11,* 509–521.

Kerr, G., & Minden, H. (1988). Psychological factors related to the occurrence of athletic injuries. *Journal of Sport and Exercise Psychology, 10,* 167–173.

Lacouture, P., Minisci, M., Gouveia, W. T., & Lovejoy, F. H. (1978). Evaluation of a community-based poison education program. *Clinical Toxicology, 13,* 623–629.

Langley, J., & Silva, P. (1982). Childhood accidents—Parents' attitudes to prevention. *Australia Paediatric Journal, 18,* 247–249.

Langlois, J. A., Wallen, B. A. R., Teret, S. P., Bailey, L. A., Hershey, J. H., & Peeler, M. O. (1991). The impact of specific toy warning labels. *Journal of the American Medical Association, 265,* 2848–2950.

Maddux, J. E., Roberts, M. C., Sledden, E. A., & Wright, L. (1986). Developmental issues in child health psychology. *American Psychology, 41,* 25–34.

Malek, M., Guyer, B., & Lescohier, I. (1990). The epidemiology and prevention of child pedestrian injury. *Accident Analysis and Prevention, 22,* 301–313.

Manheimer, D. I., & Mellinger, G. D. (1967). Personality characteristics of the child accident repeater. *Child Development, 38,* 491–514.

Matheny, A. P. (1986). Injuries among toddlers: Contributions from child, mother, and family. *Journal of Pediatric Psychology, 11,* 163–176.

Matheny, A. P. (1987). Psychological characteristics of childhood accidents. *Journal of Social Issues, 43,* 45–60.

Matheny, A. P., & Fisher, J. E. (1984). Behavioral perspectives on children's accidents. In M. L. Wolraich & D. K. Routh (Eds.), *Advances in developmental and behavioral pediatrics* (Vol. 5, pp. 221–264). Greenwich, CT: JAI Press.

McClure-Martinez, K., & Cohn, L. D. (1996). Adolescent and adult mothers' perceptions of hazardous situations for their children. *Journal of Adolescent Health, 18,* 227–231.

McFarland, L. V., Harris, J. R., Kobayashi, J. M., & Dicker, R. C. (1984). Risk factors for fireworks-related injury in Washington State. *Journal of the American Medical Association, 251,* 3251–3254.

McLoughlin, E., Clark, N., Stahl, K., & Crawford, J. D. (1977). One pediatric burn unit's experience with sleepwear-related injuries. *Pediatrics, 60,* 405–409.

Miller, R. E., Reisinger, K. S., Blatter, M. M., & Wucher, F. (1982). Pediatric counseling and subsequent use of smoke detectors. *American Journal of Public Health, 72,* 392–393.

Miller, T. R., & Galbraith, M. (1995). Injury prevention counseling by pediatricians: A benefit-cost comparison. *Pediatrics, 96,* 1–4.

Mori, L., & Peterson, L (1986). Training preschoolers in home safety skills to prevent inadvertent injury. *Journal of Clinical Child Psychology, 15,* 106–114.

Morrongiello, B. A. (1997). Children's perspectives on injury and close-call experiences: Sex differences in injury-outcome processes. *Journal of Pediatric Psychology, 22,* 499–512.

Murray, R. D., & Linscheid, T. R. (1991). Effectiveness of bicycle helmet safety intervention in schools: A comparison of student vs. parent-oriented strategies. *Children's
Environments Quarterly, 8,* 82–87.

Nadar, P. R., & Brink, S. G. (1981). Does visiting the school health room teach appropriate
or inappropriate use of health services? *American Journal of Public Health, 71,*
416–419.

National Center for Injury Prevention and Control. (1996). *Home and leisure injuries in
the United States.* Atlanta: Centers for Disease Control and Prevention.

National Committee for Injury Prevention and Control. (1989). *Injury prevention: Meeting
the challenge.* Oxford, England: Oxford University Press.

Nyman, G. (1987). Infant temperament, childhood accidents, and hospitalization. *Clinical
Pediatrics, 26,* 398–404.

O'Brien, M. (1996). Child rearing difficulties reported by parents of infants and toddlers.
Journal of Pediatric Psychology, 21, 433–446.

Osberg, J. S., & Di Scala, C. (1992). Morbidity among pediatric motor vehicle crash
victims: The effectiveness of seat belts. *American Journal of Public Health, 82,*
422–425.

Osberg, J. S., Kahn, P., Rowe, K., & Brooke, M. M. (1996). Pediatric trauma: Impact on
work and family finances. *Pediatrics, 98,* 890–897.

O'Shea, J., Collins, E., & Butler, C. (1982). Pediatric accident prevention. *Clinical Pediatrics, 21,* 290–297.

Padilla, E. R., Rohsenow, D. J., & Bergman, A. B. (1976). Predicting accident frequency
in children. *Pediatrics, 58,* 223–226.

Pearn, J. H., Wong, R. Y., Brown, J., Ching, Y. C., Bart, R., & Hammer, S. (1979).
Drowning and near drowning involving children: A five-year total population study
from the city and county of Honolulu. *American Journal of Public Health, 74,*
450–454.

Peterson, L. (1989). Latchkey children's preparation for self-care: Overestimated, underre-
hearsed and unsafe. *Journal of Clinical Child Psychology, 18,* 36–43.

Peterson, L. (1994). Child injury and abuse-neglect: Common etiologies, challenges, and
courses toward prevention. *Current Directions in Psychological Research, 8,*
116–120.

Peterson, L., Cook, S., Little, T., & Schick, B. (1991). "Mom let's me go there": The role
of environment and supervision in children's minor injuries. *Children's Environments
Quarterly, 8,* 15–23.

Peterson, L., Farmer, J., & Kashani, J. H. (1990). Parental injury prevention endeavors:
A function of health beliefs? *Health Psychology, 9,* 177–191.

Peterson, L., Farmer, J., & Kashani, J. H. (1991). The role of beliefs in parental injury
prevention efforts. In J. H. Johnson & S. B. Johnson (Eds.), *Advances in child health
psychology* (pp. 115–126). Gainesville, FL: University of Florida Press.

Peterson, L., & Roberts, M. C. (1992). Complacency, misdirection, and effective prevention
of children's injuries. *American Psychologist, 47,* 1040–1044.

Peterson, L., & Stern, B. L. (1997). Family process and child risk for injury. *Behaviour
Research and Therapy, 35,* 179–190.

Phinney, J., Colker, L., & Cosgrove, M. (1985). Literature review on the pre-school pedestrian. DOT HS—806 679. Washington: U.S. Department of Transportation, National Highway Traffic Safety Administration.

Plato, K. C., & Rasp, A. (1983). *Parental views of issues related to traffic safety education and the licensing of teenage drivers.* Olympia, WA: Washington Office of the State Superintendent of Public Instruction. (ERIC Document Reproduction Service No. ED–241 847)

Pless, I. B., & Arsenault, L. (1987). The role of health education in the prevention of injuries to children. *Journal of Social Issues, 43,* 87–104.

Poche, C., Brouwer, R., & Swearingen, M. (1981). Teaching self-protection to young children. *Journal of Applied Behavior Analysis, 14,* 169–176.

Potts, R., Martinez, I. G., & Dedmon, A. (1995). Childhood risk-taking and injury: Self-report and informant measures. *Journal of Pediatric Psychology, 20,* 5–12.

Richards, J. S., Hendricks, C., & Roberts, M. C. (1991). Prevention of spinal cord injury: An elementary education approach. *Journal of Pediatric Psychology, 16,* 595–609.

Rivara, F. P. (1982). Epidemiology of childhood injuries: A review of current research and presentation of a conceptual framework. *American Journal of the Diseases of Children, 136,* 399–405.

Rivara, F. P. (1990). Child pedestrian injuries in the United States: Current status of the problem, potential interventions and future research needs. *American Journal of Diseases of Children, 144,* 692–696.

Rivara, F., Bergman, A., LoGerfo, J., & Weiss, N. (1982). Epidemiology of childhood injuries. *American Journal of Diseases of Children, 136,* 502–506.

Rivara, F. P., Booth, C. L., Bergman, A. B., Rogers, L. W., & Weiss, J. (1991). Prevention of pedestrian injuries to children: Effectiveness of a school training program. *Pediatrics, 88,* 770–775.

Rivara, F. P., & Grossman, D. C. (1996). Prevention of traumatic deaths to children in the US: How far have we come and where do we need to go? *Pediatrics, 97,* 791–797.

Rivara, F. P., & Mueller, B. A. (1987). The epidemiology and causes of childhood injuries. *Journal of Social Issues, 43,* 13–31.

Rivara, F. P., Rivara, M. B., & Bartol, K. (1998). Dad, may I have the keys? Factors influencing which vehicles teenagers drive. *Pediatrics, 102,* e57.

Roberts, M. C. (1986). Health promotion and problem prevention in pediatric psychology: An overview. *Journal of Pediatric Psychology, 11,* 146–161.

Roberts, M. C. (1987). Public health and health psychology: Two cats of Kilkenny? *Professional Psychology: Research and Practice, 18,* 145–149.

Roberts, M. C. (1993). Special section editorial: Explicating the circumstances of nonintentional injuries in childhood. *Journal of Pediatric Psychology, 18,* 99–103.

Roberts, M. C. (1994). Prevention/promotion in America: Still spitting on the sidewalk. *Journal of Pediatric Psychology, 19,* 267–281.

Roberts, M. C., Alexander, K., & Fanurik, D. (1990). Evaluation of commercially available materials to prevent child sexual abuse and abduction. *American Psychologist, 45,* 782–783.

Roberts, M. C., Alexander, K., & Knapp, L. (1990). Motivating children to use seat belts: A program combining rewards and "Flash for Life." *Journal of Community Psychology, 18,* 110–119.

Roberts, M. C., & Broadbent, M. (1989). Increasing preschoolers' use of car safety devices: An effective program for day care staff. *Children's Health Care, 18,* 157–162.

Roberts, M. C., & Brooks, P. (1987). Children's injuries: Issues in prevention and public policy. *Journal of Social Issues, 43,* 1–12.

Roberts, M. C., Elkins, P. D., & Royal, G. P. (1984). Psychological applications to the prevention of accidents and illness. In M. C. Roberts & L. Peterson (Eds.), *Prevention of problems in childhood: Psychological research and applications* (pp. 173–199). New York: Wiley.

Roberts, M. C., & Fanurik, D. (1986). Rewarding elementary schoolchildren for their use of safety belts. *Health Psychology, 5,* 185–196.

Roberts, M. C., Fanurik, D., & Layfield, D. (1987). Behavioral approaches to prevention of childhood injuries. *Journal of Social Issues, 43,* 105–118.

Roberts, M. C., Fanurik, D., & Wilson, D. R. (1988). A community program to reward children's use of seat belts. *American Journal of Community Psychology, 16,* 395–407.

Roberts, M. C., Layfield, D. A., & Fanurik, D. (1991). Motivating children's use of car safety devices. In M. Wolraich & D. Routh (Eds.), *Advances in developmental and behavioral pediatrics* (Vol. 10, pp. 61–88). Philadelphia: Jessica Kingsley Publisher.

Roberts, M. C., Maddux, J. E., & Wright, L. (1984). The developmental perspective in behavioral health. In J.D. Matarazzo, N. E. Miller, S. M. Weiss, J. A. Herd, & S. M. Weiss (Eds.), *Behavioral health: A handbook of health enhancement and disease prevention* (pp. 56–68). New York: Wiley.

Roberts, M. C., & Turner, D. S. (1984). Preventing death and injury in childhood: A synthesis of child safety seat efforts. *Health Education Quarterly, 11,* 181–193.

Roberts, M. C., & Turner, D. S. (1986). Rewarding parents for their children's use of safety seats. *Journal of Pediatric Psychology, 11,* 25–36.

Rodriguez, J. G. (1990). Childhood injuries in the United States: A priority issue. *American Journal of Diseases of Children, 144,* 625–626.

Rosen, B. N., & Peterson, L. (1990). Gender differences in children's outdoor play injuries: A review and integration. *Clinical Psychology Review, 10,* 187–205.

Rotter, J. B. (1966). Generalized expectancies for internal versus external control of reinforcement. *Psychological Monographs, 80* (Whole no. 609).

Routledge, D., Repetto-Wright, R., & Howrath, C. (1974). The exposure of young children to accident risk as pedestrians. *Ergonomics, 17,* 457–480.

Ruch-Ross, H. S., & O'Connor, K. G. (1993). Bicycle helmet counseling by pediatricians: A random national survey. *American Journal of Public Health, 83,* 728–730.

Runyan, C. W., & Runyan, D. K. (1991). How can physicians get kids to wear bicycle helmets? A prototype challenge in injury prevention. *American Journal of Public Health, 81,* 972–973.

Sacks, J. J., Brantley, M. D., Holmgreen, P., & Rochat, R. W. (1992). Evaluation of an intervention to reduce playground hazards in Atlanta child-care centers. *American Journal of Public Health, 82,* 429–431.

Scheidt, P. C. (1988). Behavioral research toward prevention of childhood injury. *American Journal of Diseases of Children, 142,* 612–617.

Schlesinger, E. R., Dickson, D. G., Westaby, J., Lowen, L., Logrillo, V. M., & Maiwald, A. A. (1966). A controlled study of health education in accident prevention. *American Journal of Diseases of Children, 111,* 490–496.

Shaw, K. N., McCormick, M. C., Kustra, S. L., Ruddy, R. M., & Casey, R. D. (1988). Correlates of reported smoke detector usage in an inner-city population: Participants in a smoke detector give-away program. *American Journal of Public Health, 78,* 650–653.

Smith, G. S., & Falk, H. (1987). Unintentional injuries. In R. W. Ambler & N. B. Dold (Eds.), *Closing the gap: The burden of unnecessary illness* (pp. 143–163). New York: Oxford University Press.

Speltz, M., Gonzales, N., Sulzbacher, S., & Quan, L. (1990). Assessment of injury risk in young children: A preliminary study of the Injury Behavior Checklist. *Journal of Pediatric Psychology, 15,* 373–383.

Spiegel, C. N., & Lindaman, F. C. (1977). Children can't fly: A program to prevent childhood morbidity and mortality from window falls. *American Journal of Public Health, 67,* 1143–1147.

Squires, T., & Busuttil, A. (1995). Child fatalities in Scottish house fires 1980–1990: A case of child neglect. *Child Abuse and Neglect, 19,* 865–873.

Swick, K. J., & Graves, S. B. (1986). Locus of control and interpersonal support as related to parenting. *Childhood Education, 63,* 41–50.

Taylor, B., Wadsworth, J., & Butler, N., (1983). Teenage mothering: Hospitalisations and accidents during the first five years. *Archives of Disease in Childhood, 58,* 6–11.

Tertinger, D. A., Greene, B. F., & Lutzker, J. R. (1984). Home safety: Development and validation of one component of an ecobehavioral treatment program for abused and neglected children. *Journal of Applied Behavior Analysis, 17,* 159–174.

Thompson, R. S., Rivara, F. P., & Thompson, D. C. (1989). A case-controlled study of the effectiveness of bicycle safety helmets. *New England Journal of Medicine, 320,* 1361–1367.

Thuen, F. (1992). Preventing childhood accidents in the home: Parental behavior to reduce household injuries. *Scandinavian Journal of Psychology, 33,* 370–377.

U.S. Department of Health and Human Services. (1987). *Prevention of injury to children and youth: A selected bibliography.* Atlanta: Centers for Disease Control.

U.S. Department of Health and Human Services. (November, 2000). *Tracking Healthy People 2010.* Washington, DC: U.S. Government Printing Office.

Vernberg, K., Culver-Dickinson, P., & Spyker, D. (1984). The deterrent effect of poison-warning stickers. *Archives of Disease in Childhood, 138,* 1018–1020.

Vernick, J. S., Li, G., Ogaitis, S., MacKenzie, E. J., Baker, S. P., & Gielen, A. C. (1999). Effects of high school driver education on motor vehicle crashes, violations, and licensure. *American Journal of Preventive Medicine, 16,* 40–46.

Vulcan, A. P., Cameron, M. H., & Watson, W. L. (1992). Mandatory bicycle helmet use, experience in Victoria, Australia. *World Journal of Surgery, 16,* 389–397.

Wade, S. L., Borawski, E. A., Taylor, H. G., Drotar, D., Yeates, K. O., & Stancin, T. (2001). The relationship of caregiver coping to family outcomes during the initial year following pediatric traumatic injury. *Journal of Consulting and Clinical Psychology, 69,* 406–415.

Wagenaar, A. C., Maybee, R. G., & Sullivan, K. P. (1988). Mandatory seat belt laws in eight states: A time-series evaluation. *Journal of Safety Research, 19,* 51–70.

Walton, W. W. (1982). An evaluation of the Poison Prevention Packaging Act. *Pediatrics, 69,* 363–370.

Webster, D. W., & Starnes, M. (2000). Reexamining the association between child access preventing gun laws and unintentional shooting deaths of children. *Pediatrics, 106,* 1466–1469.

Weiss, B. D. (1992). Trends in bicycle helmet use by children: 1985–1990. *Pediatrics, 89,* 78–80.

Williams, A. F., & Karpf, R. S. (1982). *Teenaged drivers and fatal crash responsibility.* Washington, DC: Insurance Institute for Highway Safety. (ERIC Document Reproduction Service No. ED–221 685).

Willis, K. S. (1997). Promoting children's usage of bicycle safety helmets. Unpublished master's thesis, University of Kansas.

Wortel, E., & de Gues, G. H. (1993). Prevention of home related injuries of pre-school children: Safety measures taken by mothers. *Health Education Research, 8,* 217–231.

Wurtele, S. K., & Miller-Perrin, C. L. (1992). *Preventing child sexual abuse: Sharing the responsibility.* Lincoln, NE: University of Nebraska Press.

Yeaton, W. H., & Bailey, J. S. (1978). Teaching pedestrian safety skills to young children: An analysis and one year follow-up. *Journal of Applied Behavior Analysis, 11,* 315–329.

Young, T. L., & Zimmerman, R. (1998). Clueless: Parental knowledge of risk behaviors of middle school students. *Archives of Pediatric and Adolescent Medicine, 152,* 1137–1139.

CHAPTER 6

Substance Abuse

Oscar G. Bukstein

S ubstance use and abuse by children and adolescents remains a critical problem for modern Western culture. Despite overt public sanctions against the underage use of alcohol, tobacco, and other illicit substances, the use of psychoactive substances and other harmful of abuse is common among adolescents. The use of such psychoactive agents can lead to a variety of negative consequences for youth. The risk for substance use and abuse, the acquisition of use behaviors, and development into substance use disorders and interventions for such problems should be considered in a comprehensive manner that considers neurobiology, development, and the adolescent's environmental ecology.

DEFINITIONS

Substance use patterns by adolescents range from abstinence (i.e., nonuse), to use, to the pathological entities of abuse and dependence. Although there are a variety of labels for individuals with substance use problems, including alcoholism, addiction, and chemical dependency, the definition of substance use disorders provided in the *Diagnostic and Statistical Manual*, Fourth Edition (DSM-IV), published by the American Psychiatric Association (1994) provides the primary source for diagnoses related to substance use in adults, adolescents, and children in the United States. The DSM-IV criteria were developed for adults, and have not been established as applicable to adolescents.

Substance abuse and dependence each are, in part, defined by a maladaptive pattern of substance use. Criteria for abuse include: use resulting in inability to meet major role obligations (such as school or work absences, suspensions or expulsions from school), recurrent legal problems, an increase in risk-taking behaviors or self-exposure to hazardous situations (such as driving while intoxicated or high), and/or continued use despite having persistent social or interpersonal problems caused or worsened by substance use. A diagnosis of substance dependence includes: the presence of significant tolerance and/or withdrawal symptoms, persistent desire or unsuccessful efforts to control or stop use, giving up important activities due to use, spending increasing amounts of time in activities related to use, using for a longer time than planned, and/or use despite the existence of worsening of problems caused by substance use. More simply understood, abuse is use plus problems or negative consequences while dependence implies physiological symptoms of tolerance or withdrawal and/or a pattern of use or compulsive use of a substance despite negative consequences.

Despite similarities between adults and adolescents in the frequency of DSM-IV abuse or dependence symptoms endorsed (Lewinsohn, Rhode, & Seely, 1996), there are important differences in the most common manifestations of substance use disorders between adolescents and adults. Whereas in adults, physiologic features such as withdrawal symptoms are prominent, the most common feature of substance use disorders in adolescents is impairment in psychosocial functioning, most commonly family or other interpersonal conflict and academic failure (Bukstein & Kaminer, 1994; Martin et al., 1995). Other symptoms include reduced activities due to use, tolerance, desire to use less (frequency and amount), and using more than intended (Stewart & Brown, 1995). While tolerance (i.e., the need to use more to produce the same psychoactive effects) is frequent (up to 80%) for adolescents who abuse alcohol, tolerance appears to have a low specificity of a diagnosis of alcohol dependence in adolescents. Characteristic withdrawal symptoms and consequent medical problems are much less common in adolescents than in adults (Martin et al., 1995). *Diagnostic orphans* or adolescents with 1–2 dependence symptoms but no DSM-IV AUDs (Alcohol Use Disorders) tend to resemble those with DSM-IV alcohol abuse on such variables as level of consumption and diagnostic status at one year follow up (Pollock & Martin, 1999).

The attribution of the myriad problems observed in adolescents, such as disruptive behavior or emotional problems, who use substances remains a substantial problem. Given the high prevalence of the use of various substances among adolescents at some point in their lives, substance use per se should not be considered as evidence of a substance use disorder. All psychoactive substances, including alcohol and tobacco, are illegal for adolescents. Certain negative consequences may follow from this illegal status rather than from substance use or behaviors directly related to use. Adolescents who use substances also display a variety of other behaviors and problems (coexisting psychiatric disorders, other social deviant behaviors) which may contribute to or be the primary cause of the level of dysfunction seen in these adolescents (Bukstein & Kaminer, 1994). It is very difficult to separate the causes from the consequences of substance use in adolescents.

EPIDEMIOLOGY

Alcohol remains the substance of choice for adolescents as an overwhelming majority of adolescents report having at least one drink during adolescence. In 2000, according to the University of Michigan Monitoring the Future annual survey of high school students, over 80% of twelfth graders, over 70% of tenth graders, and over 50% of eighth graders report ever having used alcohol (University of Michigan, 2000). One in every 12 eighth graders (8.3%) reports having been drunk at least once in the past 30 days, as do a third of twelfth graders (32.3%). Under 2% (1.7) of high school seniors report daily drunkenness. Almost a quarter (22%) of eighth graders report having an alcohol drink in the preceding 30-day period and half of twelfth graders report having done so. In 1999, the Centers for Disease Control's (CDC, 2000) Youth Risk Behavior Survey (YRBS) reported that 50% of adolescents surveyed reported current alcohol use, defined as at least one or more occasions in the 30 days preceding the survey (CDC, 2000). Almost 5% (4.9%) reported having used alcohol on school property. Over a third (33.4%) of adolescents report episodic heavy drinking (at least once a month). Generally, alcohol use prevalence figures having been stable for adolescents over the past two decades.

Other than alcohol, 54% of twelfth graders and almost 27% (26.8%) of eighth graders report ever having used any illicit drug (University of Michigan, 2000). Marijuana is the most widely used of the illicit drugs with 16% of eighth graders, 32% of tenth graders, and 37% of twelfth graders indicating some use in the preceding 12-month period. Six percent of high school seniors report daily marijuana use. The CDC's YRBS reported that 7.2% of adolescents reported marijuana use on school property in 1999 (CDC, 2000).

Recently, club drugs, such as ecstasy (MDMA) and methamphetamine had been surveyed among adolescents. In 2000, the use of ecstasy continued to rise sharply. The proportion of eighth graders reporting any use of ecstasy in the preceding year rose from 1.7% in 1999 to 3.1% in 2000 (University of Michigan, 2000). Among twelfth graders, use rose from 5.6% to 8.2%. Over 50% of twelfth graders reported that they could get ecstasy fairly or very easily. Fortunately, the use of other popular illicit drugs such as inhalants, LSD, methamphetamine and Rohypnol are down in 2000 from peak levels in the mid-1990s. For most drugs, excluding alcohol, marijuana, and tobacco, the prevalence of regular use (defined as more than monthly) is less than 1–2% of adolescents at any grade level. According to the YRBS, nationwide, 3.7% of students had used illegal steroids during their lifetime. Overall, male students (5.2%) were significantly more likely than female students (2.2%) to report lifetime steroid use (CDC, 2000).

As of 2000, cigarette smoking among adolescents in the U.S. has continued to decline from a peak in the mid-1990s (University of Michigan, 2000). After reporting an almost 50% increase in the rate of smoking among younger adolescents (eighth and tenth graders), the Monitoring the Future study has documented a fairly steady decline. In 2000, 14.6% of eighth graders reported current smoking (defined as smoking at least once in the preceding 30 days) while 23.9% of tenth graders and 31.4% of twelfth graders reported current cigarette use. Approximately a quarter (24.7%) of students nationwide reported having smoked a cigarette before the age of 13 years. In 2000, 7.4%, 14%, and 20.6% of eighth, tenth, and twelfth graders reported daily cigarette use, respectively; 0.9%, 1.9%, and 3.2% of eighth, tenth, and twelfth graders reported daily smokeless tobacco, respectively.

White and Hispanic students reports a lifetime prevalence of about 82% for alcohol use as compared with 74% for African American youth. Heavy episodic use prevalence rates are 35%, 37.7%, and 18.8% for White, Hispanic, and African American students, respectively. African American students are more likely to report both lifetime and current use of marijuana than White students. For all substances, males use more than females, although the gap appears to be closing during the past 2 decades. Similarly, the gap is closing between lower levels of substance use in rural areas and higher levels in urban areas. This smaller gap may be due to increasing accessibility to all youth whether or not they live in urban or rural areas.

Unfortunately, the Monitoring the Future and CDC surveys of substance use do not indicate the prevalence of pathological use, that is, the prevalence of substance use disorders. For alcohol use disorders, community studies lifetime diagnosis of alcohol abuse range from 0.4% in the Great Smoky Mountain Study (Costello et al., 1996) to 8.2 and 9.6% in the Pittsburgh Adolescent Alcohol Research Center (Martin et al., 1995) and the National

Co-morbidity Study (Kessler et al., 1994), respectively. Lifetime diagnoses of alcohol dependence ranged from 0.6% (Costello et al., 1996) to 4.3% in the Oregon Adolescent Depression Project (Lewinsohn et al., 1996). While lifetime prevalence rates for abuse are generally higher for abuse than dependence in community studies, in clinical samples rates of alcohol dependence are greater than those for abuse.

Community surveys vary in the communities and ages surveyed, resulting in different but difficult to compare results. For example, in a community study of 15-year-old adolescents, Kashani and colleagues (1987, 1989) found a prevalence rate of 5.3% for DSM-III alcohol abuse/dependence, 3.3% for drug abuse/dependence. In another community sample of 17–19 year-olds, Reinherz and associates (Reinherz et al., 1993) reported a lifetime prevalence of 32.4% for DSM-III-R alcohol abuse and dependence and 9.8% for drug abuse/dependence. These latter figures are higher than the lifetime prevalence for adults from the Epidemiological Catchment Area Study (ECA) (Reiger, Farmer, Rae, et al., 1990). Although the extent or meaning of such high lifetime prevalence figures for adolescents is debatable, they are consistent with data suggesting higher rates of SUDs in succeeding generations (Nelson et al., 1998; Reich, Cloninger, Van Erdewegh, Rice, & Mullaney, 1988). The lower adult figures for the ECA may also be the result of poor recall for the adults.

RISK, DEVELOPMENT, AND NATURAL HISTORY

Both the risk and natural history of adolescent substance use and related problems can be viewed from a developmental perspective. An adolescent's initial experiences with psychoactive substance use most often takes place in a social setting with the use of so-called *gateway* substances such as alcohol and cigarettes that are legal for adults, and thus readily available to minors (Kandel, 1975). Factors such as curiosity, lack of parental supervision, and peer pressure may determine the risk and age of such exposure. Numerous studies have established a fairly predictable sequence or stages of substance use among adolescents (Kandel, 1975; Bukstein, 1995). Although almost all adolescents will eventually use alcohol, progressively fewer will advance to more serious level of substance use, that is, the use of marijuana, and other illicit substances such as hallucinogens, cocaine, or opiods.

While most adolescents will try one or more substances, the risk for the development of problems associated with use or substance use disorders is not equal among all adolescents. The early onset of substance use and a more rapid progression through the stages of substance use are risk factors for the development of substance abuse disorders (SUDs) (Robins & McEvoy, 1990; Robins & Przybeck, 1985). There are several major categories of risk factors for the development of problems related to substance use among adolescents.

Parent/family risk factors include parental substance use, parent beliefs, and attitudes about substance use, parent tolerance of use, lack of closeness and attachment between parent and child or adolescent, lack of parental involvement in the child's life, and lack of appropriate supervision and/or discipline (Baumrind, 1983; Kandel, Kessler, & Margulies, 1978; Wechsler & Thum, 1973). Some parent/family risk factors may affect other factors. For example, parental substance use may influence the quality of parent-child attachment or supervision, while such factors as the quality of parental supervision and involvement are environmental.

Peer-related risk factors include peer substance use, peer attitudes about substance use and greater orientation of the youth to peers (versus parents) (Kandel, Kessler, & Margulies, 1978). Although increasing orientation away from parents and family and toward peers is a developmental task of adolescence, those youth at high risk for substance use and use disorders appear to have an earlier, greater involvement with peers, at a time when their lack of maturity may not allow them to make appropriate decisions in the absence of parental guidance. The absence of an adequate level of supervision and structure from parents for these same youth can also increase the adolescents' trajectory toward deviant behavior and substance use.

Individual risk factors include early childhood characteristics such as early disruptive behavior problems, especially aggressive behavior, poor academic performance and school failure, risk-taking behaviors, and favorable beliefs, and attitudes about substance use (Brook, Linkoff, & Whiteman, 1977; Christiansen, Goldman, & Brown, 1985; Jessor & Jessor, 1977; Kandel, Kessler, & Margulies, 1978; Kellum, Simon, & Ensminger, 1980; Robins, 1980).

Twin and adoption studies have pointed to the likely contribution of genetic or constitutional factors to the risk for SUDs (Dinwiddie & Cloninger, 1991). Specific types of biologic markers or characteristics may differentiate high risk versus low risk individuals for SUDs. At risk individuals may be less sensitive to the effects of alcohol in terms of the subject's feelings of intoxication (Schuckit, 1994), or may display greater static ataxia (body sway) than low risk individuals or increased latency of the P3 component of brain-evoked potentials (Porjescz & Bergleiter, 1990; Hill, Steinhauser, & Zubin, 1987; Schuckit, 1985). Other researchers have proposed that individuals with substance use disorders obtain differential levels of reinforcement from their substance(s) of choice (Khantzian, 1985). In other words, certain people may respond in different ways to different substances of abuse. The experience of or a particular substance and its effects on the brain may serve to increase or sustain use (reinforcement) despite negative social, mental, or physical consequences. Certain behavioral traits such as impulsivity, high activity level, and irritability with a biogenetic basis may underlie a vulnerability to substance use disorders in adolescents (Tarter, 1992).

Community or neighborhood characteristics such as low socioeconomic status, high population density, physical deterioration, and high crime are associated with greater substance use in adolescence (Brook, Whiteman, Gordon, & Brook, 1990). It is difficult to know whether these community factors are a cause or effect of high rates of substance use problems in a particular community. For example, in poor, inner-city neighborhoods, many of the existing young adult male role models in the community are involved in substance use or its distribution. As poor academic performance and socioeconomic status serve to limits an inner-city adolescent's options, substance use may appear to be a normative, reasonable alternative. A number of cultural factors such as availability of substances and the mixed messages provided by the mass media may also influence substance use (Resnik, 1990).

The risk for SUDs in adolescents and the development of these disorders are similar to many other problems that are noted in youth. Children may inherit certain genetic traits that are influenced by their environment, most notably their families and later, at adolescence, by their peers. Different types of risk factors may be more significant for adolescents at specific stages of substance use. For example, peer and family factors are more critical at earlier stages of use, while individual risk factors, such as deviant behaviors and psychopathology, are likely to exert more influence at later stages of substance use (Bukstein, 1995). Although no particular risk factor or set of risk factors completely predicts substance use, or the development of use disorders in adolescents, the number of risk factors may be the best guide to prediction (Bry, 1983).

Developmental Consequences

Substance use can seriously disrupt the ability of adolescents to handle adequately other developmental tasks (Baumrind & Moselle, 1985; Newcomb & Bentler, 1988). Generally, the quantity and frequency of substance use peak in late adolescence or early adulthood, thus suggesting a maturational process. Most adolescents or young adults find that they cannot negotiate the demands and roles of adulthood while continuing a sustained pattern of substance use. Life events such as marriage, parenthood, and moving away from the adolescent subculture increase the likelihood of decreasing or discontinuation of substance use (Newcomb & Bentler, 1988). However, because some adolescents who abuse substances enter into adults roles (e.g., marriage, child-bearing) earlier than their nonsubstance abusing peers, they may experience more difficulty in successfully carrying out these adult roles or tasks.

Medical Consequences

Accidents, including driving motor vehicles and even bicycles and skateboards while intoxicated, and trauma in adolescents commonly occur under the influence of substances (Milstein & Irwin, 1987; NCHS, 1992). Alcohol is estimated to be involved in as many as 40% of adolescent drownings (Howland & Hingson, 1988). Adolescents who use and abuse substances are more likely to participate in other risk taking behaviors such as driving a motor vehicle while under the influence (NCHS, 1992). Both adolescent victims and perpetrators of violence, both with and without weapons, are commonly under the influence or have histories of SUDs (Bukstein, 1995).

Substance use is often associated with other high-risk behaviors. Early and promiscuous sexual behavior is common among adolescents, with the early onset of substance use and abuse (DiClemente & Ponton, 1993). Among currently sexually active students nationwide, 24.8% had used alcohol or drugs at last sexual intercourse. Overall, male students (31.2%) were significantly more likely than female students (18.5%) to have used alcohol or drugs at last sexual intercourse (CDC, 2000). The impairment in judgment, and the increase in impulsivity often produced by an intoxicated state, may result in unprotected and/or unsafe sexual activity and subsequent pregnancy and/or sexually transmitted diseases. Unsafe sexual practices are also common among these populations of adolescents (Rotheram-Borus, Koopman, & Ehrhardt, 1991). Although not all adolescents who use or even abuse substances are considered to be at high-risk status for HIV infection, substance use by an adolescent should prompt a thorough inquiry into specific HIV risk factors and consideration of appropriate testing. Although adolescents constitute a small percentage of the total number of individuals with HIV disease, the often long latency between HIV infection and the onset of symptoms means that many acquire HIV as adolescents (CDC, 1992). Intravenous drug and crack cocaine abusers are among the subgroups of adolescents with the highest risk for HIV (St. Louis et al., 1991). Medical complications of substance use are uncommon among adolescents (Martin et al., 1995). Long-term sequelae such as liver disease and memory problems from chronic substance use may not become apparent until well into adulthood. Those adolescents who frequently use very high quantities of substance or use acutely toxic substances may be an exception. For example, inhalants such as aromatic or halogenated hydrocarbons or other organic solvents, may produce varying levels of neurotoxicity (including acute and chronic encephalopathy) and, on occasion, cardiac arrest secondary to arrhythmia even during the initial episodes of use.

Psychiatric Co-morbidity

Psychiatric disorders are commonly associated with SUDs in youth (Bukstein, Brent, & Kaminer, 1989; Clark & Bukstein, 1998). In fact, the presence of multiple psychiatric disorders, both internalizing and externalizing types, is often the rule rather than the exception in populations of adolescents with SUDs (Bukstein, Glancy, & Kaminer, 1992; Bukstein, Brent, & Kaminer, 1989; Riggs et al., 1995). Almost all of the existing studies of psychiatric co-morbidity in adolescents with substance use disorders have been completed in clinical populations. Psychiatric co-morbidity rates vary among the clinical populations studied. For example, in a study of juvenile offenders, 81% met DSM-III-R criteria for an SUD (Neighbors, Kempton, & Forehand, 1992). Not surprisingly, among those adolescents with SUDs, 91% met criteria for conduct disorder and 58% for attention deficit hyperactivity disorder. Similar rates of disruptive behavior disorders are found in other reports of delinquent populations. Aarons and colleagues (2001) in a prevalence study across several public sectors of care in San Diego, California found 62.1% of youth in the juvenile justice system reporting a SUD diagnosis, 48% in mental health sector, 23.6% categorized as having a serious emotional disturbance in local school districts, and 19.2% in the child welfare system.

In a community study, Lewinsohn, Rhode, and Seeley (1995) found that 66% of adolescents who met DSM-III-R SUD criteria also met criteria for at least one other Axis I disorder. The Methods for the Epidemiology of child and Adolescent Mental Disorders (MECA) Study also reported a psychiatric comorbidity rate of 66% among weekly drinkers (Kandel et al., 1999). Although the level of clinical co-morbidity in the general population may not be as high as that in the clinical populations, clinical cases are those who present for treatment and constitute the first line of youth needing intervention or treatment. There are a number of relationships that have been linked with SUDs in adolescents and psychiatric disorders. Among these possible relationships are: (1) psychopathology, including deviations in temperament, as a risk factor for the subsequent development of SUDS; (see chapter 1 for a related discussion), (2) substance use or SUDs as directly causing or influencing the course of psychiatric disorders and (3) psychiatric disorders: causing or influencing the course of substance use of SUDs.

Prior to the actual development of psychopathology or SUDs, many children have deviations in temperamental traits that are likely of a biogenetic origin (Cloninger, 1987; Tarter et al., 1994). Temperament deviations have been linked with an increased risk for psychopathology and substance abuse (Reich et al., 1993). Youth having a difficult temperament in early childhood more commonly develop externalizing and internalizing behavior problems or disorders by middle childhood (Earls & Jung, 1987) and/or in adolescence (Maziade et al., 1990) when compared to children with normal temperamental traits. Researchers have noted increased behavioral activity level in both youth at high risk for substance abuse and those actually diagnosed with a substance use disorder (Tarter, Laird, & Moss, 1990; Tarter et al., 1990). Other temperament or trait deviations manifested in high risk youth include reduced attention-span-persistence (Schaeffer, Parson, & Yohman, 1984), increased impulsivity (Noll et al., 1992; Shedler & Block, 1990) and such negative affect states as irritability (Brook et al., 1990) and emotional reactivity (Chassin, Rogosch, & Barrera, 1991; Blackson, 1994). Adolescent alcoholics can be classified into two broad temperamental clusters, those with behavioral dyscontrol and hypophoria, and those with primarily negative affect (Tarter et al., 1994). These represent groups of adolescents with co-morbid disruptive behavior disorders (conduct disorder, attention-deficit hyperactivity disorder) and those with concurrent mood and/or anxiety disorders. As suggested by investigators who have found language deficits in youth affected, or at high risk for, substance use disorders, children and adolescents with learning disabilities or disorders may also show an increased incidence of co-morbidity (Bukstein & Tarter, 1998; Moss et al., 1994). Specific psychiatric disorders in childhood, including disruptive behavior disorders as well as mood or anxiety disorders confer an increased risk for the development of substance use disorders in adolescence (Bukstein, Brent, & Kaminer, 1989; Christie et al., 1988; Loeber, 1988).

Disruptive behavior disorders are the most common psychiatric disorders diagnosed in adolescents with SUDs. Conduct Disorder, including the component of aggression, usually precedes and accompanies adolescent SUDs (Huizinga & Elliot, 1981; Loeber, 1988; Milan et al., 1991). Clinical populations of adolescents with SUDs manifest rates of conduct disorder ranging from 50% to almost 80%. Although Attention Deficit Hyperactivity Disorder (ADHD) is often present in substance using and abusing youth, the observed association may be due to the high level of comorbidity between conduct disorder and ADHD (Alterman & Tarter, 1986; Barkley et al., 1990; Kaminer, 1992a; Wilens et al., 1994). The early onset of conduct disorder, aggressive behavior, in the presence of attention deficit hyperactivity disorder, may further increase the risk for later substance abuse (Loeber, 1988). Aggressive behaviors are present in many adolescents who have substance use disorders (Bukstein, 1994; Milin et al., 1991). Although many, if not most, adolescents who display aggressive behaviors have a history of such behavior prior to the onset of substance use or SUDs, the consumption of such substances as alcohol, amphetamines, and/or phencyclidine may increase the likelihood of subsequent aggressive behavior (Moss & Tarter, 1993; Tuchfield, Clayton, & Logan, 1982). The direct pharmacological effects resulting in aggression may be further exacerbated by the presence of preexisting psychopathology (e.g., ADHD, mood disorders), the use of multiple agents simultaneously, and the frequent, relative inexperience of the adolescent substance user. For example, a novice user may be more likely than an experienced user to react to specific psychoactive effects with anxiety. An inexperienced drinker may drink too rapidly, causing a rapid rise in blood alcohol level and, thus, further impairment in judgment and behavioral controls.

Mood disorders, particularly depression, frequently have onsets both preceding and consequent to the onset of substance use and SUDs in adolescents (Bukstein, Glancy, & Kaminer, 1992; Deykin, Levy, & Wells, 1987; Deykin, Bubka, & Zeena, 1992; Hovens, Cantwell, & Kiriakos, 1994). The prevalence of depressive disorders in these studies of clinical populations ranged from 24% to > 50%. Substance use disorders among adolescents are also a risk factor for suicidal behaviors, including ideation, attempted and completed suicide (Crumley, 1990; Kaminer, 1992b). Possible mechanisms for these relationships include acute and chronic effects of psychoactive substances. Adolescents who commit suicide frequently have used alcohol or other drugs at the time of suicide (Brent, Perper, & Allman, 1987). The acute substance use episode may produce transient but intense dysphoric states, disinhibition, impaired judgment, and increased level of impulsivity, or may exacerbate preexisting psychopathology, including depression or anxiety disorders (Bukstein, 1994; Schuckit, 1986).

A number of studies of clinical populations show high rates of anxiety disorders among youth with SUDs (Clark et al., 1995; Clark & Sayette,

1993). In clinical populations of adolescents with SUDs, the prevalence of anxiety disorder ranged from 7% to over 40% (Clark et al., 1995; DeMilio, 1989; Stowell & Estroff, 1992). The chronology of the onset of co-morbid anxiety and SUDs is variable, depending on the specific anxiety disorder. Social phobia usually precedes abuse, while panic and generalized anxiety disorder may more often follow the onset of SUDs (Kushner, Sher, & Beitman, 1990). Adolescents with SUDs often have a past history or current manifestation of Posttraumatic Stress Disorder (PTSD) (Clark et al., 1995; Van Hasselt et al., 1993). Bulimia nervosa is also frequently associated with adolescents having substance use disorders (Bulik, 1987; Bulik et al., 1992). SUDs are very common among individuals, especially young and chronically impaired, who are diagnosed with schizophrenia (Kutcher, Kachur, Marton, Szalai, & Jaunkalns, 1992; Regier et al., 1990).

ASSESSMENT

Children and adolescents can be assessed at several levels for substance use and related pathology and risk factors. For most health care professionals, screening is the most appropriate level of assessment. When an adolescent presents with trauma, sexually transmitted disease(s), or impaired mental status, a specific inquiry into substance use behavior is indicated. In a medical context, as opposed to a mental health or legal setting, the focus is on the health of the adolescent. Questions about substance use behavior may not be perceived as threatening. The clinician must ask, however, about the use of specific substances and potential negative consequences of use. Vague answers such as "not much" or "just a little" are not adequate; the clinician should press the adolescent to be more specific in terms of quantity, frequency and duration of use. The professional may proceed with a general inquiry into psychosocial functioning, ultimately referring for a more detailed, thorough assessment those adolescents who report a significant level of substance use along with dysfunction in one or more areas of their lives.

Most often, adolescents are referred for assessment and possible treatment following the identification of a problem such a poor school performance and/or behavior, family conflict, and violation of the law; or the occurrence of an event, such as trauma, intoxication, possession of illicit substances. Many times, substance use may not be initially identified as the reason for referral.

Although substance use behavior may be the specific target for assessment and subsequent intervention, the optimal assessment of an adolescent includes evaluation of other behavioral and environmental domains as well as risk factors for the development of substance use disorders. A multidomain, multistage assessment (Rahdert, 1991; Tarter, 1990) may be the best approach for a comprehensive assessment strategy. Examples of these domains include:

(1) substance use behaviors;
(2) psychiatric and behavior problems (including aggression and delinquency);
(3) school and/or vocational functioning;
(4) family functioning;
(5) social competency and peer relations (including social skills);
(6) leisure and recreation, and
(7) physical health or medical status.

After screening each domain via interview or instrument, each area in which there is some level of deficit or dysfunction should be more thoroughly assessed by other instruments and/or detailed inquiry or referral to another health care provider.

Substance use is a multidimensional behavior that demands a thorough evaluation of several dimensions of substance use behavior, in addition to quantity and frequency of use (Babor et al., 1991; White & Labouvie, 1989). Within the domain of substance use behavior, important dimensions include the

- *pattern of use* (quantity, frequency, onset, and types of agents used),
- *negative consequences* (school/vocational, social/peer/family, emotional/behavioral, legal and physical),
- *context of use* (time/place, peer use/attitudes, mood antecedents, consequences, expectancies, and overall social milieu) and
- *control of use* (view of use as a problem, attempts to stop or limit use, other DSM-IV dependence criteria).

The multidomain nature of substance use problems demands the cooperation of diverse professions include substance abuse counselors, teachers and other school staff, mental health professionals, and law enforcement professionals.

Although self-reports of substance use behavior have been found to be reliable in some populations, specific populations such as extremely antisocial youth may report less use than drug clinic samples (Winters et al., 1991). The clinician may attempt to discretely substantiate suspected use by reports from third parties (friends or family) or through the use of urine or blood toxicology. Some adolescents may also exaggerate their substance use patterns, especially if they feel that such a report will raise their image in the eyes of their peer group. There is no known toxicological screening tool or test for SUDs or that predicts outcomes. Regardless of the setting, the clinician should always be aware that an adolescent's report about substance us and other deviant behaves might not be accurate. Often, a survey of risk factors can provide the clinician with an index of suspicion for the presence of substance use, SUDs and related behaviors and problems. In some states, laws allow health care professionals to obtain appropriate body fluids for toxicological testing if the individual was involved in a motor vehicle accident.

A variety of instruments are available and others are being developed to assist the screening and detailed assessment of substance use and related behaviors and problems. The common use of instruments with children developed for adults, or without standardization and validation, may be inappropriate for adolescents (Winters, 1990). (The reader is referred elsewhere for a more detailed discussion of individual instruments (Leccese & Waldron, 1994; Winters, 1990; Winters & Stinchfield, 1995).) While instruments have obvious potential value in research settings, identifying targets for treatment and measuring outcomes, they are not a substitute for face-to-face clinical interviews and professional expertise and judgment.

INTERVENTIONS: PREVENTION AND TREATMENT

The principle difference between primary prevention and treatment (including secondary and tertiary prevention) interventions is usually the intensiveness of the intervention and the target population(s). Treatment is likely to be directed to small groups, including individuals and/or their families and to be more intensive in terms of the duration and frequency of the intervention modality. Both primary prevention and treatment essentially involve the targeting of risk factors, although treatment will focus more directly on substance use behavior. Another difference between primary prevention and treatment is the nature of the professionals who deliver each level of intervention. For example, teachers, law enforcement officers, laypeople including parents, or primary health care professionals such as nurses or physicians often deliver primary prevention interventions.

Prevention

The optimal intervention for adolescent substance use or use disorders is prevention. Although a consensus exists regarding the importance of prevention efforts, there is a lack of agreement of a conceptual goal for prevention, that is, "what are we attempting to prevent—use, abuse or dependence?" Although some recommend that interventions be directed at the prevention of various use patterns or consequences of substance use, a broader view of prevention includes targeting risk factors for the development of substance use or use disorders. Targeting risk factors requires a host of measures involving the educational, mental health, and welfare systems. Primary prevention efforts aimed at reducing risk factors, however, may prove to be more effective and cost efficient overall than treatment, and may influence the development of a wide range of problems and psychosocial dysfunction in children, adolescents, and their families.

Most prevention efforts are based on various theoretical models of adolescent substance use/abuse development. Social learning theorists (Bandura, 1969) propose that substance use, along with other patterns of behavior, are determined through exposure to or learning from the social environment. Most prevention interventions are based on social learning models. If one can change what youth are exposed to, then behavioral changes will follow. Social learning interventions include educational approaches, family-based interventions and community-based projects.

Educational Interventions

Educational approaches generally have three basic foci: (1) knowledge/attitude, (2) values/decision-making and (3) social competency or skills (Moskowitz, 1989). Interventions directed at knowledge and attitude change are directed at changing the knowledge and attitudes about substances, and the risks of their use, including health and social consequences, and legal sanctions. Values/decision-making interventions attempt to improve the insight of youths to adopt values on which they can base decision about their behavior. Social competency or skills interventions are based on the premise that youth need specific psychosocial skills in order to behave appropriately, prosocially. The teaching is comprised of fundamental, generalizable skills involving interpersonal communication and problem solving. In isolation from other prevention interventions, educational efforts appear to have minimal long-term effects on eventual substance use behavior.

Skills Focused Interventions

Skills focused interventions are an extension of educational interventions but usually involve smaller groups of youth in interactive sessions. Their purposes include: to improve social competency, including the ability to resist peer pressure to use substances, development of prosocial attitudes and values, development of improved problem-solving, and social communication abilities and improvements in self-esteem. The use of most skills-focused interventions have failed to result in demonstrated lasting changes in outcomes (Bukstein, 1995). One limitation to many previous efforts has been the relatively brief duration of the interventions. In implementing a skills-based prevention program based on life skills, Botvin and associates (Botvin et al., 1995) included booster sessions during the 2 years following the basic program and reported a significant reduction in substance use behavior 6 years later in groups receiving the life skills training when compared with groups of adolescents who did not receive this training.

Family-Based Interventions

Family-based prevention interventions are based on considerable research establishing the critical role of parents and other family members in the development of substance use and SUDs (Kumpfer, 1989; Szapocznik et al., 1988). Family-based interventions using both family therapy and parent management training have demonstrated a reduction of risk factors (De-Marsh & Kumpfer, 1986).

Community-Based Interventions

Community-based interventions encompass a wide variety of activities and seek to target the social environment of the specific communities where adolescents reside. Community organizations such as Mothers Against Drunk Driving (MADD) have sought to increase community awareness of adolescent substance use and related problems, to increase public support for changes in public policy and laws, and for increased law enforcement (Moskowitz & Jones, 1985). Media messages and campaigns have also sought to change the attitudes of adults and adolescents alike. Although the effectiveness of such media efforts to actually achieve persistent behavioral changes or to prevent substance use, especially in isolation from other interventions, is highly questionable, such efforts may be useful in reinforcing desired attitudes and societal norms when combined with other prevention strategies (Flay & Sobel, 1983). Several regulatory efforts, such as raising the minimum legal drinking age, have had a modest but significant effect on adolescent substance use and its consequences such as motor vehicle accidents and deaths (Moskowitz, 1989; O'Malley & Wagenaar, 1991).

Community or neighborhood characteristics such as low socioeconomic status, high population density, low population mobility, physical deterioration, and high crime are associated with high levels of substance use in adolescence (Brook et al., 1990). Thus, many costly and politically difficult efforts aimed at substantially improving the socioeconomic status of communities may ultimately have the greatest influence on substance use behaviors.

Biologic Interventions

The primary prevention of adolescent substance use and SUDs increasingly involves the identification and treatment of preexisting psychiatric disorders. These include, ADHD, mood disorders, anxiety disorders, as well as targeting deviations in temperament. In many respects, the primary prevention of substance use disorders in adolescents involves the secondary and tertiary prevention (or treatment) of psychiatric disorders in children and younger adolescents. Methods for the treatment of these psychiatric disorders include psychotropic medications and psychosocial treatments such as parent management and skills training. As many youth present with many, severe level of risk factors, intervention may need to be multimodal, that is, several diverse treatments delivered in sufficient intensity and duration over time.

Comprehensive Prevention Programs

Given the relatively poor results from the variety of types of prevention interventions discussed above, programs targeting a single risk factor or category of risk factors may be insufficient to produce real or lasting change (Battjes & Jones, 1985). Perhaps the best approach is the targeting of multiple risk factors as part of a comprehensive intervention. Such comprehensive approaches might include educational and skills interventions as well as community and media efforts. Although such an approach is costly and time-consuming, results from a recent program in Kansas City appear to be promising (Ellickson & Bell, 1990; Pentz, Dwyer, & MacKinnon, 1989). The STAR Project represents a well coordinated, communitywide prevention effort targeting several risk factors through a media campaign, school-based skills groups and a variety of other prevention projects. The comprehensive, diverse nature of the STAR project and its apparent success in reducing some indices of adolescent substance use underscores the need for comprehensive approaches to prevention that target multiple risk factors.

School-based prevention programs are a logical basis for a comprehensive approach to the prevention of substance use problems in youth. As part of a comprehensive tobacco, alcohol, and substance abuse (TAS) prevention program, schools should provide instruction about the short-term and long-term negative physiologic and social consequences of substance use, social influence on use, peer norms regarding use, and refusal skills. Successful TAS prevention programs address multiple psychosocial factors related to TAS use through the fostering of knowledge, attitudes, and skills among children and adolescents and address these factors at developmentally appropriate ages. Although curricula should be provided at grade levels, interventions in late elementary school and early middle school (grades 5–8) are particularly important due to the transitions experienced by these youth and their exposure to older youth. The curricula should be regularly reinforced throughout middle and high school as prevention results appear to dissipate over time. Studies of prevention interventions indicate that increases in the intensity and duration of programming result in increases in their effectiveness. Program delivery features should include program delivery active participation by peers, through demonstrations, modeling, and peer generated role plays.

Treatment

The primary goal for the treatment of adolescents with SUDs is achieving and maintaining abstinence from substance use. Although abstinence should remain the explicit, long-term goal for treatment, a realistic view recognizes both the chronicity of SUDs in some populations of adolescents, developmental aspects of adolescence, and the self-limited nature of substance use and substance use-related problems in other adolescent populations. Given these considerations, harm reduction may be an acceptable interim, implicit goal for treatment. Included in the concept of harm reduction is a reduction in the use and adverse effects of substances, a reduction in the severity and frequency of relapses, and improvement in one or more domains of the adolescent's functioning (e.g., academic performance or family functioning). Despite an acceptance of harm reduction as an interim goal for treatment, controlled use of any nonprescribed substance of abuse should never be an explicit goal in the treatment of adolescents. Abstinence should not be the only goal of treatment. The broad concept of rehabilitation involves targeting associated problems and domains of functioning for treatment. Interventions dealing with coexisting psychiatric and behavioral problems, family functioning, peer and interpersonal relationships, and academic functioning will produce not only general improvements in psychosocial functioning, but will most likely yield improved outcomes in the primary treatment goal of achieving and maintaining abstinence (Bukstein, 1995).

Among the important characteristics of successful treatment are sufficient duration, intensiveness and comprehensiveness, the presence of after-care or follow-up treatment(s), sensitivity to cultural, racial, and socioeconomic realities of adolescents and their families, family involvement, collaboration with social services agencies, promotion of prosocial activities and a drug-free lifestyle and involvement in self-support groups such as Alcoholics Anonymous (AA) or Narcotics Anonymous (NA) (Hser et al., 2001; Williams et al., 2000).

Despite numerous advances in research of the treatment of adult substance use disorders, there is a relative paucity of data regarding the course and correlates of treatment of adolescents. Existing studies indicate that most adolescents return to some level of alcohol or other drug abuse following treatment (Brown, Vik, & Creamer, 1989; Brown et al., 1990). Researchers have identified characteristics of adolescents in treatment as well as specific predictors of treatment outcome, including patient or adolescent characteristics, social support system variables, and program characteristics. Adolescents in substance abuse treatment begin substance use at an early age, progress rapidly to the use of hard drugs, and usually use multiple drugs (Brown, Vik, & Creamer, 1989; Brown, Mott, & Stewart, 1992; Myers & Brown, 1990).

Adolescents entering treatment often have coexisting psychiatric disorders or early personality difficulties, deviant behavior, school difficulties, including high levels of truancy, and family disruption and substance abuse (Brown, Mott, & Stewart, 1992; Bukstein, Glancy, & Kaminer, 1992; Doyle, Delaney, & Tobin, 1994). Pretreatment characteristics that predict completion of treatment by adolescents include a greater severity of alcohol problems, greater use of drugs other than alcohol marijuana and tobacco, a higher level of internalizing problems, and lower self-esteem (Doyle, Delaney, & Tobin, 1994). Preexisting psychopathology such as conduct disorder predicts noncompletion of treatment and a return to substance use (Myers & Brown, 1990).

Although such characteristics such as severity of substance use may predict short-term treatment outcomes, most longer-term outcomes may be dependent upon social and other environmental factors. This is consistent with studies of relapse among adolescent populations that suggest that relapse in adolescents is more often associated with social pressures to use, rather than situations involving negative affect, as is usually found in adult relapse (Brown et al., 1994; Vik, Grisel, & Brown, 1992). Treatment compliance as manifested by attendance at self-support or aftercare groups is associated with higher rates of abstinence and other measures of improved outcome when compared with those adolescents who did not attend such groups (Alford, Koehler, & Leonard, 1991; Myers, Brown, & Mott, 1993; Harrison & Hoffmann, 1989).

Most adolescents return to some level of substance use after treatment. However, adolescents who are abstinent following treatment, and to a lesser extent, nonabstinent treatment completers experience decreased interpersonal conflict, improved academic functioning, and increased involvement in social and occupational activities (Brown et al., 1994). Patterns of substance abuse among adolescents appear to become more stable between 6–12 months after treatment (Brown et al., 1994).

Despite the absence of well-controlled studies comparing types of treatment or treatment modalities for SUDs, reviewers of treatment outcomes have concluded that treatment can be effective and is certainly better than no treatment (Catalano et al., 1990–1991). Program characteristics that are associated with improved abstinence and lower levels of relapse include longer duration of treatment, available follow-up or after-care treatment, involvement of family, and the availability of social, support services (Fleisch, 1991; Friedman & Beschner, 1985).

Treatment planning for adolescents with substance use disorders and associated problems begins with assessment. Targets for intervention include dysfunctional domains and identified risk factors. For adolescents who are identified as substance users as opposed to those with substance use disorders, the significant risk factors or psychiatric disorders offers a useful focus for treatment. For those youth with substance use disorders, the focus of treatment become substance use and primary goal of treatment is abstinence from use. Despite the importance of targeting substance use behavior, treatment needs to attend to other dysfunctional domains in these adolescents.

Many treatment programs for adolescents are based on the 12 steps of Alcoholics or Narcotics Anonymous (AA or NA). Programs often augment group therapy and the attendance at self-support groups with self-paced work using structured booklets (Jaffe, 1990). Unfortunately, there have not been well-controlled studies of 12 step-based programs compared with other types of treatment for adolescents.

Family interventions are critical to the success of any treatment approach with adolescents with SUDs (Liddle, 1995; Stanton & Shadish, 1997; Waldron, 1997), since a number of family-related factors, such as parental substance use or abuse, poor parent-child relationships, low perceived parental support, low emotional bonding, and poor parent supervision and management of the adolescent's behavior, have been identified as risk factors for the development of substance abuse among adolescents. Although there are many approaches to family intervention, for substance abuse treatment, they have common goals: providing psychoeducation about SUDs, which decreases familial denial and resistance to treatment; assisting parents and family to initiate and maintain efforts to get the adolescent into appropriate treatment and achieve abstinence; assisting the parents and family in establishing or reestablishing structure with consistent limit-setting and careful monitoring of the adolescent's activities and behavior; and improving communication among family members.

Family therapy is the most studied modality in the treatment of adolescents with SUDs. Based on the limited number of comparative studies, outpatient family therapy appears to be superior to other forms of outpatient treatment (Deas & Thomas, 2001; Liddle & Dakof, 1995; Waldron, 1997; Williams et al., 2000). Among the forms of family therapy with support based on controlled studies are Functional Family therapy (Friedman, 1989), Multisystemic Therapy (MST) (Henggeler et al., 1991), and Family Systems Therapy (Joanning et al., 1992). Henggeler and associates' (Henggeler, Melton, & Smith, 1992) Multisystemic Therapy (MST) represents a family ecological systems approach with interventions targeting family functioning and communication, school and peer functioning and community functioning. In addressing the multidimensional nature of adolescent substance use disorders and associated problems, MST focuses on multiple targets and using many treatment techniques, as necessary, including family therapy and behavioral therapies. MST is integrative and comprehensive but targets on specific, identified areas of dysfunction. Based on its breath of potential treatment targets and its environmental focus, MST offers a compelling model for adolescent SUD treatment.

A number of cognitive behavioral treatments, including many previously used with adults (e.g., relapse prevention), have been adapted as treatment modalities for adolescents with substance use disorders (Bukstein & Van Hasselt, 1993; Marlatt & Gordon, 1985). Many cognitive-behavioral modalities, such as parent training, social skills, anger control, and problem-solving training, developed for and effective with adolescents with conduct disorder also are relevant for youth with coexisting SUDs (Kazdin, 1995). Kaminer and associates (1998) reported the effectiveness of a cognitive-behavioral model for adolescents with SUDs.

The presence of significant psychiatric comorbidity in adolescent substance abusers suggests that psychotropic medications may be used in this population. Only recently has there been research evaluating the efficacy and safety of any psychotropic medication in the treatment of adolescents with SUDs (Kaminer, 1995). Riggs and associates (Riggs et al., 1996, 1997, 1998) have conducted open trials with pemoline and bupropion for ADHD and Fluoxetine for depression in a population of drug dependent delinquents.

Pharmacotherapy or medication treatment can potentially target several problem areas including treatment of withdrawal, use to counteract or decrease the subjective reinforcing effects of illicit substance use, and treatment of comorbid psychopathology. Although clinically significant withdrawal symptoms appear to be rare in adolescents (Martin et al., 1995), there is little rationale for using different detoxification protocols, when indicated, than those for adults. The use of agents to block the reinforcing effects of various substances, as aversive agents (e.g., disulfiram) or to relieve craving during and after acute withdrawal (e.g., desipramine) has been studied in adults, but have received scant attention for adolescents (Kaminer, 1992c). Aversive pharmacological treatment with agents such as disulfiram is rare in adolescents and extreme caution should be taken in considering such therapy due to the significant potential for adverse effects with these medications and the poor compliance that is often observed in these adolescents (Myers et al., 1994). Similarly, despite the safe and effective use of the opiate antagonist naltrexone in adults to reduce cravings for alcohol, the widespread use of this agent awaits more careful study.

The most common indication for the use of psychotropic medications in the overall treatment of adolescents with SUDs is in targeting coexisting psychopathology (Bukstein, Brent, & Kaminer, 1989). Potential targets for pharmacological treatment include depression and other mood problems, ADHD, severe levels of aggressive behavior and anxiety disorders. There are studies in the literature demonstrating the efficacy of pharmacological agents prescribed for adolescents with SUDs and comorbid psychiatric disorders. Some limitations do exist in the use of psychotropic medications for adolescents with co-morbid SUDs and psychiatric disorders. General considerations, while described in general here, are discussed in more detail in other reviews (Kaminer, 1995; Rosenberg, Holttrum, & Gershon, 1994). Pharmacological approaches such as lithium (Geller et al., 1998) and serotonergic reuptake inhibitors (Cornelius et al., 2000; Deas-Nesmith et al., 1998; Riggs et al., 1997) have produced significant improvements in adolescents with SUDs and comorbid mood disorders.

Clinicians should use the same caution in considering pharmacological treatment for adolescents with comorbid SUDs and psychiatric disorders as they do with youth with psychiatric symptoms alone. The presence of SUDs or substance use may increase the potential for intentional or unintentional overdose with certain psychotropic medications, especially in combination with some substances of abuse. Some commonly used pharmacological agents, such as psychostimulants and benzodiazepines, may have inherent abuse potential.

Assessing the risk of concurrent use of various substance(s) of abuse and the pharmacotherapeutic agent is critical before prescribing any medication for an adolescent with a SUD. Informed consent should include a description of possible dangers of concurrent use of agents. The risk of abuse of a therapeutic agent either by the adolescent, his peer group or family members should prompt a thorough assessment of the risk of this outcome (e.g., past history of abuse of the agent, family/parental history of substance abuse and/ or antisocial behavior). Often, parental or adult supervision of medication administration can alleviate concerns about potential abuse. The clinician should also consider alternative agents with a lower potential for abuse. Alternatives to the Drug Enforcement Agency (DEA) Schedule II stimulants (dextroamphetamine, methylphenidate; mixed amphetamine salts) for the treatment of attention-deficit hyperactivity disorder include pemoline (Schedule IV), clonidine, tricyclic antidepressants, and bupropion. Although many anxiety symptoms or disorders in adolescents can be treated successfully with psychosocial methods such as behavior therapy, the use of tricyclic antidepressants, buspirone, or selective serotonin reuptake inhibitors are preferred over benzodiazepines. Nevertheless, as the clinician should not dismiss the use of pharmacotherapeutic agents in the treatment of adolescents with SUDs, the use of any specific agent should not be discounted until a thorough consideration of the potential benefits versus likely and possible risks is made. The clinician should carefully monitor the presence of adverse effects of pharmacotherapy and the potential relationship of these effects to ongoing substance use.

The clinical use of psychtropic agents generally involves achieving some level of abstinence or control of substance use before a more optimal assessment of psychiatric symptoms and starting pharmacological treatment. Such factors as the presence of target symptoms prior to substance abuse or during previous periods of abstinence, a family history of the targeted psychiatric disorder and past treatment failures without medication may suggest the need for a more aggressive approach.

For example, the treatment of ADHD among populations with SUDs remains problematic due to the abuse potential of CNS stimulants by the patient, family and peers (Kaminer, 1995). In addition to close supervision of medication compliance, clinicians should consider the use of effective agents with much lower abuse potential such as tricyclic antidepressants, bupropion, venlafaxine, and pemoline.

The multiple areas of possible dysfunction present in adolescents with SUDs, and the many available treatment modalities suggests a multimodal approach. The use of a concurrent combination of traditional approaches, cognitive-behavioral and family treatment and medication may prove to be the optimal intervention. Similar to prevention interventions, treatment for adolescents with SUDs may need to continue for a much longer duration to have persistent, positive effects. Despite two decades of specific treatment for adolescents with SUDs, little is known about the dose of treatment necessary for successful outcomes, nor do we know much about the specific effects of such characteristics as gender, race, and co-morbid psychopathology on outcome. Because the developmental and other treatment issue of adolescents often differ from those of adults, adolescents should have separate programs that are designed for their needs. It may be reasonable to develop programs tailored to the specific needs of such specialized adolescent treatment populations as African American or other racial groups, pregnant adolescents, gay teens, or homeless adolescents due to cultural differences and particular housing, medical needs, or other psychosocial needs.

Not all adolescents presenting for treatment of SUDs are the same, nor do they necessarily require the same treatments or level of treatment (Babor et al., 1991). Treatment matching: or matching adolescents with specific characteristics with appropriate levels of care and types of treatment modalities is a concept having received much attention in the adult literature (McLellan & Alterman, 1991). Psychiatric severity may be the best identified guide to matching (McLellan et al., 1983). Further research needs to examine the potential need to match treatments with other adolescent characteristics such as socioeconomic or racial status, family functioning or educational/vocational needs.

Recent changes in the health care system include an emphasis on lower cost ambulatory settings with only treatment failures and severe cases with co-morbidity being allowed to utilize acute hospital and other residential treatment settings (Bukstein, 1995). There exist significant differences between insurance coverage between many private and public insurance plans and these are changes almost constantly in the current managed-care environment.

SUMMARY

Substance use and substance use disorders in adolescents continue to be a major public health problem. Substance use problems are multifactoral and included prominent influences from the biology and social ecology of the adolescent. Adolescents at high risk for substance use disorders commonly have additional problem behaviors and coexisting psychiatric disorders. Substance use and use disorders may have major negative developmental consequences into later adolescence and young adulthood. Previous research and efforts at successful prevention and treatment have been limited by lack of knowledge about the risk factors and development of substance related problems in youth. As more information emerges about the development of SUDs, more effective prevention and treatment strategies are being studied and used effectively.

REFERENCES

Aarons, G. A., Brown, S. A., Hough, R. L., Garland, A. F., & Wood, P. (2001). Prevalence of adolescent substance use disorders across five sectors of care. *Journal of the American Academy of Child and Adolescent Psychiatry, 40,* 419–426.
Alford, G. S., Koehler, R. A., & Leonard, J. (1991). Alcoholic anonymous-narcotics anonymous model inpatient treatment of chemically dependent adolescents: A 2-year outcome study. *Journal of Studies on Alcohol, 52,* 118–126.
Alterman, A. I., & Tarter, R. E. (1986). An examination of selected topologies: Hyperactivity, familial and antisocial alcoholism. In M. Galanter (Ed.), *Recent developments in alcoholism* (Vol. 4, pp. 169–189). New York: Plenum.
American Psychiatric Association. (1994). *Diagnostic and Statistical Manual of Mental Disorders, 4th ed.* Washington, DC: American Psychiatric Association.
Babor, T. F., DelBoca, F., McLaney, M. A., Jacobi, B., Higgins-Biddle, & Hass, W. (1991). Just say Y. E. S.: Matching adolescents to appropriate interventions for alcohol and other drug-related problems. *Alcohol Health Research World, 15,* 77–86.
Bandura, A. (1969). *Principles of behavior modification.* New York: Holt, Rinehart and Winston.
Barkley, R. A., Fischer, M., Edelbrock, C. S., & Smallish, L. (1990). The adolescent outcome of hyperactive children diagnosed by research criteria: I. An 8-year prospective follow-up study. *Journal of the American Academy of Child and Adolescent Psychiatry, 29,* 546–557.
Battjes, R. J., & Jones, C. L. (1985). Implications of etiological research for preventative interventions and future research. In C. L. Jones & R. J. Battjes (Eds.), *Etiology of drug abuse: Implications for prevention* (pp. 269–276). Rockville, MD: Department of Health and Human Services, National Institute on Drug Abuse.

Baumrind, D. (1983). Familial antecedents of adolescent drug use: A developmental perspective. In C. L. Jones & R. J. Battjes (Eds.), *Etiology of drug abuse: Implications for prevention.* NIDA Research Monograph 56 (pp. 13–44). Rockville, MD: Department of Health and Human Services.

Baumrind, D., & Moselle, K. A. (1985). A developmental perspective on adolescent drug abuse. *Advances in Alcohol and Substance Abuse, 5,* 41–67.

Blackson, T. C. (1994). Temperament: A salient correlate of risk factors for alcohol and drug abuse. *Drug and Alcohol Dependence, 36,* 205–214.

Botvin, G., Baker, E., Dusenbury, L., Botvin, E. M., & Diaz, T. (1995). Long-term follow-up results of a randomized drug abuse prevention trial in a white middle-class population. *Journal of the American Medical Association, 273,* 1106–1112.

Botvin, G., Baker, E., Filazzola, A., & Botvin, E. M. (1990). A cognitive behavioral approach to substance abuse prevention: One year follow-up. *Addictive Behaviors, 15,* 47–63.

Brent, D. A., Perper, J. A., & Allman, C. (1987). Alcohol, firearms and suicide among youth: Temporal trends in Allegheny County, Pennsylvania, 1960 to 1983. *Journal of the American Medical Association, 257,* 3369–3372.

Brook, J. S., Linkoff, I. F., & Whiteman, M. (1977). Peer, family and personality domains as related to adolescent's drug behavior. *Psychological Reports, 41,* 1095–1102.

Brook, J. S., Whiteman, M., Gordon, A. S., & Brook, D. W. (1990). The psychosocial etiology of adolescent drug use: A family interactional approach. *General Social Psychology Monographs, 116,* 2.

Brown, S. A., D'Amico, E. J., McCarthy, D. M., & Tapert, S. F. (2001). Four-year outcomes from adolescent alcohol and drug treatment. *Journal of Studies on Alcohol, 62,* 381–388.

Brown, S. A., Mott, M. A., & Stewart, M. A. (1992). Adolescent alcohol and drug abuse. In C. E. Walter (Ed.), *Handbook of clinical child psychology* (pp. 677–693). New York: John Wiley.

Brown, S. A., Myers, M. G., Mott, M. A., & Vik, P. W. (1994). Correlates of success following treatment for adolescent substance abuse. *Applied and Preventive Psychology, 3,* 61–73.

Brown, S. A., Vik, P. N., & Creamer, V. (1989). Characteristics of relapse following adolescent substance abuse treatment. *Addictive Behaviors, 14,* 291–300.

Brown, S. A., Vik, P. W., McQuaid, J. R., Patterson, T., Irwin, M. R., & Grant, I. (1990). Severity of psychosocial stress and outcome of alcoholism treatment. *Journal of Abnormal Psychology, 99,* 344–348.

Bry, B. H. (1983). Predictive drug abuse: Review and reformulation. *Journal of the Addictions, 18,* 223–233.

Bukstein, O. G. (1994). Substance abuse. In M. Hersen, R. T. Ammerman, & L. A. Sisson (Eds.), *Handbook of aggressive and destructive behavior in psychiatric patients* (pp. 445–468). New York: Plenum.

Bukstein, O. G. (1995). *Adolescent substance abuse: assessment, prevention, and treatment.* New York: Wiley InterScience.

Bukstein, O. G., Brent, D. A., & Kaminer, Y. (1989). Comorbidity of substance abuse and other psychiatric disorders in adolescents. *American Journal of Psychiatry, 146,* 1131–1141.

Bukstein, O., Glancy, L. J., & Kaminer, Y. (1992). Patterns of affective comorbidity in a clinical population of dually-diagnosed substance abusers. *Journal of the American Academy of Child and Adolescent Psychiatry, 31,* 1041–1045.

Bukstein, O. G., & Kaminer, Y. (1994). The nosology of adolescent substance abuse. *The American Journal on Addictions, 3,* 1–13.

Bukstein, O. G., & Tarter, R. E. (1998). Substance use disorders in children and adolescents. In E. Coffey (Ed.), *Textbook of pediatric neuropsychiatry.* New York: American Psychiatric Press.

Bukstein, O. G., & Van Hasselt, V. B. (1993). Alcohol and drug abuse. In A. S. Bellack & M. Hersen (Eds.), *Handbook of behavior therapy in the psychiatric setting* (pp. 453–475). New York: Plenum.

Bulik, C. M. (1987). Drug and alcohol use by bulimic women and their families. *American Journal of Psychiatry, 144,* 1604–1606.

Bulik, C. M., Sullivan, P. F., Epstein, L. H., Weltzin, T., & Kaye, W. (1992). Drug use in women with anorexia and bulimia. *International Journal of Eating Disorders, 11,* 213–225.

Catalano, R. F., Hawkins, J. D., Wells, E. A., Miller, J., & Brewer, D. (1990–1991). Evaluation of the effectiveness of adolescent drug abuse treatment, assessment of risks for relapse, and promising approaches for relapse prevention. *International Journal of Addictions, 25,* 1085–1140.

Centers for Disease Control. (1992). Selected behaviors that increase risk for HIV infection among high school students vs. 1990. *Morbidity and Mortality Weekly Report (MMWR), 41,* 231–240.

Centers for Disease Control. (2000). Youth risk behavior surveillance—Untied States, 1999. *Morbidity and Mortality Weekly Report (MMWR), 49,* 1–96.

Chassin, L., Rogosch, F., & Barrera, M. (1991). Substance use and symptomatology among adolescent children of alcoholics. *Journal of Abnormal Psychology, 4,* 449–463.

Christiansen, B. A., Goldman, M. S., & Brown, S. A. (1985). The differential development of adolescent alcohol expectancies may predict adult alcoholism. *Addictive Behaviors, 10,* 299–306.

Christie, K. A., Burke, J. D., Regier, D. A., Rae, D. S., Boyd, J. H., & Locke, B. Z. (1988). Epidemiologic evidence for early onset of mental disorders and higher risk of drug abuse in young adults. *American Journal of Psychiatry, 145,* 971–975.

Clark, D. B., & Bukstein, O. G. (1998). Psychopathology in adolescent alcohol abuse and dependence. *Alcohol Health and Research World, 22,* 117–121.

Clark, D. B., Bukstein, O. G., Smith, M. G., Kaczynski, N. A., Mezzich, A. C., & Donovan, J. E. (1995). Identifying anxiety disorders in adolescents hospitalized for alcohol abuse or dependence. *Psychiatric Services, 46,* 618–620.

Clark, D. B., & Sayette, M. A. (1993). Anxiety and the development of alcoholism. *The American Journal on Addictions, 2,* 56–76.

Cloninger, C. R. (1987). Neurogenetic adaptive mechanisms in alcoholism. *Science, 236,* 410–415.

Cornelius, J. R., Salloum, I. M., Haskett, R. F., Daley, D. C., Cornelius, M. D., Thase, M. E., et al. (2000). Flouxetine versus placebo in depressed alcoholics: A 1-year follow-up study. *Addictive Behaviors, 25,* 307–310.

Costello, J. E., Angold, A., Burns, B. J., Stangl, D. K., Tweed, D. L., Erkanli, A., & Wotrthman, C. M. (1996). The smoky Mountains study of youth: Goals, design, methods, and the prevalence of DSM-II-R disorders. *Archives of General Psychiatry, 53*, 1129–1136.

Crumley, F. E. (1990). Substance abuse and adolescent suicidal behavior. *Journal of the American Medical Association, 263*, 3051–3056.

Deas, D., & Thomas, S. E. (2001). An overview of controlled studies of adolescent substance abuse treatment. *American Journal on Addictions, 10*, 178–189.

Deas-Nesmith, D., Campbell, S., & Brady, K. T. (1998). Substance use disorders in adolescent in-patient psychiatric populations. *Journal of the National Medical Association, 90*, 233–238.

DeMarsh, J., & Kumpfer, K. L. (1986). Family-oriented interventions for the prevention of chemical dependency in children and adolescents. In S. Griswold-Ezekoye, K. L. Kumpfer, & W. J. Bukowski (Eds.), *Children and chemical abuse: Prevention and intervention* (pp. 117–151). New York: Haworth.

DeMilio, L. (1989). Psychiatric syndromes in adolescent substance abusers. *American Journal of Psychiatry, 146*, 1212–1214.

Deykin, E. Y., Buka, S. L., & Zeena, T. H. (1992). Depressive illness among chemically dependant adolescents. *American Journal of Psychiatry, 149*, 1341–1347.

Deykin, E. Y., Levy, J. C., & Wells, V. (1987). Adolescent depression alcohol and drug abuse. *American Journal of Public Health, 77*, 178–182.

DiClemente, R. J., & Ponton, L. E. (1993). HIV-related risk behaviors among psychiatrically hospitalized adolescents and school-based adolescents. *American Journal of Psychiatry, 150*, 324–325.

DiClemente, R. J., Wingood, G. M., Crosby, R,. Sionean, C., Cobb, B., Harrington, K., et al. (2001). Parental monitoring: Association with adolescents' risk behaviors. *Pediatrics, 107*(6), 1363–1368.

Dinwiddie, S. H., & Cloninger, C. R. (1991). Family and adoption studies in alcoholism and drug addiction. *Psychiatric Annals, 21*, 206–214.

Doyle, H., Delaney, W., & Trobin, J. (1994). Follow-up study of young attenders at an alcohol unit. *Addiction, 89*, 183–189.

Drug Enforcement Administration. (1995). *Methylphenidate review document.* Washington, DC: DEA Office of Diversion Control, Drug and Chemical Evaluation Section.

Earls, F., & Jung, K. (1987). Temperament and home environment characteristics in the early development of child psychopathology. *Journal of the American Academy of Child Psychiatry, 26*, 491–498.

Ellickson, P. L., & Bell, R. M. (1990). Drug prevention in junior high: A multi-site longitudinal test. *Science, 16*, 1299–1305.

Flay, B. R., & Sobel, J. L. (1983). The role of mass media in preventing adolescent substance abuse. In T. J. Glynn, C. G. Luekefeld, & J. P. Ludford (Eds.), *Preventing adolescent drug abuse: Intervention strategies.* NIDA Research Monograph No. 47 (pp. 5–35). Washington, DC: U.S. Government Printing Office.

Fleisch, B. (1991). *Approaches in the treatment of adolescents with emotional and substance abuse problems.* DHSS Pub. No. (ADM) 91–1744. Washington, DC: U.S. Government Printing Office.

Friedman, A. S., & Beschner, G. M. (Eds.). (1985). *Treatment services for adolescent substance abusers.* DHSS Pub. No. (ADM) 85–1342. Washington, DC: U.S. Government Printing Office.

Friedman, A. S., & Utada, A. (1989). A method for diagnosing and planning the treatment of adolescent drug abusers (The Adolescent Drug Abuse Diagnosis [ADAD] Instrument). *Journal of Drug Education, 19,* 285–312.

Geller, B., Cooper, T. B., Sun, K., Zimermann, B., Frazier, J., Williams, M., & Heath, J. (1998). Double-blind and placebo-controlled study of lithium for adolescent bipolar disorders with secondary substance dependency. *Journal of the American Academy of Child and Adolescent Psychiatry, 37,* 171–178.

Grella, C. E., Hser, Y., Joshi, V., & Rounds-Bryant, J. (2001). Drug treatment outcomes for adolescents with comorbid mental and substance use disorders. *Journal of Nervous and Mental Disease, 189,* 384–392.

Harrison, P. A., & Hoffmann, N. (1989). *CATOR report: Adolescent treatment completers one year later.* St Paul, MN: Chemical Abuse/Addiction Treatment Outcome Registry.

Henggeler, S. W., Melton, L. A., & Rodrgue (1991). Effects of multisystemic therapy on drug use and abuse in serious juvenile offenders: A progress report from two outcome studies. *Family Dynamics of Addiction Quarterly, 1,* 40–51.

Henggeler, S. W., Melton, G. B., & Smith, L. A. (1992). Family preservation using multisystemic therapy: An effective alternative to incarcerating serious juvenile offenders. *Journal of Consulting and Clinical Psychology, 66,* 953–961.

Hill, S. Y., Steinhauser, S. R., & Zubin, J (1987). Biological markers for alcoholism: A vulnerability model conceptualization. In P. C. Rivers (Ed.), *Alcohol and addictive behavior* (pp. 207–256). Lincoln, NE: University of Nebraska Press.

Hovens, J., Cantwell, D. P., & Kiriakos, R. (1994). Psychiatric comorbidity in hospitalized adolescent substance abusers. *Journal of the American Academy of Child and Adolescent Psychiatry, 33,* 476–483.

Howland, J., & Hingson, R. (1988). Alcohol as a risk factor for drownings: A review of the literature (1950–1985). *Accidents and Annals of Prevention, 20,* 19–20.

Hser, Y., Grella, C. E., Hubbard, R. L., Hsieh, S., Fletcher, B. W., Brown, B. S., & Anglin, M. D. (2001). An evaluation of drug treatments for adolescents in 4 U.S. cities. *Archives of General Psychiatry, 58,* 689–695.

Huizinga, D., & Elliot, D. S. (1981). *A longitudinal study of drug use and delinquency in a national sample of youth: An assessment of causal order. Project report No. 16, A national youth study.* Boulder, CO: Behavioral Research Institute.

Jaffe, S. (1990). *Step workbook for adolescent chemical dependency recovery.* Washington, DC: American Academy of Child and Adolescent Psychiatry.

Jessor, R., & Jessor, S. (1977). *Problem behavior and psychosocial development: A longitudinal study of youth.* New York: Academic Press.

Joanning, H., Quinn, W., Thomas, F., & Mullen, R. (1992). Treating adolescent drug abuse: A comparison of family system therapy, group therapy and family drug education. *Journal of Marital and Family Therapy, 18,* 345–356.

Kaminer, Y. (1992a). Clinical implications of the relationship between attention-deficit hyperactivity disorder and psychoactive substance use disorders. *The American Journal on Addictions, 1,* 257–264.

Kaminer, Y. (1992b). Psychoactive substance abuse and dependence as a risk factor in adolescent-attempted and -completed suicide. *The American Journal on Addictions, 1,* 21–29.

Kaminer, Y. (1992c). Desipramine facilitation of cocaine abstinence in an adolescent. *Journal of the American Academy of Child and Adolescent Psychiatry, 31,* 312–317.

Kaminer, Y. (1995). Issues in the pharmacological treatment of adolescent substance abuse. *Journal of Child and Adolescent Psychopharmacology, 5,* 93–106.

Kaminer, Y., Blitz, C., Burleson, J. A., Kadden, R. M., & Rounsaville, B. J. (1998). Measuring treatment process in cognitive-behavioral and interactional group therapies for adolescent substance abusers. *Journal of Nervous and Mental Disease, 186,* 407–413.

Kaminer, Y., Burleson, J. A., Blitz, C., Sussman, J., & Rounsaville, B. J. (1998). Psychotherapies for adolescent substance abusers: A pilot study. *Journal of Nervous and Mental Disease, 186,* 684–690.

Kandel, D. (1975). Stages in adolescent involvement in drug use. *Science, 190,* 912–914.

Kandel, D. B., Kessler, R. C., & Margulies, R. Z. (1978). Antecedents of adolescent initiation into stages of drug use: A developmental analysis. In D. B. Kandel (Ed.), *Longitudinal research on drug use: Empirical findings and methodological issues* (pp. 73–99). Washington, DC: Hemisphere (Halstead-Wiley).

Kandel, D. B., Johnson, J. G., & Bird, H. R. (1999). Psychiatric comorbidity among adolescents with substance use disorders: Findings from the MECA study. *Journal of the American Academy of Child and Adolescent Psychiatry, 38,* 693–699.

Kashani, J. H., Carlson, G. A., Beck, N. C., Hoeper, E. W., Corcoran, C. M., McAllister, J. A., Fallahi, C., Rosenberg, T. K., & Reid, J. C. (1987). Depression, depressive symptoms, and depressed mood among a community sample of adolescents. *American Journal of Psychiatry, 144,* 931–933.

Kashani, J. H., Orvaschel, H., Rosenberg, T. K., & Reid, R. C. (1989). Psychopathology in a community sample of children and adolescents: A developmental perspective. *Journal of the American Academy of Child and Adolescent Psychiatry, 28,* 701–706.

Kazdin, A. E. (1995). *Conduct disorder* (2nd ed.). Newbury Park, CA: Sage.

Kellam, S. G., Simon, M., & Ensminger, M. D. (1980). Antecedents in first grade of teenage drug use and psychological well-being: A ten year community-wide prospective study. In D. Ricks & B. Dohrenwend (Eds.), *Origins of psychopathology: Research and public policy.* Cambridge: Cambridge University Press.

Kessler, R. C., McGonagle, K. A., Zhao, S., Nelsen, C. B., Hughes, M., Eshleman, S., Wittchen, H-U., & Kendler, K. S. (1994). Lifetime and 12-month prevalence of DSM-II-R psychiatric disorders in the United States: Results from the national comrobidity survey. *Archives of General Psychiatry, 51,* 8–19.

Khantzian, E. J. (1985). The self-medication hypothesis of addictive disorders: Focus on heroin and cocaine dependence. *American Journal of Psychiatry, 142,* 1246–1259.

Kumpfer, K. L. (1989). Prevention of alcohol and drug abuse: A critical review of risk factors and prevention strategies. In D. Shaffer, I. Phillips, & N. B. Enzer (Eds.), *Prevention of mental disorders, alcohol and other drug use in children and adolescents* (pp. 309–272). Rockville, MD: U.S. Department of Health and Human Services.

208   *Preventable Conditions*

Kushner, M. G., Sher, K. J., & Beitman, B. D. (1990). The relation between alcohol problems and anxiety disorders. *American Journal of Psychiatry, 147*, 685–695.

Kutcher, S., Kachur, E., Marton, P., Szalai, J., & Jaunkalns, R. (1992). Substance abuse among adolescents with chronic mental illnesses: A pilot study of descriptive and differentiating features. *Canadian Journal of Psychiatry, 37*, 428–431.

Leccese, M., & Waldron, H. B. (1994). Assessing adolescent substance use: A critique of current measurement instruments. *Journal of Substance Abuse Treatment, 11*, 553–563.

Lewinshohn, P. M., Rohde, P., & Seeley, J. R. (1996). Alcohol consumption in high school adolescents: Frequency of use and dimensional structure of associated problems. *Addiction, 91*, 375–390.

Liddle, H. A., & Dakof, G. A. (1995). Family-based treatment for adolescent drug use: State of the science In E. Rahdert & D. Czechowicz (Eds.), *Adolescent Drug Abuse: Clinical Assessment and Therapeutic Interventions* (pp. 218–254). National Institute on Drug Abuse Research Monograph 156. Rockville, MD: NIDA.

Loeber, R. (1988). Natural histories of conduct problems, delinquency and associated substance use. In B. B. Lahey & A. E. Kazdin (Eds.), *Advances in Clinical Child Psychology* (Vol. 11, pp. 73–124). New York: Plenum.

Marlatt, G. A., & Gordon, J. R. (1985). *Relapse prevention*. New York: Guilford Press.

Martin, C. S., Arria, A. M., Mezzich, A. C., & Bukstein, O. G. (1993). Patterns of polydrug use in adolescent alcohol abusers. *American Journal of Drug and Alcohol Abuse, 19*, 511–522.

Martin, C. S., Kaczynski, N. A., Maisto, S. A., Bukstein, O. G., & Moss, H. B. (1995). Patterns of DSM-IV alcohol abuse and dependence symptoms in adolescent drinkers. *Journal of Studies on Alcohol, 56*, 672–680.

Maziade, M., Caron, C., Cote, P., Boutin, P., & Thivierge, J. (1990). Extreme temperament and diagnosis. A study in a psychiatric sample of consecutive children. *Archives of General Psychiatry, 47*, 477–484.

McLellan, A. T., & Alterman, A. I. (1991). *Patient treatment matching: A conceptual and methodological view with suggestions for future research in national institute on drug abuse, improving drug abuse treatment*. Washington, DC: U.S. Department of Health and Human Services.

McLellan, A. T., Luborsky, L., Woody, G. E., O'Brien, C. P., & Druley, K. A. (1983). Predicting response to alcohol and drug abuse treatment: Role of psychiatric severity. *Archives of General Psychiatry, 40*, 620–628.

Milin, R., Halikas, J. A., Meller, J. E., & Morse, C. (1991). Psychopathology among substance abusing juvenile offenders. *Journal of the American Academy of Child and Adolescent Psychiatry, 30*, 569–574.

Milstein, S. G., & Irwin, C. E. (1987). Accident-related behaviors in adolescents: A biopsychosocial view. *Alcohol, Drugs and Driving, 4*, 21–29.

Moskowitz, J. M. (1989). The primary prevention of alcohol problems: A critical review of the research literature. *Journal of Studies on Alcohol, 50*, 54–88.

Moskowitz, J. M., & Jones, R. (1985). Evaluating the effects of parent groups on the correlates of adolescent substance abuse. *Journal of Psychoactive Drugs, 17*, 173–178.

Moss, H. B., Kirisci, L., Gordon, H. W., & Tarter, R. E. (1994). A neuropsychological profile of adolescent alcoholics. *Alcoholism, Clinical and Research Experience, 18,* 159–163.

Moss, H. B., & Tarter, R. E. (1993). Substance abuse, aggression and violence: What are the connections? *The American Journal on Addictions, 2,* 149–160.

Myers, M. G., & Brown, S. A. (1990). Coping responses and relapse among adolescent substance abusers. *Journal of Substance Abuse, 2,* 177–190.

Myers, M. G., Brown, S. A., & Mott, M. A. (1993). Coping as a predictor of adolescent substance abuse treatment outcome. *Journal of Substance Abuse, 5*(1), 15–29.

Myers, M. G., Brown, S. A, & Mott, M. A. (1995). Preadolescent conduct disorder behaviors predict relapse and progression of addiction for adolescent alcohol and drug abusers. *Alcoholism, Clinical and Experimental Research, 19,* 1528–1536.

Myers, W. C., Donaue, J. E., & Goldstein, M. R. (1994). Disulfiram for alcohol use disorders in adolescents. *Journal of the American Academy of Child and Adolescent Psychiatry, 33,* 484–489.

National Center for Health Statistics. (1992). *Advance Reports of Final Mortality Statistics, 1990 monthly vital statistics.* Report 41, (Suppl 7), 1–52.

Neighbors, B., Kempton, T., & Forehand, R. (1992). Co-occurrence of substance use with conduct, anxiety, and depression disorders in juvenile delinquents. *Addictive Behaviors, 17,* 379–386.

Nelson, C. B., Health, A. C., & Kessler, R. C. (1998). Temporal progression of alcohol dependence symptoms in the U.S. household population: Results from the National Comorbidity Survey. *Journal of Clinical and Consulting Psychology, 66,* 474–483.

Newcomb, M. D., & Bentler, P. M. (1988). *Consequences of adolescent drug use.* Newbury Park, CA: Sage.

Noll, R. B., Zucker, R. A., Fitzgerald, H. E., & Curtis, W. J. (1992). Cognitive and motoric functioning of sons of alcoholic fathers and controls: The early childhood years. *Developmental Psychology, 28,* 665–675.

O'Malley, P. M., & Wagenaar, A. C. (1991). Effects of minimum drinking age laws on alcohol use, related behaviors and traffic crash involvement among American youth: 1976–1987. *Journal of Studies on Alcohol, 52,* 478–491.

Pentz, M. A., Dwyer, J. H., & MacKinnon, D. P. (1989). A multicommunity trial for primary prevention of adolescent drug abuse. *Journal of the American Medical Association, 261,* 3259–3266.

Pollock, N. K., & Martin, C. S. (1999). Diagnostic orphans: Adolescents with alcohol symptoms who do not qualify for DSM-IV abuse or dependence diagnoses. *American Journal of Psychiatry, 156,* 897–901.

Porjescz, B., & Begleiter, H. (1990). Event-related potentials in individuals at risk for alcoholism. *Alcohol, 7,* 465–469.

Rahdert, E. (Ed.). (1991). *The Adolescent Assessment and Referral System Manual.* DHHS Publication No. (ADM) 91–1735. Rockville, MD: National Institute on Drug Abuse.

Regier, D. A., Farmer, M. E., Rae, D. S., Locke, B. Z., Keith, S. J., Judd, L. L., & Goodwin, F. R. (1990). Comorbidity of mental disorders with alcohol and other drug abuse. *Journal of the American Medical Association, 264,* 2511–2518.

Reich, T., Cloninger, C. R., Van Eerdewegh, P., Rice, J. P., & Mullaney, J. (1988). Secular trends in the familial transmission of alcoholism. *Alcoholism, Clinical and Experimental Research, 12*, 458–464.

Reich, W., Earls, F., Frankel, O., & Shayka, J. (1993). Psychopathology in children of alcoholics. *Journal of the American Academy of Child and Adolescent Psychiatry, 32*, 995–1002.

Reinherz, H. Z., Giaconia, R. M., Lefkowitz, E. S., Pakiz, B., & Frost, A. K. (1993). Prevalence of psychiatric disorders in a community population of older adolescents. *Journal of the American Academy of Child and Adolescent Psychiatry, 32*, 369–377.

Resnik, H. (Ed.). (1990). *Youth and drugs: Society's mixed messages.* Rockville, MD: Office for Substance Abuse Prevention, U.S. Department of Health and Human Services.

Riggs, P. D., Baker, S., Mikulich, S. K., Young, S. E., & Crowley, T. J. (1995). Depression in substance-dependent delinquents. *Journal of the American Academy of Child and Adolescent Psychiatry, 34*, 764–771.

Riggs, P. D., Leon, S. L., Mikulich, S. K., & Pottle, L. C. (1998). An open trial of bupropion for ADHD in adolescents with substance use disorders and conduct disorder. *Journal of the American Academy of Child and Adolescent Psychiatry, 12*, 1271–1278.

Riggs, P. D., Mikovich, S. K., Coffman, L. M., & Crowley, T. J. (1997). Fluoexetine in drug-dependant delinquents with major depression: An open trial. *Journal of Child and Adolescent Psychopharmacology, 7*, 87–95.

Riggs, P. D., Thompson, L. L., Mikulich, S. K., Whitmore, E. A., & Crowley, T. J. (1996). An open trial of pemoline in drug-dependant delinquents with attention-deficit hyperactivity disorder. *Journal of the American Academy of Child and Adolescent Psychiatry, 35*, 1018–1024.

Robins, L. N. (1980). The natural history of drug abuse. In D. J. Lehier, M. Sayers, & H. W. Pearson (Eds.), Evaluation of treatment of drug abusers. *Acta Psychiatrica Scandanvia*(Suppl 284), 7–20.

Robins, L. N., & McEvoy, L. (1990). Conduct problems as predictors of substance abuse. In L. N. Robins & M. Rutter (Eds.), *Straight and devious pathways from childhood to adulthood* (pp. 182–204). Cambridge, England: Cambridge University Press.

Robins, L. N., & Przybeck, T. R. (1985). Age of onset of drug use as a risk factor in drug and other disorders. In C. L. Jones & R. J. Battjes (Eds.), *Etiology of drug abuse: Implications for prevention* (pp. 178–192). Rockville, MD: Department of Health & Human Services, National Institute on Drug Abuse.

Rosenberg, D., Holttrum, J., & Gershon, S. (1994). *Child and adolescent psychopharmacology.* Philadelphia: Saunders.

Rotheram-Borus, M. J., Koopman, C., & Ehrhardt, A. A. (1991). Homeless youths and HIV infection. *The American Psychologist, 46*, 1188–1197.

Schaeffer, K., Parson, O., & Yohman, J. (1984). Neuropsychological differences between male familial alcoholics and nonalcoholics. *Alcoholism, Clinical and Experimental Research, 8*, 347–351.

Schuckit, M. A. (1984). Subjective responses to alcohol in sons of alcoholics and control subjects. *Archives of General Psychiatry, 41*, 879–884.

Schuckit, M. A. (1985). Ethanol induced changes in body sway in men at high alcoholism risk. *Archives of General Psychiatry, 42,* 375–379.

Schuckit, M. A. (1986). Genetic and clinical implications of alcoholism and affective disorder. *American Journal of Psychiatry, 143,* 140–147.

Schuckit, M. A. (1994). Alcohol sensitivity and dependence. *EXS, 71,* 341–348.

Shedler, J., & Block, J. (1990). Adolescent drug use and psychological health: A longitudinal inquiry. *The American Psychologist, 45,* 612–630.

Spooner, C., Mattick, R. P., & Noffs, W. (2001). Outcomes of a comprehensive treatment program for adolescents with a substance-use disorder. *Journal of Substance Abuse Treatment, 20,* 205–213.

Stanton, M. D., & Shadish, W. R. (1997). Outcome, attention, and family couples treatment for drug abuse: A meta-analysis and review of the controlled, comparative studies. *Psychological Bulletin, 122,* 170–191.

St. Louis, M. E., Conway, G. A., Haymancr, Miller, C., Pederson, L. R., & Dondero, T. J. (1991). Human immunodeficiency virus infection in disadvantaged adolescents. *Journal of the American Medical Association, 266,* 2387–2391.

Stewart, D. G., & Brown, S. A. (1995). Withdrawal and dependency symptoms among adolescent alcohol and drug abusers. *Addiction, 9,* 627–635.

Stowell, R. J., & Estroff, T. W. (1992). Psychiatric disorders in substance-abusing adolescent inpatients: A pilot study. *Journal of the American Academy of Child and Adolescent Psychiatry, 31,* 1036–1040.

Szapocznik, J., Kurtines, W. M., Foote, F. H., Perez-Vidal, A., & Hervis, O. (1983). Conjoint versus one-person family therapy: Some evidence for the effectiveness of conducing family therapy through one person. *Journal of Clinical and Consulting Psychology, 5,* 889–899.

Szapocznik, J., Kurtines, W. M., Foote, F. H., Perez-Vidal, A., & Hervis, O. (1986). Conjoint versus one-person family therapy: Some evidence for the effectiveness of conducing family therapy through one person with drug-abusing adolescents. *Journal of Clinical and Consulting Psychology, 54,* 95–397.

Szapocznik, J., Perez-Vidal, A., Briskman, A. L., Foote, F. H., Santisteban, D., & Hervis, O. (1988). Engaging adolescent drug abusers and their families in treatment. *Journal of Clinical and Consulting Psychology, 56,* 552–557.

Tarter, R. E. (1990). Evaluation and treatment of adolescent substance abuse: A decision tree method. *American Journal of Drug and Alcohol Abuse, 16,* 1–46.

Tarter, R. E. (1992). Prevention of drug abuse: Theory and application. *The American Journal on Addictions, 1,* 2–20.

Tarter, R. E., Kirisci, L., Hegedus, A., Mezzich, A., & Yanyukov, M. (1994). Heterogeneity of adolescent alcoholism. In T. A. Babor, V. Hesselbrock, R. E. Meyer, & W. Shoemaker (Eds.), *Types of alcoholics: Evidence from clinical, experimental and genetic research* (pp. 172–180). New York: New York Academy of Science.

Tarter, R. E., Laird, S. B., & Moss, H. B. (1990). Neuropsychological and neurophysiological characteristics of children of alcoholics. In M. Windel & J. S. Searles (Eds.), *Children of alcoholics: Critical perspectives* (pp. 73–98). New York: Guilford Press.

Tarter, R. E., Laird, S. B., Mostefa, K., Bukstein, O. G., & Kaminer, Y. (1990). Drug abuse severity in adolescents is associated with magnitude of deviation in temperamental traits. *British Journal of Addictions, 85,* 1501–1504.

Tuchfeld, B. S., Clayton, R. R., & Logan, J. A. (1982). Alcohol, drug use and delinquent and criminal behaviors among male adolescents and young adults. *Journal of Drug Issues, 2*, 185–198.

University of Michigan. (2000). *2000 Monitoring the Future Survey.* Ann Arbor: Institute for Social Research.

Van Hasselt, V. B., Herson, M., Null, J. A., Ammerman, R. T., Bukstein, O. G., McGillivray, J., et al. (1993). Drug abuse prevention for high-risk African American children and their families: A review and model program. *Addictive Behaviors, 18*, 213–234.

Vik, P. W., Grisel, K., & Brown, S. A. (1992). Social resource characteristics and adolescent substance abuse relapse. *Journal of Adolescent Chemical Dependency, 2*, 59–74.

Waldron, H. B. (1997). Adolescent substance abuse and family therapy outcome. A review of randomized trials. In T. H. Ollendick & R. J. Prinz (Eds.), *Advances in clinical child psychology* (Vol. 19). New York: Plenum.

Wechsler, H., & Thum, D. (1973). Teenage drinking, drug use, and social correlates. *Quarterly Journal of Studies on Alcohol, 34*, 1220–1227.

White, H. R., & Labouvie, E. W. (1989). Towards the assessment of adolescent problem drinking. *Journal of Studies on Alcohol, 50*, 30–37.

Wilens, T. E., Biederman, J., Spencer, T. J., & Frances, R. J. (1994). Comorbidity of attention-deficit disorder and psychoactive substance use disorders. *Hospital and Community Psychiatry, 45*, 421–435.

Williams, C. D., & Adams-Campbell, L. L. (2000). Addictive behaviors and depression among African Americans residing in a public housing community. *Addictive Behaviors, 25*, 45–56.

Winters, K. C. (1990). The need for improved assessment of adolescent substance involvement. *Journal of Drug Issues, 20*, 487–502.

Winters, K. C., & Stinchfield, R. D. (1995). Current issues and future needs in the assessment of adolescent drug abuse. In E. Rahdert & D. Czechowicz (Eds.), *Adolescent drug abuse: Clinical assessment and therapeutic interventions* (pp. 218–254). Research Monograph 156. Rockville, MD: National Institute on Drug Abuse.

Winters, K. C., Stinchfield, R. D., Henly, G. A., & Schwartz, R. H. (1991). Validity of adolescent self-report of alcohol and other drug involvement. *International Journal of Addictions, 25*, 1379–1395.

CHAPTER 7

Obesity: Nongenetic Influences in Childhood and Adolescence

Laura L. Hayman

The development and expression of obesity is influenced by the interaction of genetic and nongenetic factors. A review of the National Health and Nutrition Examination Surveys from 1963–1994 indicates a significant increase in overweight from the preschool years through adolescence (Troiano & Flegal, 1998). Very recent data from the National Longitudinal Survey of Youth (Strauss & Pollack, 2001) indicate a significant increase in overweight in children (4–12 years of age) during 1986–1998. The pattern and trend, similar to that observed for adults (Kuller, 1999), suggest a fundamental shift in the determinants of energy balance in children and youth in the United States. Collectively, life span data point to the importance of population-based/public health strategies, with emphasis on the nongenetic (potentially modifiable) influences on obesity. Toward this goal, the purposes of this chapter are to (1) present an overview of the epidemiology of obesity; (2) examine the nongenetic, potentially modifiable factors that contribute to the development and expression of obesity in childhood and adolescence; (3) examine developmental trends in the emergence of obesity-cardiovascular risk factor (CVD) associations; and, (4) identify specific areas for future research focused on individual and population-based approaches to primary prevention. In this chapter, nongenetic influences are defined as potentially modifiable behaviors and environments that contribute to the development and expression of obesity in childhood and adolescence. Conceptualized

This chapter was adapted and reprinted with permission from Fletcher, G. F., Grundy, S. M., & Hayman, L. L. (Eds.). (1999). *Obesity: Impact on Cardiovascular Disease* (pp. 75–90). Originally published by Futura Publishing, Armonk, New York, a Blackwell Publishing Imprint.

within a developmental contextual life span framework (Lerner, 1979, 1987, 1998), emphasis is placed on individual behaviors relevant to obesity (i.e., dietary intake and physical activity) and the environments (i.e., family, school, community) in which they develop and are maintained.

EPIDEMIOLOGY OF OBESITY: AN OVERVIEW

Recent data from the Behavioral Risk Factor Surveillance System (BRFSS) Centers for Disease Control and Prevention (CDC) (Mokdad et al., 2001), consistent with other population-based surveys, indicate a dramatic increase in the prevalence of overweight and obesity in U.S. adults (18 years of age and older). Results from this telephone survey of 184,450 participants conducted in all 50 states in 2000 indicate a 61% increase in the prevalence of obesity (defined as body/mass index [BMI] $>/= 30$ kg/m^2) since 1991. The BRFSS results indicated that 56.4% of U.S. adults (65.5% of men and 47.6% of women) were overweight (defined as BMI $>/= 25$ kg/m^2). Noteworthy is the concomitant 49% increase in the prevalence of self-reported Type 2 diabetes. Evidence from several recent studies of adults (Ford, Williamson, & Liu, 1997; Resnick, Valsania, Halter, & Lin, 2000) support earlier observations (Barrett-Connor, 1985; Pi-Sunyer, 1993) indicating that obesity and weight gain are associated with an increased risk of Type 2 diabetes. Other adverse health outcomes including dyslipidemias, hypertension, and coronary artery disease observed by Pi-Sunyer (1993) and in numerous clinical studies were not examined in this survey.

With emphasis on the modifiable determinants of obesity and diabetes, the BRFSS examined leisure-time physical activity (LTPA) and consumption of fruits and vegetables. Twenty-seven percent of participants did not engage in any LTPA and another 28.2% were not regularly active. Only 24.4% consumed fruits and vegetables five or more times daily. Noteworthy is that only 42.8% of obese participants who had a routine health exam in the prior year were advised by health care professionals to lose weight. Consistent with other national initiatives, Mokdad and colleagues conclude with emphasis on the need for multicomponent individual and public health strategies designed to prevent and manage obesity and overweight.

As observed in several surveys using a variety of criteria, the prevalence of overweight and obese U.S. children and youth is also increasing. Specifically, data from the most recent National Health and Nutrition Examination Survey (NHANES III) demonstrate that the number of overweight children has increased among all age, race, and sex groups since the NHANES II survey (Troiano, Flegal, Kuczmarski, Campbell, & Johnson, 1995). In the NHANES III cohort, approximately 11% of U.S. children were overweight (defined by the age- and sex-specific 95th percentile of BMI); an additional 14% were considered at risk (BMI between the 85th and 95th percentile). Other recent data generated from a national network of pediatric primary care practices (the Practice Partner Research Network) indicate a prevalence rate of 18–20% (Gauthier, Highner, & Ornstein, 2000). A recent study of overweight prevalence among third and sixth grade children in New York City reported rates of 15%–22% (Melnick, Jesaitis, Wales, & Bonam, 1998). Prevalence and trend data generated from the National Longitudinal Survey of Youth (NLSY) provide additional insight regarding sociodemographic characteristics and overweight children (Strauss & Pollack, 2001). The study population consisted of 4–12 year-old children born to women enrolled in the NLSY. Results indicated a significant and steady increase (from 1986–1998) in overweight prevalence among African American, Hispanic, and White children. By 1998, the prevalence of overweight children increased to 21.5% among African Americans, 21.8% among Hispanics, and 12.3% among non-Hispanic Whites. Consistent with NHANES III data, overweight children were significantly heavier in 1998 compared with 1986. The number of children with BMI greater than the 85th percentile increased significantly among African American and Hispanic children only. Regional and economic disparities among children with BMIs above the 85th percentile were also observed. In 1986, for example, overweight prevalence among upper-income White girls and lower-income African American and Hispanic boys was highly similar; by 1998 overweight prevalence had increased slightly to 8.7% among upper-income White girls and substantially and significantly (to 27.4%) among lower income African American and Hispanic boys (Strauss & Pollack, 2001). Winkleby, Robinson, Sundquist, and Kraemer (1999) also observed ethnic differences in BMI levels (and other CVD risk factors) among girls who participated in NHANES III. Specifically, Black and Mexican-American girls had significantly higher levels than their white counterparts.

Taken together, prevalence and trend data point to the urgent need for public health approaches designed to prevent the continuing epidemic of overweight and obese children and youth in the U.S. As suggested by Strauss and Pollack (2001) culturally competent prevention and treatment strategies combined with multilevel policy change are necessary to increase physical activity and healthful eating patterns, modifiable determinants of obesity and overweight.

PARTITIONING THE GENETIC AND NONGENETIC INFLUENCES

As illustrated above, body/mass index (BMI) has been used as a surrogate measure of obesity in epidemiologic surveys of adults (Kuller, 1999). The National Institutes of Health (NIH) National, Heart, Lung, and Blood Institute (NHLBI) (1998) recently advanced criteria for defining overweight and obesity in adults based on BMI. Similarly, recent population-based surveys of children and adolescents, including NHANES III, define overweight by the age- and sex-specific 95th percentile of BMI (Troiano & Flegal, 1998). Recent recommendations from a Pediatric Expert Committee support the use of BMI and suggest an in-depth health assessment for children and youth with BMI >/= the 95th percentile for age and sex (Barlow & Dietz, 1998). A comprehensive discussion of the methodologic issues and challenges in defining and measuring obesity in children and youth is beyond the scope of this chapter. In quantifying genetic and nongenetic influences; however, the method of measurement (i.e., BMI, triceps skinfold) is an important consideration.

Substantial research has focused on quantifying the genetic influences on obesity using a variety of paradigms and methods (Meyer & Stunkard, 1994). Methodologic limitations notwithstanding, twin and twin-family studies have been used extensively and provide most of the available data. By design, the results of these studies also provide indirect estimates of nongenetic influences. The classical and widely used approach to the analysis of twin data compares the similarity of identical or monozygotic (MZ) twins, who share all their genes, with fraternal or dizygotic (DZ) twins, who share (on average) half of their genes (Falconer, 1989). Based on this principle, the estimate of heritability (h^2) is calculated as twice the difference between the MZ and DZ intraclass correlation coefficients: $[h^2 = 2(r_{MZ} - r_{DZ}]$. In this approach, heritability (h^2) is defined as the proportion of variation in the characteristic accounted for by genetic factors in the population under study. Important to emphasize is that heritability estimates are specific to the population under study and must be viewed and interpreted accordingly. Across studies, these estimates have been shown to vary as a function of the sociodemographic characteristics of the population under study, the indicator and method of measurement of obesity, and analytic method used to quantify heritability (Meyer & Stunkard, 1994). Although minimal longitudinal data exist, estimates computed for the same population over time indicate that the magnitude of the estimate varies across the lifespan (Meyer, unpublished data; Stunkard, Foch, & Hrubec, 1986). In addition, h^2 is based on the assumption that only additive genetic effects and shared common family environmental effects influence intrapair similarity. Thus, h^2, derived using the classical approach, is subject to biases in the presence of genetic dominance or epistasis (intraloci or interloci interactions) (Meyer & Stunkard, 1994). Nonadditive genetic influences lower the DZ intraclass correlation to less than one half the MZ correlation; the end result is overestimation of the genetic influences.

One method for addressing some of the limitations in the classical twin approach and estimating nongenetic influences is the co-twin control or matched pair analyses of MZ twins. Comparisons within genetically identical MZ twin pairs remove all genetic variability. Thus, if intrapair differences in a characteristic exist (i.e., BMI), they must be attributable to environmental or potentially modifiable influences. Newman and colleagues (1990) applied this approach in matched co-twin analyses of 250 Caucasian, male MZ twins from the National Heart, Lung, and Blood Institute (NHLBI) Twin Study. The study was designed to examine the cross-sectional and longitudinal nongenetic influences of obesity (BMI) on risk factors for CVD (lipids and lipoproteins, blood pressure, glucose intolerance). In both analyses, results indicated significant obesity-CVD risk factor associations. At midlife (42–55 years of age), heavier MZ co-twins had significantly higher levels of systolic and diastolic blood pressure, glucose (1-hr-postload), total cholesterol, low-density lipoprotein cholesterol (LDL-C), and triglycerides and lower levels of high-density lipoprotein cholesterol (HDL-C) than their genetically identical, lighter co-twin. Similar results were obtained in longitudinal analyses of weight change during adulthood (from mean age of 20 to mean age of 48 years) and risk factor status at middle age. These results suggest that associations between adult obesity and CVD risk are influenced by behaviors and environmental exposures that occur later in life and provide additional support for weight reduction efforts during adulthood.

DEVELOPMENTAL TRENDS IN OBESITY-CVD RISK FACTOR ASSOCIATIONS

Application of the co-twin matched pair analyses to data collected as part of the Delaware Valley Twin Study (DVTS) (Hayman, Meininger, Stashinko, Gallagher, & Coates, 1988; Meininger et al., 1988) provided a unique opportunity to examine developmental trends in the nongenetic influences of obesity on risk factors for CVD (Hayman, 1995). Specifically, the purpose of this longitudinal study was to examine the nongenetic influences of obesity (BMI and triceps skinfolds) on risk factors for CVD (the lipid profile, systolic and diastolic blood pressure) during two phases of development: the school-age years (Phase 1) and adolescence (Phase 2). The influence of change in obesity (amount of gain in BMI from the school-age years to adolescence) on risk factors for CVD was also examined. The Phase 1 sample consisted of a panel of 73 Caucasian, 6–11-year-old MZ twin pairs identified as potential participants for the longitudinal DVTS through public and private schools in the Philadelphia metropolitan area. Mean age of twin participants at Phase 1 was 8.5 years; the mean age at Phase 2 was 12.5 years. The median interval between Phases was 40 months. In Phase 2, 77% (n = 56 twin pairs) of the original Phase 1 MZ cohort was retained in the study. Zygosity was determined on the basis of blood group antigens including Kell, Duffy, Kidd, ABO, Rh, MNSs, P, and Lewis. If co-twins were concordant on every antigen tested, they were classified as an MZ pair. Additional procedural and measurement details for the DVTS are described elsewhere (Hayman, Meininger, Coates, et al., 1995; Hayman, Meininger, Stashinko, et al., 1988; Meininger et al., 1988, 1998).

Significant mean intrapair differences in each of three measures of obesity were observed in both phases of development. In Phase 1, the mean intrapair difference in weight was 2.4 kg and the mean intrapair difference in height was 0.635 cm. The lighter co-twin was, on average, slightly taller than the heavier co-twin. Similarly, in Phase 2 (adolescence), significant mean intrapair differences in each of the measures of obesity were observed. The mean intrapair differences in weight and height were 2.38 kg and 0.33 cm, respectively. These results indicate significant environmental influences on obesity during the school-age years and adolescence. In previous analysis of MZ and DZ twins in this cohort at Phase 1 (Meininger, 1988), the amount of variance explained by genetic factors was slightly less than 50%. Taken together, these results suggest substantial environmental influences on obesity in this cohort at school age. Noteworthy, in both phases of development, obesity-CVD risk factor associations were observed. Specifically, in Phase 1, intraindividual associations of obesity and atherogenic lipids emerged; heavier co-twins demonstrated higher (5 mg/dl) levels of total and LDL-cholesterol and apolipoprotein-B than their lighter co-twin counterparts. The clinical significance remains to be determined; however, these results are consistent with studies of singletons (Khoury, 1980; NHLBI Growth & Health Study Research Group, 1992; Webber, 1979). The DVTS results, however, suggest that nongenetic influences contribute to the emergence of obesity-CVD risk factor associations during this developmental period.

In adolescence, Phase 2 of the DVTS, obesity-lipid associations were also observed. Specifically, in matched-pair regression analyses of Phase 2 data (Hayman, 1995), obesity was defined as the intrapair difference (between heavier and lighter co-twins) in body/mass index (Rohrer Index). Dependent variables were the intrapair differences in levels of other CVD risk factors. Results indicated that nongenetic influences of obesity contribute to the nongenetic variability in HDL-cholesterol (beta = −0.33, p < .01) and total triglyceride (beta = 0.31, p < .02), accounting for 11% and 10%, respectively, of the nongenetic variance in these risk factors at Phase 2. Adding to the environmental hypothesis were the results of the longitudinal analyses indicating significant intrapair differences in change in obesity (defined as the amount of gain in the Rohrer Index). This change in obesity was associated with total triglyceride (p < .006) accounting for 14% of the variance in this risk factor (Hayman, 1995). These results are consistent with Newman's observations regarding the nongenetic influences on obesity (Newman, 1990). Taken together, the results support the matched-pair analyses as a viable approach for examining nongenetic influences. Most importantly, the results emphasize the role of potentially modifiable behaviors and environments in the development and expression of obesity across the life span and point to the importance of developmental transitions as critical periods for preventive interventions.

Additional longitudinal analyses of data collected from the DVTS cohort support the matched pair results and emphasize obesity as part of the CVD risk profile (Hayman, Meininger, Gallagher, et al., 1995). Specifically, remeasurements of CVD risk factors were conducted later in adolescence (Phase 3); the mean age was 15.5 years and the median P2–P3 interval was 30 months. Seventy-seven twin-pairs (n = 154 participants) were retained in the sample at P3. Stepwise regression analyses were conducted to determine the predictors of lipids and lipoproteins at Phase 3. For these analyses, twin pairs were split and assigned randomly to group 1 or group 2; this procedure allowed for independence of observations and provided the opportunity to cross validate the findings. Obesity (BMI) or P1–P3 change in BMI and the respective P1 lipid values explained a significant portion of the variance in atherogenic lipids and HDL-cholesterol with R2 ranging from 0.21 for HDL-C to 0.50 for total and LDL-C. These results were consistent for both twin groups. As discussed by Obarzanek (1999), these results are consistent with numerous observational studies of obesity-CVD risk factor associations in singletons.

Intraindividual clustering of risk factors in children and adults is well established; similarly, obesity and change in obesity are recognized determinants of adverse lipid profiles across the life span. From a developmental perspective, questions remain regarding the temporal sequence of obesity-CVD risk factor clustering. Toward that goal, in a recent study, Tershakovec and colleagues (1998) examined age-related changes in CVD risk factors of hypercholesterolemic (HC) children (nonfasting TC = 176 mg/dl; mean of two fasting LDL-C levels = >/= 80th age- and sex-specific percentile). Specifically, the sample for this cross-sectional study of 4–10 year-old Caucasian children consisted of n = 227 HC and n = 80 nonhypercholesterolemic children (NHC). In addition to the lipid profile, risk factors measured were skinfolds (biceps, triceps, suprailiac, subscapular), percent weight-for-height median (WHM), systolic blood pressure, and insulin levels (HC only). Results indicated that HC had a greater percent WHM, greater skinfold thickness measures, and higher systolic blood pressure than their NHC counterparts. Analysis of variance (ANOVA) by age group with three interaction terms (age group, gender, and TC) was conducted for the anthropometric measures. A significant age interaction demonstrated that the HC group's larger suprailiac and sum of skinfold measures were expressed in the 8.0–9.9-year-old children but not in the 4.0–5.9 year-olds. For both HC and NHC, systolic blood pressure was associated with the measures of adiposity; in the HC group, insulin levels were also associated with adiposity. As observed in a study of children with familial combined hypercholesterolemia (Shamir et al., 1996), these results suggest that children with HC have greater body fat. The results also suggest that the expression of the hypercholesterolemia precedes the expression of increased body fat; and, altered insulin and blood pressure levels are expressed in association with increased body fat in children with HC. These results question the commonly held view that excess adiposity is a causative factor that precedes the phenotypic expression of dyslipidemias in children. As Tershakovec and colleagues (1998) conclude, these results require replication with diverse samples and reexamination in longitudinal studies. As noted by Daniels (1998), if these results are confirmed, the mechanisms underlying the age-related differences in the TC-adiposity relationship still remain to be explicated.

Obesity is a well established risk factor for Type 2 diabetes; both are now recognized as risk factors for CVD (NCEP, 2001). Because of the documented increased prevalence of Type 2 diabetes in children and youth (Pinhas-Hamiel et al., 1996) the American Diabetes Association (ADA) convened an expert panel to address some of the unanswered questions concerning epidemiology, classification and prevention of Type 2 diabetes (ADA, 2000). Obesity was identified in the panel report as a prevalent characteristic observed in children with Type 2 diabetes. Although the panel acknowledged the need for additional research on the determinants of Type 2 diabetes in children and youth, testing was recommended (beginning at age 10) for all children with a BMI >/= 85th age- and sex-specific percentile and have a family history of the disease or signs of insulin resistance (IR), or conditions associated with IR (acanthosis nigricans, hypertension dyslipidemia) or belong to a certain race/ethnic group (American Indians, African Americans, Hispanic Americans, Asians/South Pacific Islanders). Strategies for primary prevention of Type 2 diabetes were highlighted by the panel with emphasis on modifiable lifestyle factors such as physical activity, nutrition and obesity.

Collectively, the results of the DVTS and epidemiologic and clinical studies of children and adolescents suggest substantial nongenetic (potentially modifiable) influences on obesity, emphasize its importance as part of the CVD risk profile, and point to the need for individual and population-based approaches to primary prevention.

HEALTH BEHAVIORS: MODIFIABLE INFLUENCES ON OBESITY

Health behaviors, particularly patterns of dietary intake and physical activity, are generally viewed as modifiable influences on obesity. These health behaviors develop within the context of the family environment and are influenced by many extrafamilial factors. Substantial research has examined the independent and combined influences of these health behaviors on the development of obesity across the life span. Hill and Kriketos (1999) present an informative discussion on energy expenditure and obesity with emphasis on these modifiable influences. Although available data are equivocal, they do suggest that dietary intake and physical activity interact to influence the energy balance equation and the obesity-CVD risk profile in childhood and adulthood (Epstein, Kuller, et al., 1989; Epstein, Valoski, et al., 1994; Hill & Kriketos, 1999).

Dietary Intake/Eating Behaviors

Consistent with the emphasis on primary prevention of obesity, recent research attention has focused on infancy, particularly the totality of infant feeding experiences including socialization of food preferences and self-regulation of eating behaviors. In a recent comprehensive review of this literature, Birch and Fisher (1998) emphasize the importance of the family environment including the influence of parenting practices and eating behaviors on the development of these behaviors in their offspring. For example, food preferences as determinants of children's intake, may be linked with early infant feeding practices that are under parental control (Sullivan & Birch, 1994). Breast-feeding has been the recommended method of infant feeding because of the numerous, well-established physiological and psychological benefits. Recent data suggest, however, that early food preferences may be influenced by method of feeding (Birch & Fischer, 1998; Sullivan & Birch, 1994). Breast-fed infants have exposure to a variety of flavors reflecting maternal diet transmitted through human milk. In contrast, formula-fed infants have experience with a single flavor. Data from Sullivan and Birch (1994), consistent with other reports (Capretta, 1975), suggest that breast-fed infants demonstrate greater acceptance of new foods during the transitional period of weaning. The long-term influences of these early infant feeding experiences, however, remain to be clarified. Further, as Birch and Fisher emphasize, whether infants differing in familial risk for obesity also differ in their responsiveness to flavors or in their responsiveness to solid food is unknown. This is a fertile area for future research. Using a gene/environment interaction paradigm, this type of inquiry could provide unique information regarding family-focused modifiable influences in individuals at high risk for obesity.

As discussed by Obarzanek (1999), familial aggregation of obesity has been investigated extensively. Similar to CVD, familial aggregation of obesity is attributed to both shared genes and shared (common) family environment. The mechanisms through which the family environment operates to influence health behaviors associated with obesity (including patterns of dietary intake and physical activity) remain to be clarified; however, available data provide some insight and direction for future research. In a recent review of the available literature on families and health actions, Baranowski (1997) presents data to support a model of family reciprocal determinism. Derived from social cognitive theory and consistent with developmental-contextualism (Lerner, 1998), this model emphasizes the dynamic interaction of person and environment in the development and acquisition of health behaviors, particularly eating behaviors. Applied to families and health actions, emphasis is placed on parental modeling and reinforcement of health behaviors as well as the influence of other important developmental contexts including school, peers, and the media. By definition, and partially supported by available data, the model also suggests that children influence the health behaviors of their parents (Knight & Grantham-McGregor, 1985; Nader et al., 1982).

Data from several sources support components of Baranowski's (1997) model and suggest the family as a unit of analysis and intervention. For example, data from several studies including the Framingham Children's Study (Oliveria, 1992) and the Princeton School District Study (Laskarzewski, 1980), indicate concordance in the dietary patterns of parents and children. Concordance, estimated by correlation analysis, is relatively low across studies and appears to vary as a function of age of the child, family role (i.e., mother, father) ethnicity of the family, and nutrients or foods analyzed (Baranowski, 1997; Laskarzewski, 1980; Oliveria, 1992). Results of a recent study of fat preferences and consumption in preschool children add to this database by demonstrating significant associations between parental BMI and children's fat preferences ($r = 0.75$). In this study, Fisher and Birch (1995) also observed significant associations between parental BMI and children's fat intake ($r = 0.67$). Noteworthy is that children were offered a single menu consisting of 32% energy as fat; children's fat intakes actually ranged from 25–41%. Taken together and placed in the context of other studies (Eck, 1992; Michela & Contento, 1986) these results suggest that children's preferences for and consumption of fat may be influenced by familial factors including the availability of and exposure to high-fat foods (Fisher & Birch, 1995).

Results from a very recent crossover trial, designed to determine whether individual variation in cholesterol response to dietary modification (margarine versus butter) is a familial trait, support and extend earlier observations (Denke, Adams-Huet, & Nguyen, 2000). Specifically, results from this 2-period, 5-week crossover dietary trial of 46 families (with 2 biological parents and >/= 2 children aged 5 or older) indicate that family membership explained 19% of the variability in response (percent change in low density lipoprotein [LDL-C] levels) for adults and children together and 40% in children separately. In the separate prediction model for children, family membership accounted for 26% of the variation while significant covariates of response, BMI and change in cholesterol ester ratio (CE) explained 26% of the variation. Denke and colleagues concluded that individual variation in response to a cholesterol-lowering diet is a familial trait and body weight (BMI) is an important modifiable factor that influences response.

In the context of modifiable influences on obesity, the family emerges as an important determinant of relevant health behaviors and should be considered as a unit of analysis in future research. Although familial patterns of dietary intake and eating behaviors have received more research attention than physical activity (discussed below), lacking are data on the specific mechanisms through which these behaviors are acquired and transmitted within multi-generational families. Further, most of the available data have been generated from studies of white, middle-class families. With emphasis on population-based approaches and primary prevention, future research should target families of diverse sociocultural-economic backgrounds. Since obesity is influenced by energy intake and expenditure, future research on modifiable influences should have a conjoint focus (i.e., patterns of dietary intake and physical activity).

Physical Activity

Developmental trends in physical activity in children and adolescents in the United States argue convincingly for additional research on the determinants of this behavior. Data from the 1992 National Health Interview Survey—Youth Risk Behavior Survey (U.S. Department of Health & Human Services, 1996) indicate substantial declines in physical activity in both males and females during the transition from childhood to adolescence. This decrement has been observed in numerous studies and is particularly pronounced in females (Centers for Disease Control & Prevention, 1996; Ross & Pate, 1987; Sallis, 1993). Population-based data on temporal trends are lacking; however, the age-related downward trend in the prevalence of participation in physical activity combined with scattered data on the prevalence of sedentary activities (Dietz & Strasburger, 1991) and potential benefits of decreasing these behaviors (Epstein et al., 1997) underscore the need for additional research.

Individual and contextual/environmental factors have been linked with physical activity in children and adolescents. As Kohl and Hobbs (1998) observed in a recent comprehensive review of this literature, most of the available data have been generated from cross-sectional studies. Thus, the temporal relationships between these factors and patterns of activity in children and adolescents remain to be clarified. In addition, between-study differences in operational definitions and methods of measurement of physical activity make it difficult to compare results across studies. These limitations notwithstanding, individual factors associated with physical activity include age, gender, physical fitness, health status, self-efficacy, knowledge and attitudes, education, and socioeconomic status (Kohl & Hobbs, 1998; Sallis, 1993). Some of these factors (i.e., self-efficacy) (Reynolds et al., 1990) are more amenable to modification than others (i.e., age, gender). Data are inconclusive; however, they suggest that individual factors are influenced by developmental contexts/environments including the family (parental influences, competing attentions) (Biddle & Goudas, 1996; Reynolds et al., 1990; Sallis et al., 1988; Zakarain et al., 1994), school (peer influences, programs, and policies) (Arbeit et al., 1992; Kelder et al., 1995), and community (available facilities, safety issues, and policies) (Butcher, 1995; Gottlieb & Chen, 1985; Stucky-Ropp & DiLorenzo, 1993). Thus, using paradigms that allow for examination of individual and environmental factors (both main effects and interactions) would optimize the information yield and provide more specific direction for preventive interventions.

Daniels (1999) argues convincingly for both individual and population-based approaches to increasing physical activity in children and youth with emphasis on some of these family and community factors. Adding to this database with implications for primary prevention of obesity are recent data from NHANES III (Andersen et al., 1998) and accumulated data on the potential multidimensional role of schools in promoting healthy lifestyles and preventing obesity (McGinnis, 1993; Resnicow & Robinson, 1997). Specifically, Andersen and colleagues used data from NHANES III to determine cross-sectional prevalence rates of daily television watching habits and weekly bouts of vigorous physical activity in this nationally representative sample of U.S. children aged 8–16 years. The relationship between BMI, body fatness, and bouts of vigorous activity and television watching were also examined. Eighty percent of children reported 3 or more bouts of vigorous activity each week; however, the rate was lower in non-Hispanic Black and Mexican-American girls (69% and 73%, respectively). Twenty-six percent of U.S. children watched 4 or more hrs of television per day while 67% watched at least 2 hrs per day. Most importantly, boys and girls who watched >/= 4 or more hrs per day had the highest skinfold thicknesses and BMIs while children who viewed </= 1 hr per day had the lowest BMIs. Non-Hispanic Black children reported the highest prevalence rates (42%) of this sedentary activity. These population-based data confirm that vigorous activity among ethnic minority children is lower than among non-Hispanic White children. As Andersen and colleagues conclude, these results have important implications for the design and implementation of school and community-based interventions aimed at increasing physical activity in children and youth.

Schools have been suggested as critical, captive environments for promoting the adoption of healthy behaviors, including patterns of physical activity and dietary intake. Data from CDC suggest, however, that substantial efforts are necessary in order for schools to optimize this potential. For example, participation in all types of physical activity decreases as age or grade in school increases. Centers for Disease Control data also indicate that only 19% of all high school students are physically active for 20 minutes or more,

5 days a week. Further, daily enrollment in physical education classes declined from 42% to 25% among high school students between 1991–1995 (U.S. Department of Health & Human Services, 1996). School-based research initiatives including the Child and Adolescent Trial for Cardiovascular Health (CATCH) (Luepker et al., 1996) and the Cardiovascular Health in Children (CHIC) study (Harrell et al., 1996) emphasize the school as a viable, feasible, and effective environment for changing health behaviors in ethnically diverse children and youth. The CATCH Trial targeted the individual health behaviors and the modification of the school environment including the curriculum and educational materials, teacher training, and on-site consultation (Luepker, 1996). Students' moderate to vigorous physical activity (in school) increased from 37.4% at baseline to 51.9% postintervention (Luepker et al., 1996). Thus, a major lesson learned from CATCH, supported by results of other school-based studies (Arbeit et al., 1992; Harrell et al., 1996; Resnicow & Robinson, 1997) was demonstrating that changing school environments can result in changing health behaviors of children. Adding to this database, CHIC results also suggest that a short-term (8-week) classroom-based intervention can be effective in reducing cardiovascular risk factors (including levels of serum total cholesterol) in elementary school children (Harrell et al., 1996). Longitudinal studies are necessary, however, to determine adherence over time particularly throughout the adolescent transition.

CONCLUSIONS

Obesity is a highly prevalent chronic condition that results from an imbalance in energy intake and expenditure. Genetic and nongenetic factors interact across the lifespan to influence the development, expression, and maintenance of obesity. Developmental trends indicate the emergence of obesity-CVD risk factor associations early in life and point to the importance of an integrated profile approach to cardiovascular health with emphasis on primary prevention of obesity (Gidding et al., 1996; Strong et al., 1992; Williams et al., in press). The current epidemic of obesity in the United States indicates an urgent need for effective high-risk and population-based approaches to prevention and management with emphasis on the potentially modifiable influences including health behaviors and the environments in which they develop and are maintained. Although many questions remain unanswered, available data emphasize the potential role of the family and school environments in the development and maintenance of health behaviors including patterns of dietary intake and physical activity. Developmentally appropriate and culturally competent population-based strategies are recommended to reduce the public health burden of obesity. Toward that goal, a multidisciplinary research agenda that includes and emphasizes health behaviors and relevant sociocultural-environmental factors within and across diverse populations is suggested.

REFERENCES

American Diabetes Association (ADA). (2000). Type 2 diabetes in children and adolescents. *Pediatrics, 105*(3), 671–680.

Andersen, R. E., Crespo, C. J., Bartlett, S. J., Cheskin, L. J., & Pratt, M. (1998). Relationship of physical activity and television watching with body weight and level of fatness among children: Results from the Third National Health and Nutrition Examination Survey. *Journal of the American Medical Association, 279*(12), 938–942.

Arbeit, M. L., Johnson, C. C., Mott, D. S., Harsha, D. W., Nicklas, R. A., Webber, L. S., & Berenson, G. S. (1992). The Heart Smart cardiovascular school health promotion: Behavior correlates of risk factor change. *Preventive Medicine, 21*(1), 18–32.

Baranowski, T. (1997). Families and health actions. In D. S. Gochman (Ed.), *Handbook of health behavior research: Vol 1. Personal and social determinants* (pp. 179–206). New York: Plenum.

Barlow, S. E., & Dietz, W. H. (1998). Obesity evaluation and treatment: Expert committee recommendations. *Pediatrics Electronic Pages, 102*(3), e29.

Barrett-Connor, E. L. (1985). Obesity, atherosclerosis, and coronary artery disease. *Archives of Internal Medicine, 103*, 1010–1019.

Biddle, S., & Goudas, M. (1996). Analysis of children's physical activity and its association with adult encouragement and social cognitive variables. *Journal of School Health, 66*(2), 75–78.

Birch, L. L., & Fischer, J. O. (1998). Development of eating behaviors among children and adolescents. *Pediatrics, 101*(Suppl), 539–548.

Bouchard, C., Perusse, L., Leblanc, C., Tremblay, A., & Theriault, G. (1988). Inheritance of the amount and distribution of body fat. *International Journal of Obesity, 12*(3), 205–215.

Butcher, J. (1995). Longitudinal analysis of adolescent girls' participation in physical activity. *Sociological Sports Journal, 2*, 130–143.

Capretta, P. I., Petersik, I. T., & Steward, D. I. (1975). Acceptance of novel flavours is increased after early experience of diverse tastes. *Nature, 254*, 689–691.

Centers for Disease Control and Prevention. (1996). Youth risk behavior surveillance—United States, 1995. *MMWR. Morbid Mortal Weekly Report, 45*, 1–63.

Daniels, S. R. (1998). Overweight and cholesterol elevation: Which is the chicken and which is the egg? *Journal of Pediatrics, 132*, 383–384.

Daniels, S. R. (1999). Prevention of obesity. In G. Fletcher, S. F. Grundy, & L. L. Hayman (Eds.), *Obesity: Impact on cardiovascular disease* (pp. 91–111). New York: Futura.

Denke, M. A., Adams-Huet, B., & Nguyen, A. T. (2000). Individual cholesterol variation in response to a margarine- or butter-based diet. *Journal of the American Medical Association, 284*(21), 2740–2747.

Dietz, W. H., & Strasburger, V. C. (1991). Children, adolescents and television. *Current Problems in Pediatrics, 1,* 8–31.

Eck, L. H., Klesges, R. C., Hanson, C. L., & Slawson, D. (1992). Children at familial risk for obesity: An examination of dietary intake, physical activity and weight status. *International Journal of Obesity and Related Metabolic Disorders, 16*(2), 71–78.

Epstein, L. H., Kuller, L. H., Wing, R. R., Valoski, A., & McCurley, J. (1989). The effect of weight control on lipid changes in obese children. *American Journal of Diseases of Children, 143*(4), 454–457.

Epstein, L. H., Saelens, B. F., Myers, M. D., & Vito, D. (1997). Effects of decreasing sedentary behaviors on activity choice in obese children. *Health Psychology, 16*(2), 107–113.

Epstein, L. H., Valoski, A., Wing, R. R., & McCurley, J. (1994). Ten-year outcomes of behavioral family-based treatment for childhood obesity. *Health Psychology, 13*(5), 373–383.

Falconer, D. S. (1989). *Introduction to quantitative genetics.* New York: Wiley.

Fisher, J. O., & Birch, L. L. (1995). Fat preferences and fat consumption of 3–5-year-old children are related to parental adiposity. *Journal of the American Dietetic Association, 95,* 759–764.

Ford, E. S., Williamson, D. F., & Liu, S. (1997). Weight change and diabetes incidence: Findings from a national cohort of US adults. *American Journal of Epidemiology, 146,* 214–222.

Gauthier, B. M., Highner, J. M., & Ornstein, S. (2000). High prevalence of overweight children and adolescents in the Practice Partner Research Network. *Archives of Pediatric and Adolescent Medicine, 154,* 625–628.

Gidding, S. S., Leibel, R. L., Daniels, S. R., Rosenbaum, M., Van Horn, L., & Marx, G. R. (1996). Understanding obesity in youth. A statement for healthcare professionals from the Committee on Atherosclerosis and Hypertension in the Young of the Council on Cardiovascular Disease in the Young and the Nutrition Committee, American Heart Association. *Circulation, 94*(12), 3383–3387.

Gottlieb, N. H., & Chen, M. S. (1985). Sociocultural correlates of childhood sporting activities: Their implications for heart health. *Social Science and Medicine, 21*(5), 533–539.

Harrell, J. S., McMurray, R. G., Bangdiwala, S. I., Frauman, A. C., Gansky, S. A., & Bradley, C. B. (1996). Effects of a school-based intervention to reduce cardiovascular disease risk factors in elementary-school children: The Cardiovascular Health in Children (CHIC) study. *Journal of Pediatrics, 128*(6), 797–805.

Hayman, L. L., Meininger, J. C., Coates, P. M., & Gallagher, P. R. (1995a). Nongenetic influences of obesity on risk factors for cardiovascular disease during two phases of development. *Nursing Research, 44*(5), 277–283.

Hayman, L. L., Meininger, J. C., Gallagher, P. R., & Napolitano, J. (1995b). Tracking of the lipid profile from childhood to adolescence. *Circulation, 92*(8), 767.

Hayman, L. L., Meininger, J. C., Stashinko, E. E., Gallagher, P. R., & Coates, P. M. (1988). Type A behavior and physiological cardiovascular risk factors in school-age twin children. *Nursing Research, 37,* 290–296.

Hill, J. O., & Kriketos, A. D. (1999). Energy expenditure and obesity. In G. Fletcher, S. F. Grundy, & L. L. Hayman (Eds.), *Obesity: Impact on cardiovascular disease* (pp. 247–259). New York: Futura.

Kelder, S. H., Perry, C. L., & Peters, R. J. (1995). Gender differences in the Class of 1989 Study: The school component of the Minnesota Heart Health Program. *Journal of Health Education, 26*(Suppl), 36–34.

Khoury, P., Morrison, J. A., Kelly, K., Mellies, M., Horvitz, R., & Glueck, C. J. (1980). Clustering and interrelationships of coronary heart disease risk factors in school-children, ages 6–19. *American Journal of Epidemiology, 112*(4), 524–538.

Knight, J., & Grantham-McGregor, S. (1985). Using primary school children to improve child-rearing practices in rural Jamaica. *Child: Care, Health, and Development, 11,* 81–90.

Kohl, H. W., & Hobbs, K. E. (1998). Development of physical activity behaviors among children and adolescents. *Pediatrics, 101*(Suppl.), 549–554.

Kuller, L. H. (1999). The epidemiology of obesity in adults in relationship to cardiovascular disease. In G. Fletcher, S. F. Grundy, & L. L. Hayman (Eds.), *Obesity: Impact on cardiovascular disease* (pp. 3–29). New York: Futura.

Laskarzewski, P., Morrison, J. A., Khoury, P., Kelly, K., Glatfelter, L., Larsen, R., & Glueck, C. J. (1980). Parent-child nutrient intake interrelationships in school children ages 6 to 19: The Princeton School District Study. *American Journal of Clinical Nutrition, 33*(11), 2350–2355.

Lerner, R. M. (1998). Theories of human development: Contemporary perspectives. In W. Damon (Ed. In-Chief) & R. M. Lerner (Vol. Ed.), *The handbook of child psychology: Vol. 1. Theoretical models of human development* (5th ed., pp. 1–24). New York: Wiley.

Luepker, R. V., Perry, C. L., McKinlay, S. M., Nader, P. R., Parcel, G. S., Stone, E. J., Webber, L. S., Elder, J. P., Feldman, H. A., Johnson, C. C., et al. (1996). Outcomes of a field trial to improve children's dietary patterns and physical activity: The Child and Adolescent Trial for Cardiovascular Health (CATCH) collaborative group. *Journal of the American Medical Association, 275*(10), 768–776.

McGinnis, J. M. (1993). The year 2000 initiative: Implications for comprehensive school health. *Preventive Medicine, 22,* 493–498.

Meininger, J. C., Hayman, L. L., Coates, P. M., & Gallagher, P. R. (1988). Genetics or environment? Type A behavior and other cardiovascular risk factors in twin children. *Nursing Research, 37*(6), 341–346.

Meininger, J. C., Hayman, L. L., Coates, P. M., & Gallagher, P. R. (1998). Genetic and environmental influences on cardiovascular disease risk factors in adolescents. *Nursing Research, 47*(1), 11–18.

Melnick, T. A., Jesalitis, A. T., Wales, K. R., & Bonam, S. B. (1998). Prevalence of overweight among third and sixth grade children—New York City, 1996. *MMWR, Morbidity, Mortality Weekly Report, 47,* 980–984.

Meyer, J. M., Bodurtha, J. N., & Eaves, L. J. Tracking genetic and environmental effects on adolescent BMI: The MCV twin study. (Unpublished data.)

Meyer, J. M., & Stunkard, A. J. (1994). Twin studies of human obesity. In C. Bouchard (Ed.), *The genetics of obesity* (pp. 63–78). Boca Raton: CRC Press.

Michela, J. L., & Contento, I. R. (1986). Cognitive, motivational, social, and environmental influences on children's food choices. *Health Psychology, 5,* 209–230.

Mokdad, A. H., Bowman, B. A., Ford, E. S., Vinicor, F., Marks, J. S., & Koplan, J. P. (2001). The continuing epidemics of obesity and diabetes in the United States. *Journal of the American Medical Association, 286*(10), 1195–1200.

Nader, P. R., Perry, C., Maccoby, N., Solomon, D., Killen, J., Telch, M., & Alexander, J. K. (1982). Adolescent perceptions of family health behavior: A tenth grade educational activity to increase family awareness of a community cardiovascular risk reduction program. *Journal of School Health, 52*(8), 372–377.

National Cholesterol Education Program (NCEP). (2001). Executive Summary of the Third Report of the National Cholesterol Education Program (NCEP) Expert Panel on Detection, Evaluation, and Treatment of High Blood Cholesterol in Adults (Adult Treatment Panel III). *Journal of the American Medical Association, 285*(19), 2486–2497.

National Heart, Lung, and Blood Institute Growth and Health Study Research Group. (1992). Obesity and cardiovascular disease risk factors in black and white girls: The NHLBI Growth and Health Study. *American Journal of Public Health, 82*(12), 1613–1620.

Newman, B., Selby, J. V., Quesenberry, C. P., Jr., King, M. C., Friedman, G. D., & Fabsitz, R. R. (1990). Nongenetic influences of obesity on other cardiovascular disease risk factors: An analysis of identical twins. *American Journal of Public Health, 80*(6), 675–678.

NHLBI Growth and Health Study Research Group: Obesity and cardiovascular disease risk factors in black and white girls: The NHLBI Growth and Health Study. (1992). *American Journal of Public Health, 82,* 1613–1620.

Obarzanek, E. (1999). Obesity in children, adolescents and families. In G. Fletcher, S. F. Grundy, & L. L. Hayman (Eds.), *Obesity: Impact on cardiovascular disease* (pp. 31–53). New York: Futura.

Oliveria, S. A., Ellison, R. C., Moore, L. L., Gillman, M. W., Garrahie, E. J., & Singer, M. R. (1992). Parent-child relationships in nutrient intake: The Framingham Children's Study. *American Journal of Clinical Nutrition, 56*(3), 593–598.

Pinhas-Hamiel, O., Dolan, L. M., Daniels, S. R., Standiford, D., Khoury, P. R., & Zeitler, P. (1996). Increased incidence of non-insulin dependent diabetes mellitus among adolescents. *Journal of Pediatrics, 128*(5), 608–615.

Pi-Sunyer, F. X. (1993). Medical hazards of obesity. *Archives of Internal Medicine, 119,* 655–660.

Resnick, H., Valsania, P., Halter, J., & Lin, X. (2000). Relation of weight gain and weight loss on subsequent diabetes risk in overweight adults. *Journal of Epidemiology and Community Health, 54,* 596–602.

Resnicow, K., & Robinson, T. N. (1997). School-based cardiovascular disease prevention studies: Review and synthesis. *Annals of Epidemiology*(Suppl. 7), 14–31.

Reynolds, K. D., Killen, J. D., Bryson, S. W., Maron, D. J., Taylor, C. B., Maccoby, N., & Farquhar, J. W. (1990). Psychosocial predictors of physical activity in adolescents. *Preventive Medicine, 19*(5), 541–551.

Ross, J. G., & Pate, R. R. (1987). The National Children and Youth Fitness Study. II: A summary of the findings. *Journal of Physical Education and Recreational Dance, 58,* 51–56.

Sallis, J. F. (1993). Epidemiology of physical activity and fitness in children and adolescents. *Critical Review of Food, Science & Nutrition, 33,* 403–408.

Sallis, J. F., Patterson, T. L., Buono, M. J., Akins, C. J., & Nader, P. R. (1988). Aggregation of physical activity habits in Mexican-American and Anglo families. *Journal of Behavioral Medicine, 11*(1), 31–41.

Selby, J. V., Newman, B., Quesenberry, C. P., Jr., Fabsitz, R. R., Carmelli, D., Meaney, F. J., & Slemenda, C. (1990). Genetic and behavioral influences on body fat distribution. *International Journal of Obesity, 14*(7), 593–602.

Shamir, R., Tershakovec, A. M., Gallagher, P. R., Liacouras, C. A., Hayman, L. L., & Cortner, J. A. (1996). The influence of age and relative weight on the presentation of familial combined hyperlipidemia in childhood. *Atherosclerosis, 121,* 85–91.

Strauss, R. S., & Pollack, H. A. (2001). Epidemic increase in childhood overweight, 1986–1998. *Journal of the American Medical Association, 286*(22), 2845–2848.

Strong, W. B., Deckelbaum, R. J., Gidding, S. S., Kavey, R. E., Washington, R., Wilmore, J. H., & Perry, C. L. (1992). Integrated cardiovascular health promotion in childhood. A statement for health professionals from the Subcommittee on Atherosclerosis and Hypertension in Childhood of the Council on Cardiovascular Disease in the Young, American Heart Association. *Circulation, 85*(4), 1638–1650.

Stucky-Ropp, R. C., & DiLorenzo, T. M. (1993). Determinants of exercise in children. *Preventive Medicine, 22,* 880–889.

Stunkard, A. J., Foch, T. T., & Hrubec, Z. (1986). A twin study of human obesity. *Journal of the American Medical Association, 256*(1), 51–54.

Sullivan, S. A., & Birch, L. L. (1994). Infant dietary experience and acceptance of solid foods. *Pediatrics, 93,* 271–277.

Tershakovec, A. M., Jawad, A. F., Stallings, V. A., Cortner, J. A., Zemel, B. S., & Shannon, B. M. (1998). Age-related changes in cardiovascular disease risk factors of hypercholesterolemic children. *Journal of Pediatrics, 132*(3 pt. 1), 414–420.

Troiano, R. P., Flegal, K. M., Kuczmarski, R. J., Campbell, S. M., & Johnson, C. L. (1995). Overweight prevalence and trends for children and adolescents: The National Health and Nutrition Examination Surveys, 1963–1991. *Archives of Pediatric and Adolescent Medicine, 149,* 1085–1091.

Troiano, R. P., & Flegal, K. M. (1998). Overweight children and adolescents: Description, epidemiology and demographics. *Pediatrics, 101*(Suppl.), 497–504.

U.S. Department of Health and Human Services. (1996). *Physical Activity and Health: A Report of the Surgeon General.* Atlanta: Author.

Webber, L. S., Voors, A. W., Srinivasan, S. R., Frerichs, R. R., & Berenson, G. S. (1979). Occurrence in children of multiple risk factors for coronary artery disease: The bogalusa heart study. *Preventive Medicine, 8*(3), 407–418.

Williams, C. L., Hayman, L. L., Daniels, S. R., Robinson, T. N., Steinberger, J., Paridon, S., & Bazarre, T. (in press). Integrated cardiovascular health promotion in childhood: A statement for health professionals from the committee on atherosclerosis, hypertension, and obesity in youth (AHOY) of the Council on Cardiovascular Disease in the Young, American Heart Association. *Circulation.*

Winkleby, M. A., Robinson, T. N., Sundquist, J., & Kraemer, H. C. (1999). Ethnic variation in cardiovascular disease risk factors among children and young adults: Findings from the Third National Health and Nutrition Examination Survey, 1988–1994. *Journal of the American Medical Association, 281*(11), 1006–1013.

Zakarain, J. M., Hovell, M. F., Hofstetter, C. R., Sallis, J. F., & Keating, K. J. (1994). Correlates of vigorous exercise in a predominately low SES and minority high school population. *Preventive Medicine, 23*(3), 314–321.

CHAPTER 8

Reducing Sexually Transmitted Diseases Among African American Youth

Loretta Sweet Jemmott, John B. Jemmott, III, and Emma J. Brown

A dolescence is a time of experimentation as young people strive to develop their identity in preparation for adulthood. For many young people, it is also a time of sexual experimentation. Unfortunately, the consequences often include sexually transmitted diseases (STDs) such as human immunodeficiency virus (HIV) infection, which causes acquired immune deficiency syndrome (AIDS). The goals of this chapter are to: (1) present an epidemiologic overview of STDs with emphasis on HIV infection among adolescents; (2) describe a cognitive behavioral approach for reducing adolescents' risk for STDs especially HIV infection; (3) present strategies for health care practitioners who intervene with children and adolescents to reduce their risk for STDs; and, (4) describe implications for the screening, management and treatment of STDs among adolescents.

EPIDEMIOLOGIC PERSPECTIVES: SEXUALLY TRANSMITTED DISEASES

Sexually transmitted diseases (STDs) refer to the more than 25 infectious organisms (including HIV) transmitted primarily through sexual activity, including anal and vaginal intercourse (CDC, 2001). Although considerable progress was made in decreasing the incidence and complications of STDs in the 1990s, STDs remain at epidemic levels in the United States. Recent data from the Centers for Disease Control and Prevention (CDC), similar to earlier reports, indicate gender, age, social-economic, geographic, and racial/ ethnic disparities in incidence and STD-associated complications (CDC, 2001). Noteworthy in this context (and discussed below) are the high rates of STDs observed among adolescents, particularly among minority youth. Adolescents are increasingly at risk for STDs including HIV infection because of their sexual behaviors. A national survey revealed that 48% of adolescents, both male and female, had engaged in sexual intercourse by age 16 (Leigh, Morrison, Trocki, et al., 1994). More recent data from the CDC (CDC, 1998) indicate that 61% of all high school seniors have had sexual intercourse and approximately 50% are currently sexually active. In addition, the Committee on Adolescence of the American Academy of Pediatrics (AAP-COA, 1994) estimated that 25% of adolescents will contract STD by the time they graduate from high school. Recent data from CDC (2001) indicate that approximately 25% of new cases of STDs occur among adolescents. Currently, sexually active adolescents have the highest rates of gonorrhea, syphilis, and pelvic inflammatory disease of any age group (AAP-COA, 1994; CDC, 1999). Although the use of latex condoms can reduce substantially the risk of STDs (CDC, 1988; Stone, Grimes, & Magder, 1986), most sexually active adolescents do not use condoms consistently (Jemmott & Jemmott, 1990; Jemmott & Jemmott, 1992; Jemmott, Jemmott, & Hacker, 1992; Jemmott, Jemmott, & Fong, 1992; Keller et al., 1991). In addition, national surveys of adolescents have consistently indicated that a greater proportion of African American compared with whites or Hispanics report that they are sexually active (CDC, 1991; Hofferth & Hayes, 1987; Kann et al., 1996), even when socioeconomic background is statistically controlled (Hofferth, Kahn, & Baldwin, 1987). Other data indicate that African American and Hispanic adolescents are less likely than White adolescents to use condoms at first sexual intercourse (Sonenstein et al., 1989). Consistent with recent CDC data, earlier reports also indicate that STDs are 2 to 3 times more common among low-income individuals residing in urban areas than among people of higher income or those who live in suburban communities (Cates, 1987; Hatcher et al., 1994; Jones et al., 1986).

There are important consequences of STDs. The immediate consequences of STDs can be physical discomfort and embarrassment. However, STDs are often asymptomatic, particularly in females and the consequences for females are more substantial than those for men. These more long-term consequences for women include pelvic inflammatory disease, infertility, cervical cancer, ectopic pregnancy, chronic pelvic pain, and infections passed on to newborns (CDC, 1995).

EPIDEMIOLOGIC PERSPECTIVES: HIV/AIDS

Although significant progress has been made in the treatment of AIDS during the past 2 decades, available prevalence and trend data suggest the need for continued emphasis on prevention strategies. The proportion of different population groups affected by HIV/AIDS has changed over time. Comparing the 1980s to the 1990s, for example, the proportion of AIDS cases among White men who have sex with White men (MSM) declined while the proportion of AIDS cases among women and men increased in select racial and ethnic groups, especially among African Americans and Hispanics (CDC, 2001). Half of all new HIV infections in the United States now occur in individuals between the ages of 13–24 (Futterman, Chabon, & Hoffman, 2000). Females account for more than half of new cases in adolescents, and approximately 75% of new infections in adolescent females occur via heterosexual transmission. Among adolescent males, at least two thirds of HIV transmissions occur via male-to-male sex (CDC, 1999). The exact number of adolescents infected with HIV in the United States is unknown, however, because currently no representative population-based studies estimating HIV seroprevalence in adolescents have been conducted.

The risk of sexually transmitted HIV infection is especially great among African American and Hispanic adolescents. For instance, although Blacks comprise 12% of the U.S. population, they represent 36% of persons with AIDS, and Hispanics, who comprise 11% of the U.S. population, represent 18% of persons with AIDS (CDC, 1997a). The disproportionate impact of AIDS on African Americans is particularly marked among adolescents. HIV surveillance data on civilian applicants for military service (CDC, 1990) and HIV surveillance data on entrants to Job Corps, a job-training program for urban and rural disadvantaged adolescents 16–21 years of age (CDC, 1990), converge to indicate higher HIV seroprevalence rates among African American and Latino adolescents than among their White counterparts.

Taken together, the available prevalence and trend data support the need for effective prevention strategies focused on reducing the risk for STDs. Public health approaches that consider cultural, developmental, and sociodemographic determinants of STD, as suggested in *Healthy People 2010* (CDC, 2001), are needed to reduce the risk and burden of STDs. As described in the next section of this chapter, theoretically derived behavioral interventions are a central and essential component of both individual and population-based approaches to STD risk reduction.

THEORETICAL FRAMEWORK: A COGNITIVE BEHAVIORAL APPROACH

At present there is no cure for AIDS, nor is there a vaccine to prevent HIV infection. Because the risk of HIV infection among adolescents is related to personal behavior, behavioral interventions are the only viable strategy to reduce this risk. Although it might be argued that behavior change interventions are essential for the prevention of HIV only until a vaccine or treatment is developed, these authors believe that such interventions will be essential well beyond that time. Despite effective, inexpensive, and easily accessible treatments for many STDs, epidemics of gonorrhea, chlamydia, and primary syphilis have prevailed among adolescents in recent years. This would suggest that an exclusive focus on physiologic, medical approaches is unlikely to be effective in controlling the sexual transmission of HIV. Hence, behavior change interventions are required.

Fortunately, progress has been made in identifying effective behavioral interventions to reduce adolescents' risk of sexually transmitted HIV infection (Interventions to Prevent HIV Risk Behaviors, 1997; Kalichman, Carey, & Johnson, 1996; Kim, Stanton, Dickersin, & Galbraith, 1997; Marin, 1995). These behavioral interventions can also be also be applied to reduce the risk of other STDs. An increasing number of researchers support the view that intervention approaches based on formative research with members of the study population and on a solid theoretical framework are most effective in changing HIV risk-associated sexual behavior. By measuring the theoretical mediators of intervention-induced behavior change, a better understanding of risk behavior has emerged.

The research described herein has drawn upon Social Cognitive Theory (Bandura, 1986, 1989), the Theory of Reasoned Action (Ajzen & Fishbein, 1980; Fishbein & Ajzen, 1975), and its extension, the Theory of Planned Behavior (Ajzen, 1991; Jemmott, Jemmott, & Hacker, 1992; Madden, El-len, & Ajzen, 1992). These theories and models highlight the importance of beliefs, outcome expectancy, perceived norms, skills, self-efficacy, and intentions as determinants of HIV risk-associated behavior. The Theory of Planned Behavior provides a particularly useful way of organizing much of the literature on determinants of HIV risk-associated behavior. Interventions to reduce HIV risk-associated behavior should affect these behaviors by affecting the variables that, according to the theory of planned behavior, are determinants of such behavior. The theory of planned behavior holds that specific behavioral intentions are the sole direct determinants of behaviors. Consider, for instance, the behavior of condom use. As shown in Figure 8.1, the theory would predict that the chief determinant of whether adolescents use condoms is their intention to use condoms. Several studies provide evi-

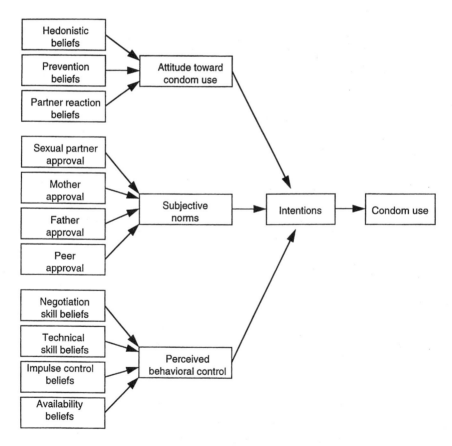

FIGURE 8.1 The theory of planned behavior applied to condom use.

dence that intentions are strong predictors of behavior, including condom use (Ajzen, 1991; Fisher, Fisher, & Rye, 1995; Sheppard, Hartwick, & Warshaw, 1988).

The theory further holds that individuals' behavioral intentions have three determinants: attitudes toward the behavior, subjective norms regarding it, and perceived behavioral control over it. Attitudes toward the specific behavior are individuals' evaluations of the behavior as positive or negative. Subjective norms regarding the behavior are individuals' perceptions of whether significant others approve of their engaging in the behavior. Perceived behavioral control has to do with the individual's confidence that he or she can perform the behavior. It reflects past experiences as well as anticipated impediments, obstacles, resources, and opportunities, and has affinity with the social cognitive theory construct of perceived self-efficacy (Bandura, 1986, 1989).

Attitude toward condom use is determined by behavioral beliefs about the consequences of using condoms. Such beliefs are conceptually similar to the social cognitive theory construct of outcome expectancy. Three types of behavioral beliefs have received considerable attention. First, there is *prevention belief*—the belief that the use of condoms can prevent pregnancy, STD, and HIV infection (Jemmott, Jemmott, Spears, Hewitt, & Cruz-Collins, 1992). Studies have also focused on *hedonistic beliefs*, which are beliefs about the consequences of condom use on sexual enjoyment (Jemmott & Jemmott, 1992; Jemmott, Jemmott, Spears, et al., 1992; NIMH Multisite HIV Prevention Trial, 1997). There is considerable evidence that such beliefs are associated with intentions to use condoms and self-reported condom use (Catania, Dolcini, et al., 1989; Jemmott & Jemmott, 1992; Valdiserri, Arena, Proctor, & Bonati, 1989). A third type of behavioral belief is *partner reaction belief*—the belief that ones' sexual partner would react favorably to their effort to use condoms (Jemmott & Jemmott, 1992).

According to the theory of planned behavior, subjective norms are determined by normative beliefs, or whether specific significant referents approve or disapprove of the behavior. In the case of condom use, the key referents would certainly include sexual partners. Other referents who are sources of normative influence for adolescents' sexual behavior include peers, parents, and other family members (DiClemente, 1991; Di Clemente et al., 2001; Fisher, Misovich, & Fisher, 1992; Fox & Inazu, 1980; Hofferth & Hayes, 1987; Milan & Kilmann, 1987).

Perceived behavioral control is determined by control beliefs about the factors that would facilitate or thwart a person's ability to perform the behavior. Four control beliefs have emerged reducing risky sexual behavior: *Avail-*

ability beliefs (adolescents' confidence that they can have condoms available when needed), *impulse control beliefs* (adolescents' confidence that they can control themselves enough to use condoms when they are sexually excited), *negotiation beliefs* (adolescents' confidence that they can persuade their sexual partners to use condoms), and *technical skill beliefs* (adolescents' ability to use condoms with facility and "without ruining the mood").

Attitudes, subjective norms, perceived behavioral control, and intentions do not constitute an exhaustive list of the potential influences on behavior. Other variables may also affect behavior; however, according to the theory of planned behavior, the effects of these *external variables* on behavior and intentions are mediated by their effects on the attitudinal component, the normative component, the perceived control component, or all three. In this way, the theory can accommodate variables that are external to it. Such external variables might include gender, socioeconomic status, race, personality, and cultural variables. A key external variable in the program of research described in this chapter is an HIV risk-reduction behavioral intervention. The interventions are designed to influence adolescents' behaviors by influencing those psychological constructs that, according to the theory of planned behavior, should predict behavior. Specifically, the interventions are primarily designed to influence adolescents' behavioral beliefs and control beliefs regarding specific HIV risk-associated sexual behaviors (Jemmott, Jemmott, & McCaffree, 1995).

APPLICATION OF COGNITIVE BEHAVIORAL THEORY: HELPING ADOLESCENTS REDUCE THEIR RISK OF HIV INFECTION

Over the past 15 years Jemmott and colleagues have conducted a program of research on HIV risk-reduction among inner-city adolescents. The goals of this research have been to (1) develop theory-based, culturally-sensitive, developmentally appropriate strategies to reduce HIV risk-associated sexual behaviors among African American adolescents, (2) elucidate the social psychological factors that underlie HIV risk-associated sexual behaviors, (3) answer practical questions about the most effective way to implement HIV risk-reduction interventions with African American adolescents, and (4) disseminate effective research-based behavioral interventions to community-based organizations, schools, and others concerned with the health of ethnic minority youth. This research has addressed several key questions: Can theory-based interventions change the HIV risk-associated sexual behavior of ethnic minority adolescents? Does matching the gender of facilitator and participant enhance intervention effects? Can culturally sensitive interventions be effective when implemented by facilitators who do not share the ethnic group membership of participants? Are adult or peer facilitators more effective? Is an emphasis on abstinence or condom use more effective in reducing unprotected sexual intercourse? In this section, three studies are described to answer those questions. This research has emphasized risk of HIV infection, but it is also relevant to STD prevention more broadly.

Intervening with African American Male Adolescents

The initial work was a randomized controlled trial with inner-city African American male adolescents (Jemmott, Jemmott, & Fong, 1992). This answers the first question, can theory-based interventions change the HIV risk-associated sexual behavior of ethnic minority adolescents? The focus was on this study population for several reasons. Inner-city African American male adolescents are at high risk of STD, however, most research on adolescents' sexual behavior has focused on female adolescents. What makes the paucity of data on African American male adolescents troublesome is that the male condom—the primary method of protection from sexually transmitted infection—must be used by males. Besides an interest in the efficacy of an HIV risk-reduction intervention, the researchers were also interested in whether the gender of the facilitator who implemented the intervention would moderate the efficacy of the intervention. It is often assumed that it is important to match the genders of participants and facilitators to maximize the efficacy of an intervention. Accordingly, African American male adolescents would be assumed to be more receptive to behavior change recommendations if they come from African American male facilitators, as compared with African American female facilitators.

The participants in the trial were 157 African American male adolescents (mean age, 14.6 years) in Philadelphia, Pennsylvania, who volunteered for a weekend program. Preintervention measures indicated that 83.0% of respondents reported having experienced sexual intercourse at least once. The adolescents were randomly assigned to an HIV risk-reduction condition or to a control condition and to a small group of about six boys led by a specially trained male or female African American facilitator. Adolescents in the HIV risk-reduction condition received an intensive 5-hr intervention comprised of videotapes, games, exercises, and small group discussions.

To control for Hawthorne effects, to reduce the likelihood that effects of the HIV risk-reduction intervention could be attributed to nonspecific features, including group interaction and special attention (Cook & Campbell, 1979), adolescents randomly assigned to the control condition also received a 5-hr intervention. Structurally similar to the HIV risk-reduction intervention, it involved culturally and developmentally appropriate videotapes, exercises, and games focused on career opportunities. Although career-opportunity-intervention participants did not learn about AIDS, given the high unemployment among inner-city African American adolescent men, the goal was to provide information that would be valuable to them as they planned their futures.

There were significant effects of the HIV intervention on the theoretical mediator variables. Postintervention analyses revealed that the adolescents who received the HIV risk-reduction intervention scored higher in AIDS knowledge, lower in attitudes toward HIV risk-associated sexual behavior, lower in intentions to engage in HIV risk-associated sexual behavior, higher in hedonistic beliefs favorable to condom use, and higher in perceived self-efficacy to use condoms than did the adolescents in the control condition. About 96% of the adolescents were retained at 3-month follow-up. Adolescents who had received the HIV risk-reduction intervention reported engaging in significantly fewer HIV risk-associated behavior in the previous 3 months than did those in the control condition. They had sexual intercourse less often, had fewer partners, used condoms more consistently, had fewer occasions of sexual intercourse without using a condom, and had a lower incidence of anal intercourse. Surprisingly, there was no consistent effect of the gender of the facilitator. It was expected that effects of the HIV risk-reduction intervention would be enhanced with African American male facilitators. Consistent with this, the HIV risk-reduction intervention caused a greater increase in postintervention AIDS knowledge among participants who had a male facilitator than among those who had a female facilitator, however, this interaction was not evident on intentions and attitudes regarding risky behavior. In addition, the effects of the HIV risk-reduction intervention on sexual behavior were significantly stronger with female facilitators than with male facilitators. This study indicates that a relatively brief intervention can have impact on theory-based mediators of behavior change and self-reported sexual risk behavior among African American adolescents.

Matching Facilitator and Participant on Race and Gender

The second study focused on practical questions about the best way to intervene with inner-city African American adolescents. Therefore, in a second randomized controlled trial, the efficacy of this intervention with a younger group of adolescents was tested. These authors reasoned that it was particularly important to intervene with young adolescents because, once established, habitual nonuse of condoms may be a very difficult behavior to modify. In addition, practical and theoretical questions about intervening with inner-city African American adolescents were also addressed. The issue of gender of facilitator was also pursued further. Hence, the possibility of an effective theory-based, culture sensitive HIV intervention when the race and gender of participants and facilitators are *not* matched or when the groups are not homogeneous on gender was also examined (Jemmott, Jemmott, Fong, & McCaffree, 1999).

A second issue of interest was the race of the facilitator. The hypothesis that an intervention with African American adolescents would be more effective if the facilitator were African American, as compared with white was tested. Matching the race/ethnicity of facilitators and intervention participants may be incorporated in a more general approach of using culturally sensitive intervention strategies (Mays & Cochran, 1988; Peterson & Marin, 1988). Another issue the researchers addressed was the gender composition of the group. Interventions dealing with sexual behavior of adolescents may be more effective if implemented in single-sex groups. The advantage of single-sex groups may be greater for female adolescents. Thus, whether the effectiveness of the intervention varied depending on whether the groups were single gender or both male and female adolescents was tested.

The participants in this randomized controlled trial were 496 inner-city African American adolescents who volunteered for a weekend program. The sample was 54% female with a mean age of 13.1 years. Slightly more than 55% of the respondents reported having sexual intercourse at least once and 30.2% reported having sexual intercourse in the previous 3 months. About 17.7% of respondents reported ever having anal intercourse, and 8.3% reported such involvement in the previous 3 months. Adolescents were randomly assigned to either an HIV intervention or a structurally similar control condition. In addition, participants were randomized to a small group that was either homogeneous or heterogeneous in gender and led by a male or female facilitator who was African American or White. In this study the control condition received a general heath promotion intervention that focused on health problems related to behavior, but unrelated to sexual behavior. These health problems included cardiovascular disease, hypertension, breast cancer, and colon cancer—significant causes of morbidity and mortality among African Americans (AHA, 2000; CDC, 2001; Gillum, 1982; Page & Asire, 1985).

The findings indicated that the HIV intervention had significant effects on the theoretical variables it was designed to influence. The adolescents who received the HIV intervention had greater HIV knowledge, more favorable behavioral beliefs about condoms, greater perceived self-efficacy to use condoms, and stronger condom-use intentions postintervention than did those in the control condition. Most of these effects were sustained through a 6-month follow-up. Although, for the most part, the means were in the predicted direction, analyses on behavior reported at the 3-month follow-up revealed no significant difference in reported sexual behavior between the HIV risk-reduction condition and the control condition. A 6-month follow-up on 93% of the original participants revealed that those who received the HIV intervention reported less HIV risk-associated sexual behavior, including less unprotected sexual intercourse and a lower incidence of anal intercourse, than did their counterparts in the control condition. Consistent with the Jemmott, Jemmott, and Fong (1992) study, self-reported sexual behavior and changes in self-reported behavior were unrelated to scores on a standard measure of social desirability response bias.

Analyses to examine whether the effects of the intervention varied as a function of the race of the facilitator, the gender of the facilitator, the gender of the participants, and the gender composition of the intervention groups were conducted. The results were nonsignificant. The effects of the HIV intervention were about the same regardless of the race of the facilitator, the gender of the facilitator, the gender of the participants, and the gender composition of the intervention group. The interactions did not affect self-reported HIV risk-associated behavior, intentions, HIV risk-reduction knowledge, behavioral beliefs, or perceived self-efficacy. Moreover, they did not affect facilitators' reports of how the participants reacted to the intervention or participants' own reports of their reactions to the interventions: how much they liked it, how much they talked, and how much they felt they learned.

In short, instead of specificity of intervention effects, overwhelming evidence for the generality of intervention effects was demonstrated (Jemmott, Jemmott, Fong, & McCaffree, 1999). Thus, this study demonstrated that risk behavior can be reduced among young adolescents and that the effects of a theory-based, culturally-sensitive intervention generalize across implementation by facilitators varying in race and gender and groups varying in gender composition. It may be that public schools, health clinics, community-based organizations, and other organizations that are implementing HIV prevention programs may not have to be concerned about matching the characteristics of the facilitators and the audience, or implementing single-gender groups, if the content of the intervention is appropriate for the audience (e.g., culturally sensitive), if the intervention is highly structured, and if the facilitators are trained to implement the intervention according to the protocol.

Varying the Message and the Messenger

The third study was a randomized controlled trial designed to test the effects of two types of HIV risk-reduction messages, abstinence and safer sex, delivered by two types of messengers, adult and peer facilitators (Jemmott, Jemmott, & Fong, 1998). Sexual transmission of HIV is tied to unprotected sexual intercourse—that is, sexual intercourse without the use of a latex condom. Thus, to reduce the risk of sexually transmitted HIV infection, a behavioral intervention must reduce the frequency of unprotected sexual intercourse. This can be achieved in two ways: (1) the abstinence strategy, which focuses on reducing the frequency of sexual intercourse, and (2) the safer sex strategy, which focuses on increasing the frequency of condom use. Whether abstinence or safer sex should be the focus of intervention efforts has been vigorously debated among public health experts, educators, parents, and other advocates for youth. This study considered the efficacy of both intervention approaches. It was reasoned that an abstinence intervention would have the best chance of being effective with young sexually inexperienced adolescents. Accordingly, in this study the focus was on a younger age group than in our previous studies.

The study also examined the relative efficacy in delivering HIV risk-reduction messages of two types of intervention or messengers—peers as opposed to adults. It is often asserted that interventions for adolescents may be especially efficacious if peers implement them (Rickert, Jay, & Gottlieb, 1991; Slap, Plotkin, Khalid, Michelman, & Forke, 1991). Peer facilitators may be better at establishing rapport, credibility, and trust with adolescents. On the other hand, adult facilitators may be efficacious. Owing to adults' experience and maturity, adolescents may respect them more and may perceive them to be more credible sources of information about sex. A second goal of this study, then, was to compare the efficacy of peers and adults in implementing HIV risk-reduction interventions with young adolescents.

The program participants were 659 sixth and seventh grade inner-city African American students from public middle schools. The mean age of the sample was 11.8 years, 53% were female. Despite the young mean age of the sample, preintervention questionnaire responses indicated that 25.2% reported having had sex at least once, with 15.4% reported having had sex in the past 3 months. Few respondents (1.6%) reported having sexual relationships with a person of their own gender. Participants were randomly assigned to one of three interventions, and to a group composed of (6–8) adolescents led by an adult facilitator or two peer co-facilitators. Each intervention consisted of eight 1-hr modules implemented on two consecutive Saturdays. Slightly more than 98% of the participants attended the second day of the interventions. The abstinence intervention mentioned condom use, but stressed delaying the initiation of sexual intercourse and reducing the frequency of sexual intercourse. The safer sex intervention indicated that abstinence is the best choice, but stressed that adolescents should use condoms if they decide to have sexual intercourse. A general health promotion intervention similar to the one previously described served as the control condition.

The adult facilitators (mean age: 40 years) were male or female; the peer co-facilitators (mean age: 6 years) were 2 males, 2 females, or 1 male and 1 female. Facilitators were believed to be capable of implementing any of the interventions. They were randomly assigned to be trained to implement one of the three interventions. In this way, facilitator characteristics were randomized across intervention conditions. The results, accordingly, cannot be attributed to characteristics of the facilitators as opposed to the intervention content.

The interventions had significant effects on the theoretical mediator variables they were designed to influence. The adolescents who received the safer sex intervention scored significantly higher in condom-use knowledge, believed more strongly that condoms can prevent pregnancy, STD, and HIV, believed more strongly that using condoms would not interfere with sexual enjoyment, and reported greater self-efficacy for using condoms than did those in the control condition. Most importantly, there were also significant effects of the HIV interventions on self-reported sexual behavior. At the 3-month follow-up session there was a 96% return rate, 94% at 6-month follow-up, and 93% at 12-month follow-up. Abstinence intervention participants were less likely to report having sexual intercourse in the 3 months after intervention than were control condition participants, but not at 6- or 12-month follow-up. Safer sex intervention participants reported more frequent condom use than did control condition participants at all follow-ups. There were interactions between preintervention sexual experience and the interventions. Among adolescents who reported sexual experience at baseline, safer sex intervention participants reported less frequent sexual intercourse at 6- and 12-month follow-up than did control and abstinence intervention and less frequent unprotected intercourse at all follow-ups than did control condition. There were no differences in intervention effects with adult facilitators as compared with peer co-facilitators. The results also did not differ as a function of gender of facilitator or matching gender of facilitator and gender of participant. Again, in this study self-reported sexual behavior and changes in self-reported behavior were unrelated to scores on a standard measure of social desirability response bias.

One common argument against AIDS education programs that emphasize condom use has been that they encourage adolescents to engage in sexual activity. Adolescents who received the safer sex intervention that emphasized condom use, were not more likely to report having sexual intercourse at the follow-ups than were adolescents in the control condition. Indeed, among adolescents who reported preintervention sexual experience, those in the safer sex condition reported less frequent sexual intercourse than did those in the control condition at the 6-month and 12-month follow-ups, thus providing evidence *contrary* to the common belief that sex education increases sexual activity. Moreover, safer sex intervention participants who did report having sexual intercourse reported using condoms more frequently than did their counterparts in the control condition at all three follow-ups.

This study suggests that intensive theory-based culturally sensitive interventions designed to influence mediators of risk behavior, including HIV knowledge, behavioral beliefs, self-efficacy, and skills, whether implemented by adult facilitators or peer co-facilitators, can reduce the HIV risk-associated sexual behavior among inner-city African American adolescents. It also suggests that safer sex interventions may be especially effective with sexually experienced adolescents and may have longer lasting effects than abstinence interventions. Thus, if the goal is to curb unprotected sexual intercourse among adolescents who are already sexually experienced, then safer sex interventions may hold the most promise.

Collectively, results from this ongoing multidisciplinary program of research have influenced clinical practice (described below) in delineating theoretically derived behavioral interventions focused on HIV risk reduction. A unique outcome of this research, *Be Proud! Be Responsible!* (BPBR) (Jemmott, Jemmott, & McCaffree, 1996), has been adopted by CDC as one of four HIV interventions for youth in its *Programs That Work* project (DASH, 1997). In addition, the efficacy and effectiveness of the BPBR curriculum is currently being examined in an ongoing randomized clinical trial with suburban and inner-city youth of diverse racial/ethnic and socioeconomic backgrounds (Borawski, Hayman, Adams-Davis, Robbins, & Green, 1999).

IMPLICATIONS FOR STD RISK REDUCTION INTERVENTIONS

Because condoms can reduce the risk of STDs, clinicians must be aware of the determinants of condom use among adolescents The review of the literature suggests that interventions to increase African American adolescents' use of condoms need to address hedonistic beliefs regarding the consequences of safer sex practices for sexual enjoyment. For example, Jemmott, Jemmott, Spears, and colleagues (1992) found that an intervention that incorporated hedonistic beliefs was especially effective at changing intentions to use condoms. Jemmott and Jemmott (1992) reported evidence that changes in hedonistic beliefs were a mediator of changes in intentions to use condoms. Thus, interventions should attempt to weaken this common belief that sexual enjoyment is curtailed if condoms are used.

Quite apart from adolescents' beliefs about condoms, HIV risk-reduction interventions need to address the reactions of adolescents' sexual partner, particularly the sexual partner's approval or disapproval of safer sex practices, including abstinence. Unlike many health behavior interventions, HIV risk-reduction interventions have to take into account the fact that the adolescent may not have complete control over the targeted behavior. Protected sexual intercourse is interpersonal behavior and hence the sexual partner's beliefs are important. Trust is an issue that often arises during intervention group discussions regarding convincing sexual partners to use condoms. Asking a partner to use condoms may suggest to the partner that the adolescent does not trust the partner. This is particularly likely if the partner has an established or long-term relationship with the adolescent. In contrast it may be easier to establish condom use at the beginning of new relationships. Clearly, HIV risk-reduction interventions have to take this barrier to condom use into account.

Several studies also suggested that interventions should address skills and perceived self-efficacy. Although skills and perceived self-efficacy are likely to be correlated—people who have the skills are also likely to feel efficacious—they are not identical and it is unclear which of the two is more important to behavior change. A number of types of skills and efficacy have been highlighted in the literature. Perhaps the most widely recognized type of skill or perceived efficacy is *negotiation or resistance skill*—the ability of the adolescent to convince a sexual partner to practice protected sexual intercourse or to resist partner pressure to practice unprotected sexual intercourse. Much less attention has been paid to *technical skill* in condom use, particularly skill at using condoms without ruining the mood. This type of skill, however, may be just as important as negotiation skill (Jemmott, Jemmott, & Hacker, 1992). HIV risk-reduction interventions must teach adolescents how to use condoms. It is not enough to simply tell them they should use condoms. By increasing technical skill at using condoms it may be possible to allay the adolescents' sexual partner's concerns about the adverse impact of condom use on sexual enjoyment. Clearly, if an adolescent successfully negotiates condom use, but then implements it in a clumsy manner, the experience may decrease the likelihood that the adolescent will attempt to use condoms in the future or may make it more difficult to negotiate future use with that sexual partner. Role plays are one way to enhance negotiation skills; condom exercises can be used to rehearse use of condoms. Because of the importance of negotiation and technical skills and perceived self-efficacy it is important to use well-trained facilitators who are comfortable with sexual matters. A facilitator who is uncomfortable with sexual matters may give the skills short shrift. Yet these skills are a critical feature of the intervention.

The goal of STD and HIV risk-reduction interventions is to decrease unprotected sexual intercourse so as to reduce risk of exposure to an STD, especially HIV. Empirical evidence does not clarify whether the best strategy to accomplish this goal is to stress decreases in sexual activity (e.g., abstinence) or to stress the consistent use of condoms during sexual activity. Although interventions should emphasize that the decision to practice abstinence or to have sexual intercourse is one that the adolescent has to make, they should make clear that abstinence is an acceptable choice that many adolescents make and that abstinence is the only way to eliminate completely the potential for sexually transmitted HIV infection. In addition, interventions should emphasize that adolescents who decide to have sexual intercourse should use condoms to reduce their risk of sexually transmitted infection. The issue of birth control may arise. Adolescents are often far more concerned about pregnancy than about STDs, though this may be changing. Adolescents may believe that condoms are unnecessary because of the use of contraceptive pills. It should be emphasized that both pregnancy prevention *and* STD prevention are important, that even if the female partner uses contraceptive pills, it is still necessary to use a latex condom to prevent sexually transmitted infection.

ASSESSMENT OF STDS IN CHILDREN AND ADOLESCENTS

Health providers who work with children and adolescents must be aware of the need to assess and screen for STDs in these populations (AAP-COA,

2001). Children who are suspected victims of sexual abuse should be evaluated for STDs, however, the assessment of the psychological, social, and legal aspects of childhood sexual assault or abuse is beyond the scope of this chapter. Therefore, the focus of this next section is on the physical evaluation of STDs among children and sexually active adolescents. The recommended frequency of STD screening for sexually active adolescents is annually while STD screening for at risk adolescents (those who are sex workers, homeless, incarcerated, gay males, and pregnant) is more frequent perhaps, every 6 months (AAP-COA, 1994).

The American Academy of Pediatrics (1997) suggests that preadolescents with genital, anal, or perineal ulcers; perineal pruritus; condyloma acuminata; or vaginitis and dysuria and children suspected of being victims of sexual abuse, rape, or incest are also in need of STD screening. STD screening includes history taking, physical examination, and laboratory tests. Sexual abuse is the most common cause of gonorrhea and must be considered a cause of chlamydia and acquired primary and secondary syphilis in preadolescents (CDC, 1993). AAP (1997) suggested that 20% of girls and 10% of boys will have been sexually abused by adulthood. The definition of child sexual abuse is "contact or interaction between a child and an adult when the child is used for the sexual stimulation of the adult or another person" (AAP, 1997, p. 112). There are laws in all states and territories of the United States that mandate the reporting of suspected or confirmed child abuse. Hence, health care providers must contact the child protective services of their respective state if they suspect sexual abuse among pediatric patients.

Because of the likelihood of sexual abuse and the potential for additional medical and legal investigations, evaluation of STDs in children must include the collection of cultures. The isolation of C. Trachomatis cells in cultures confirmed by microscopic identification are recommended for chlamydia diagnosis, while standard culture systems for the isolation of N. Gonorrhea confirmed by biochemic, enzyme substrate, and serologic is recommended for gonorrhea diagnosis. Nonculture tests are not recommended because of the possibility of false positive test results (CDC, 1993).

Health care providers who work with adolescents must first create nonjudgmental and respectful atmospheres that provide confidentiality (AAP-COA, 1994; AAP-COA, 2001; Scott, 1996). Laws concerning consent and confidentiality for HIV care and treatment vary from state to state; thus, it is essential that health care providers are familiar with the laws of the state in which they practice (AAP-COA, 2001). Noteworthy is that public health statues and legal precedents allow for medical evaluation and treatment of minors (defined as less than 18 years of age) for selected categorical illnesses/ conditions (particularly STDs) without parental consent. Currently, not every state has explicitly defined HIV infection as one for which assessment or treatment of a minor may proceed without parental consent (AAP-COA, 2001). Nevertheless, the confidentiality of the communication and treatment proposed should be verbally stated as well as written, as adolescents are more likely to honestly divulge sensitive information such as sexual and drug use history when they are aware of the confidential nature of the health care encounters (Scott, 1996). All STD evaluations must include a detailed sexual history and a cursory assessment of drug use patterns, particularly focusing on the use of alcohol and drugs in conjunction with sexual intercourse. These preliminary data will guide the STD screening procedure.

Health care providers can best establish rapport with adolescents by using the first few minutes of the encounter to provide introductory conversation and to assure adolescents about the confidentiality of the information, results of the examination and/or treatment with the exception of sexual abuse. An overview of what will take place during the encounter (inquiry of sexual and drug history, physical evaluation, and treatment if warranted) must be provided. It may be helpful to inform adolescents that some of the discussion could be sensitive, but that the behaviors discussed are not unusual for adolescents (Scott, 1996).

Next, in a nonjudgmental manner, a thorough sexual history needs to be obtained. Aspects of the sexual history include sexual active status, age of initiation, sexual orientation or preference, frequency of sexual intercourse, type of sex (oral, vaginal, anal), use of contraception with method, condom use status with frequency of use (male and/or female), number of partners (one, multiple, or serial) (AAP-COA, 1994; Scott, 1996), alcohol or other drugs in conjunction with sexual activity, and current or past sexual abuse (assault, rape, incest). A detailed alcohol and drug history may be warranted for some adolescents.

Information collected from the sexual history is used, in part, to guide the physical evaluation. Additional inquiries about frequency of urination and the presence of pain, genital discharge, pruritus, or skin lesions are necessary either during the taking of the history or during the physical examination (AAP-COA, 1994). Scott (1996) suggested that the physical examination is an idea teaching tool for anatomy, adolescent growth and development, and self-examination (for example, self-breast examination and testicular examination). According to AAP-COA (1994), it is necessary to include the following in the actual examination of adolescent suspected of having an STD:

1. A complete visualization of the body
2. Inspection of the skin for rashes and bruise.
3. Examination of the throat, joints, and abdomen
4. Inspection and palpation of males' urethral to assess for the presence of discharge. Discharge is collected using a urethral swab for microscopical examination, culture, and other diagnostic testing when found.
5. Examination of males' rectum to assess for prostatitis
6. Examination of females' genitalia using Papanicolaou smear (pap smear)
7. Examination of females' vaginal secretions for chlamydia and gonorrhea
8. Inspection and palpation of the pelvic in females with unexplained abdominal pain to rule out pelvic inflammatory disease.

In addition, all sexually active males and females should routinely be evaluated for gonorrhea or chlamydia using microscopic examination, cultures, urine leukocytes esterase analysis (male), DNA probes, and/or immunofluorescent antibody screening. Refer to the American Academy of Pediatrics, Committee of Adolescence (1994) *Sexually Transmitted Disease* and American Academy of Pediatrics (1997) *Report of the Committee on Infectious Diseases*, 24th Edition, for complete information on the laboratory assessment of all STDs.

MANAGEMENT OF STDS IN CHILDREN AND ADOLESCENTS

The first task of managing STDs in these populations is to increase their access to care (Scott, 1996). As a group, adolescents in the United States are least likely to have access to health care and they have the lowest rate of primary care visits (Klein et al., 1993). Access to care is a major obstacle for asymptomatic males (Shafer et al., 1993).

Providing sexually active adolescents with educational information about: (1) their genital anatomy and (2) safer sexual methods is another important management strategy. Adolescent females should be informed that their vaginal area and larger perineal may increase their risk of STDs and HIV infection because of the blood rich mucosa lining. Health care providers must explain to their sexually active adolescent clients that they are at risk for STDs/HIV even when they use condoms consistently, but especially when they do not use condoms or use condoms inconsistently. It must be stressed that this risk exists even when the adolescents think that they are in long-term monogamous relationships unless both partners were evaluated for STDs/HIV and received negative results which were mutually verified.

After a thorough evaluation for STDs and the educational intervention, medicinal treatment is given when warranted and based upon age, weight, and other criteria (AAP, 1997; AAP-COA, 2001; CDC, 1993). Because each STD has a specific treatment protocol, the detailed treatment guidelines for STDs and HIV/AIDS are not outlined in this chapter. AAP has made available on their web site (www.pediatrics.org) detailed documents including the evidence base for treatment of STDs including HIV/AIDS. For example, guidelines for the use of combination regimens of antiretroviral medications, designed to reduce AIDS-related symptomology and prolong survival, are available (www.hivatis.org). Other comprehensive sources for treatment recommendations include the American Academy of Pediatrics (1997) *Red Book: Report of the Committee on Infectious Diseases*, 24th Edition and The Centers for Disease Control and Prevention (1993) *Sexually Transmitted Diseases Treatment Guidelines*.

CONCLUSIONS

Major components of effective clinical management of STDs include screening, diagnosis and treatment, risk reduction counseling and education, identification and treatment of partners, and access to quality laboratory services for STDs. Screening allows for the detection of infected persons who would otherwise remain undetected, develop complications of STDs, and transmit the infection to their sex partners. In order to prevent or treat STDs effectively, it is important that health care providers develop knowledge and awareness of sexual health issues and become comfortable discussing them. This will enable optimal utilization of clinical opportunities to effectively counsel patients regarding healthy sexual behaviors, and therefore improve clinical care for STDs. Communicating effectively with patients regarding sexual health is a particularly critical skill for health care providers, however, most clinicians are not adequately trained in communication and counseling skills (Eng & Butler, 1997).

Focusing on prevention is crucial. Clinicians should emphasize prevention because averting illness is desirable, many STDs are incurable, and STD-related complications may be irreversible. Effective prevention programs are usually the result of extensive research and evaluation. Areas of prevention-related research that should be emphasized include determinants of sexual behavior and sustained behavior change; determinants of initiation of sexual intercourse among adolescents; influence of social and other community-related factors on risk of STDs, interventions to improve condom use and reduce high risk behavior; effectiveness of sexual risk behavior assessment and counseling; biomedical interventions that do not rely primarily on individual behaviors, such as vaccines, female-controlled prevention methods; cost-effectiveness of interventions, methods for preventing STDs among disenfranchised populations, interventions for preventing STDs among persons of all sexual orientation and methods to assess prevention programs effectiveness.

There is ample evidence of the risk of sexually transmitted HIV infection among inner-city African American adolescents. Much less progress has been made toward scientific knowledge regarding how to reduce this risk. One common argument against STD and HIV risk-reduction education programs for adolescents and children has been that exposing them to information about sex will encourage them to engage in sexual activity. These data, however, provide some evidence that the *opposite* may be true. Adolescents who received the HIV risk-reduction intervention were *less* likely to engage in sexual activity, and those who did were more likely to engage in safe sexual activity. Thus, the fear that providing adolescents with information about STDs and AIDS will result in greater sexual activity is perhaps simply a fear. Given the widely recognized potential risk of pregnancy and STDs, including HIV, among inner-city adolescents, particularly African Americans and Latinos, the findings that relatively brief but intensive intervention can have significant impact on sexual risk behavior and theory-based mediators of such behavior among African American inner-city adolescents are encouraging.

REFERENCES

American Academy of Pediatrics. (1997). *Red book. Report of the Committee on Infectious Diseases* (24 ed.). Illinois: Author.

American Academy of Pediatrics, Committee on Adolescence. (1994). Sexually transmitted disease. *Pediatrics, 94,* 568–572.

American Academy of Pediatrics, Committee on Adolescence. (1999). Contraception and adolescents. *Pediatrics, 104,* 1161–1166.

American Academy of Pediatrics, Committee on Adolescence (2001). Adolescents and human immunodeficiency virus infection: The role of the pediatrician in prevention and intervention. *Pediatrics, 107*(1), 188–190.

American Academy of Pediatrics, Committee on Pediatric AIDS. (2000). Education of children with human immunodeficiency virus infection. *Pediatrics, 105,* 1358–1360.

American Heart Association. (2000). Heart and Stroke Statistical Update. Dallas, TX: Author.

Ajzen, I. (1991). The theory of planned behavior. *Organizational Behavior and Human Decision Processes, 50,* 179–211.

Ajzen, I., & Fishbein, M. (1980). *Understanding attitudes and predicting social behavior.* Englewood Cliffs, NJ: Prentice-Hall.

Bandura, A. (1986). *Social foundations of thought and action: A social cognitive theory.* Englewood Cliffs, NJ: Prentice-Hall.

Bandura, A. (1989). Perceived self-efficacy. In V. M. Mays, G. W. Albee, & S. F. Schneider (Eds.), *Primary prevention of AIDS: Psychological approaches* (pp. 128–141). Newbury Park, CA: Sage.

Becker, M. H. (Ed.). (1974). The health belief model and personal health behavior. *Health Education Monographs, 2* (No. 4).

Borawski, E., Hayman, L. L., Adams-Davis, K., Robbins, F., & Green, S. (1999). *Taking Be Proud! Be Responsible! To the Suburbs.* Grant Narrative, RO1 HD 38456.

Catania, J. A., Dolcini, M. M., Coates, T. J., Kegeles, S. M., Greenblatt, R. M., Puckett, S., Corman, M., & Miller, J. (1989). Predictors of condom use and multiple partnered sex among sexually-active adolescent women: Implications for AIDS-related health interventions. *Journal of Sex Research, 26,* 514–524.

Catania, J. A., Kegeles, S. M., & Coates, T. J. (1990). Towards an understanding of risk behavior: An AIDS risk reduction model (ARRM). *Health Education Quarterly, 17,* 53–72.

Cates, W. Jr. (1987). Epidemiology and control of sexually transmitted diseases: Strategic evolution. *Infectious Disease Clinics of North America, 1,* 1–23.

Centers for Disease Control and Prevention. (1988). Condoms for the prevention of sexually transmitted diseases. *MMWR. Morbidity and Mortality Weekly Report, 37,* 133–137.

Centers for Disease Control and Prevention. (1990). *National HIV seroprevalence surveys: Summary of results. Data from serosurveillance activities through 1989.* Atlanta, GA: U.S. Department of Health and Human Services.

Centers for Disease Control and Prevention. (1991). Premarital sexual experience among adolescent women—United States, 1970–1988. *MMWR. Morbidity and Mortality Weekly Report, 39,* 929–932.

Centers for Disease Control and Prevention. (1997a). *HIV/AIDS Surveillance Report, 9*(No. 1), 1–37.

Centers for Disease Control and Prevention. (1997b). *Sexually Transmitted Disease Surveillance, 1996.* Atlanta, GA: U.S. Department of Health and Human Services, Public Health Services.

Centers for Disease Control and Prevention. (1998). Youth risk behavior surveillance— United States, 1997. *MMWR, Morbidity, Mortality Weekly Report, 47*(SS-3), 1–89.

Centers for Disease Control and Prevention. (2001). *Healthy People 2000 Final Review.* U.S. Department of Health and Human Services, Public Health Service, National Center for Health Statistics, Hyattsville, Maryland. (DHHS Publication No. 01–0256).

Cook, T., & Campbell, D. (1979). *Quasi-experimentation: Design and analysis for field settings*. Chicago.

Crowne, D., & Marlowe, D. (1964). *The approval motive*. New York: Wiley.

DiClemente, R. J. (1991). Predictors of HIV-preventive sexual behavior in a high-risk adolescent population: The influence of perceived peer norms and sexual communication on incarcerated adolescents' consistent use of condoms. *American Journal of Adolescent Health, 12*, 385–390.

DiClemente, R. J., Wingood, G. M., Crosby, R., Sionean, C., Cobb, B., Harrington, K., Davies, S., Hook, E. W., & Oh, M. K. (2001). Parental monitoring: Association with adolescents' risk behaviors. *Pediatrics, 107*(6), 1363–1368.

Eng, T., & Butler, W. (1997). *The Hidden Epidemic: Confronting Sexually Transmitted Diseases*. The Committee of Prevention and Control of Sexually Transmitted Diseases, Institute of Medicine. Washington, DC: National Academy Press.

Fishbein, M., & Ajzen, I. (1975). *Belief, attitude, intention and behavior*. Boston: Addison-Wesley.

Fisher, J. D., Fisher, W. A., Williams, S. S., & Malloy, T. E. (1994). Empirical tests of an information-motivation-behavioral skills model of AIDS preventive behavior. *Health Psychology, 13*, 238–250.

Fisher, J. D., Misovich, S. J., & Fisher, W. A. (1992). Impact of perceived social norms on adolescents AIDS risk behavior and prevention. In R. DiClemente (Ed.), *Adolescents and AIDS: A generation in jeopardy* (pp. 117–135). Newbury Park, CA: Sage.

Fisher, W. A., Fisher, J. D., & Rye, B. J. (1995). Understanding and promoting AIDS-preventive behaviors: Insights from the theory of reasoned action. *Health Psychology, 14*, 255–264.

Fox, G. L., & Inazu, J. K. (1980). Patterns and outcomes of mother-daughter communication about sexuality. *Journal of Social Issues, 36*, 7–29.

Futterman, D., Chabon, B., & Hoffman, N. D. (2000). HIV and AIDS in adolescents. *Pediatric Clinics of North America, 14*, 171–188.

Gillum, R. F. (1982). Coronary heart disease in Black populations. I. Mortality and morbidity. *American Heart Journal, 104*, 839–843.

Hansen, W. B., Graham, J. W., Wolkenstein, B. H., & Rohrbach, L. A. (1991). Program integrity as a moderator of prevention program effectiveness: Results for fifth-grade students in the adolescent alcohol prevention trial. *Journal of Studies on Alcohol, 52*(6), 568–579.

Hatcher, R. A., Trussell, J., Stewart, F., Stewart, G. K., Kowal, D., Guest, F., Cates, Jr., W., & Policar, M. S. (1994). *Contraceptive technology, Sixteenth revised edition*. New York: Irvington Publishers, Inc.

Hofferth, S. L., & Hayes, C. D. (Eds.). (1987). *Risking the future: Adolescent sexuality, pregnancy, and childbearing, Volume 2*. Washington, DC: National Academy Press.

Hofferth, S., Kahn, J., & Baldwin, W. (1987). Premarital sexual activity among U.S. teenage women over the past three decades. *Family Planning Perspectives, 19*(20), 46–53.

Janz, N. K., & Becker, M. H. (1984).The health belief model: A decade later. *Health Education Quarterly, 11*, 1–47.

Jemmot, J. B., III, & Jemmott, L. S. (2000). HIV risk reduction behavioral interventions with heterosexual adolescents. *AIDS, 14*(2), 40–52.

Jemmott, J. B. III, Jemmott, L. S., & Fong, G. T. (1992). Reductions in HIV risk-associated sexual behaviors among Black male adolescents: Effects of an AIDS prevention intervention. *American Journal of Public Health, 82*, 372–377.

Jemmott, J. B., Jemmott, L. S., & Fong, G. (1998) Abstinence and safer sex HIV risk reduction interventions for African American adolescents: A randomized controlled trial. *Journal of the American Medical Association, 279*(19), 1529–1536.

Jemmott, J. B. III, Jemmott, L. S., Fong, G. T., & McCaffree, K. (1999). Reducing HIV risk-associated sexual behavior among African-American adolescents: Testing the generality of intervention effects. *American Journal of Community Psychology, 27*(2), 161–187.

Jemmott, J. B. III, Jemmott, L. S., & Hacker, C. I. (1992). Predicting intentions to use condoms among African American adolescents: The theory of planned behavior as a model of HIV risk associated behavior. *Journal of Ethnicity and Disease, 2*, 371–380.

Jemmott, J. B. III, Jemmott, L. S., Spears, H., Hewitt, N., & Cruz-Collins, M. (1992). Self-efficacy, hedonistic expectancies, and condom-use intentions among inner-city Black adolescent women: A social cognitive approach to AIDS risk behavior. *Journal of Adolescent Health, 13*, 512–519.

Jemmott, L. S., & Jemmott, J. B. III. (1990). Sexual knowledge, attitudes, and risky sexual behavior among inner-city Black male adolescents. *Journal of Adolescent Research, 5*, 346–369.

Jemmott, L. S., & Jemmott, J. B. III. (1992). Increasing condom-use intentions among sexually active inner-city Black adolescent women: Effects of an AIDS prevention program. *Nursing Research, 41*, 273–279.

Jemmott, L. S., Jemmott, J. B., & McCaffree, K. (1995). *Be Proud! Be Responsible!: Strategies to Empower Youth to Reduce Their Risk for AIDS.* New York: Select Media.

Jones, E. F., Forrest, J. D., Goldman, N., Henshaw, S., Lincoln, R., Rosoff, J. I., Westoff, C. F., & Wulf, D. (1986). *Teenage pregnancy in industrialized countries.* New Haven, CT: Yale University Press.

Kalichman, S. C., Carey, M. P., & Johnson, B. T. (1996). Prevention of sexually transmitted HIV infection: A meta-analytic review of the behavioral outcome literature. *Annals of Behavioral Medicine, 18*(1), 6–15.

Kann, L., Warren, C., Harris, W., Collins, J., Williams, B., Ross, J., Kolbe, L., & State and Local YRBSS coordinators. (1996). Youth risk behavior surveillance—United States, 1995. *CDC Surveillance Summaries, Mortality and Morbidity Weekly Report, 45*(No. SS–4), 1–84.

Keller, S. E., Barlett, J. A., Schleifer, S. J., Johnson, R. L., Pinner, E., & Delaney, B. (1991). HIV-relevant sexual behavior among a healthy inner-city heterosexual adolescent population in an endemic area of HIV. *Journal of Adolescent Health, 12*, 44–48.

Kim, N., Stanton, B., Li, X., Dickersin, K., & Galbraith, J. (1997). Effectiveness of the 40 adolescent AIDS risk-reduction interventions: A quantitative review. *Journal of Adolescent Health, 20*, 204–215.

Klein, J. D., Slap, G. B., Elster, A. B., & Cohn, S. E. (1993). Adolescents and access to health care. *Bulletin of the New York Academy of Medicine, 70,* 219–234.

Leish, B. C., Morrison, D. M., Trocki, K., & Temple, M. T. (1994). Sexual behavior of American adolescents: Results from a U.S. national survey. *Journal of Adolescent Health, 15*(2), 117–125.

Madden, T. J., Ellen, P. S., & Ajzen, I. (1992). A comparison of the theory of planned behavior and the theory of reasoned action. *Personality and Social Psychology Bulletin, 18,* 3–9.

Marin, B. V. (1995). *Analysis of AIDS prevention among African Americans and Latinos in the United States.* Washington, DC: Office of Technology Assessment.

Mays, V. M., & Cochran, S. D. (1988). Issues in the perception of AIDS risk and risk reduction activities by Black and Hispanic/Latina women. *The American Psychologist, 43,* 949–957.

Milan, R. J., & Kilmann, P. R. (1987). Interpersonal factors in premarital contraception. *Journal of Sex Research, 23,* 289–321.

NIMH Multisite HIV Prevention Trial. (1997). NIMH Multisite HIV Prevention Trial: A randomized, controlled evaluation of risk reduction interventions. *Science.*

Page, H. S., & Asire, A. J. (1985). *Cancer rates and risks* (3rd ed.) (NIH Publication No. 85–691). Bethesda, MD: National Institutes of Health.

Peterson, J. L., & Marin, G. (1988). Issues in the prevention of AIDS among Black and Hispanic men. *The American Psychologist, 11,* 871–877.

Rickert, V. I., Jay, M. S., & Gottlieb, A. (1991). Effects of a peer-counseled AIDS education program on knowledge, attitudes, and satisfaction of adolescents. *Journal of Adolescent Health, 12,* 38–43.

Rosenstock, I. M., Strecher, V. J., & Becker, M. H. (1988). Social learning theory and the health belief model. *Health Education Quarterly, 15,* 175–183.

Scott, M. A. (1996). Reducing the risks: Adolescents and sexually transmitted diseases. *Nurse Practitioner Forum, 7,* 23–29.

Shafer, M. A., Shelton, J. F., Ekstrand, M., Keogh, J., Gee, L., DiGiorgio-Haas, L., Shalwitz, J., & Schachter, J. (1993). Relationship between drug use and sexual behaviors and the occurrence of sexually transmitted disease among high-risk male youth. *Sexually Transmitted Diseases, 20,* 307–313.

Sheppard, B. H., Hartwick, J., & Warshaw, P. R. (1988). The theory of reasoned action: A meta-analysis of past research with recommendations for modifications and future research. *Journal of Consumer Research, 15,* 325–343.

Slap, G., Plotkin, S., Khalid, N., Michelman, D., & Forke C. (1991). A human immunodeficiency virus peer education program for adolescent females. *Journal of Adolescent Health, 12,* 434–442.

Solomon, M. Z., & DeJong, W. (1989). Preventing AIDS and other STDs through condom promotion: A patient education intervention. *American Journal of Public Health, 79,* 453–458.

Sonenstein, F. L., Pleck, J. H., & Ku, L. C. (1989). Sexual activity, condom use and AIDS awareness among adolescent males. *Family Planning Perspectives, 21*(4), 152–158.

Stone, K. M., Grimes, D. A., & Magder, L. S. (1986). Personal protection against sexually transmitted diseases. *American Journal of Obstetrics and Gynecology, 155,* 180–188.

Tanner, W. M., & Pollack, R. H. (1988). The effect of condom use and erotic instructions on attitudes toward condoms. *Journal of Sex Research*, *25*, 537–541.
Valdiserri, R. O., Arena, V. C., Proctor, D., & Bonati, F. A. (1989). The relationship between women's attitudes about condoms and their use: Implications for condom promotion programs. *American Journal of Public Health*, *79*, 499–503.

PART 4

Conclusion

CHAPTER 9

Social and Health Policy: Influences on Child and Adolescent Health

Antonia M. Villarruel, Jennifer Moore, and
Julie Sochalski

Any discussion of the development, health, and well-being of children
and adolescents is not complete without taking into account the
influence of the social, cultural, economic, and political contexts on
the health behaviors and outcomes of the nation's youth. Strategies to reduce
rates of behavior-based morbidity and mortality among children and adolescents will undoubtedly be less than successful if the contexts that influence
unhealthy behaviors and poor health outcomes are ignored. Consequently,
the development of broad based strategies to address the health needs of
youth must begin with the identification and understanding of the contextual
or environmental factors that influence health outcomes.

Several theorists have explicated the interactive and interdependent relationship between the contextual influences and human development. Lerner
(1992) proposed that multiple levels of organization are involved in human
life and development. He theorized the relation between the structure and
function of variables from these multiple levels was one of dynamic interactionism. That is, both the structure and function of variables from any level
of organization are influenced by those from other levels. Similarly, Bronfren-
brenner (1979) described individuals and families as interdependent with the
environments in which they live; that is, the broader social, economic, and
political systems. As an example, economic necessity and changes in societal

attitudes regarding women's place in the workforce has resulted in an increase in the number of employed mothers. Coupled with factors such as shrinking family networks and increased family mobility, the necessity for childcare options that are independent of family networks has increased. The impact of ineffective and limited child care options on employment and both national and local economies has led to public and private policies to facilitate access to affordable and quality child care.

The importance and interaction among contextual factors and health outcomes have also been recognized. Social policy, poverty, neighborhood environments, and discrimination are some aspects of the environment that have been linked with health, morbidity, and mortality. Link and Phelan (1996) contended that social conditions expose people to risk factors that cause disease and disease patterns in populations. The prevention of those risk factors will subsequently cause changes in social patterns and thus influence disease or health outcomes. Similarly, underlying the relation between social policy and health, De Leeuw (1989) posited that social policy is the largest determinant of health. This relationship is evident in considering the leading health risk for children today—poverty. Poverty limits access to adequate nutrition and resources for child development while increasing exposure to unhealthy environments. The mutual influence between health, social patterns, and social policy is an example of dynamic interactionism.

An example of the relationships between health, individual behavior, and the contextual elements of the environment can further be illustrated with the issue of youth violence. Unintentional injuries, homicides, and suicides are leading causes of death among youth 18–24 years of age (Singh & Su, 1996b). Although there is a downward trend in deaths related to unintentional injuries in this age group, death as a result of interpersonal violence, especially as it involves handguns, has risen within the last 2 decades (Sells & Blum, 1996a). Individual variables such as youths' grade point average, deviant behavior, perceived risk of untimely death, history of victimization or witnessing violence, and family variables such as parent/family connectedness, recent family suicide attempts, and household access to guns have been associated with youth violence (Resnick et al., 1997).

Researchers have also described a relationship between firearm violence and factors such as accessibility to firearms, legislative controls related to firearm access, and school and neighborhood environments (Cohall, Mayer, Cohall, & Walter, 1991; Earls, 1991; Singh & Su, 1996a; Vaughn et al., 1996). The concentration of youth violence in poor communities characterized by limited economic opportunities, and the collapse of social institutions, including schools, warrants the examination of interventions at the school, family, community, and policy level. Clearly, changes in the social, cultural, and economic circumstances that foster violent behavior are needed to address this important health problem (Vaughan et al., 1996).

Health risk, protective, and promotion behavior patterns begin in early childhood and are influenced by the family, social, economic, and political environments. Thus, effective interventions to support health promoting and protective behavior should be implemented at several levels. These interventions should be directed toward strengthening individual knowledge and skills, promoting community education, changing organizational practices, and influencing policy and legislation (National Institute of Nursing Research [NINR], 1993).

In this chapter, an overview of the current and projected demographic, social, and economic context of children and families in the United States is provided. Within this context, current child health care policies, specifically, as they relate to Medicaid coverage are examined. An analysis of current policies for creating environments that support and promote children's health will be discussed.

THE ENVIRONMENTAL CONTEXT OF CHILDREN AND YOUTH IN THE UNITED STATES

Changing Demographic Profile

Children represent a significant segment of the U.S. population. In 2000 children under 18 years of age comprised 28.6% of the U.S. population (U.S. Census Bureau, 2001a). Although the percentage of the child population will remain stable by the year 2010, the number of children is expected to increase from 70.4 million in 2000 to 77.2 million in 2002 (U.S. Department of Health and Human Services [DHHS], 2001). Although the proportion of children in the U.S. has been stable over time, there has been marked increase in racial and ethnic diversity. Consistent with overall population trends, there have been dramatic shifts in the racial and ethnic composition of this age group. Since 1980, according to the U.S. Bureau of the Census (2001a), the percentage of children who are non-Hispanic White has steadily decreased. This trend is expected to continue. For example, in 2000, 63% of children in the U.S. were non-Hispanic White. This percentage is projected to decrease to 54% by the year 2020. Conversely, the percentage of Blacks, Hispanics, and Asian Americans has increased steadily since 1980. Conversely, no growth in the percentage of Native American children has occurred, and further, this trend is also expected to continue.

Population trends suggest that the numbers of Hispanic and Asian American children will continue to increase. In 2000 (U.S. Census Bureau, 2001a) the percentage of Black, Hispanic, and Asian American children was estimated at 15%, 9%, and 2%, respectively; by the year 2020 it is projected to be 32.4%, 35.7%, and 21.8%, respectively. Initial projections estimated that Hispanic children would be the largest minority group by the year 2010. Figures released from the Census Bureau in 1995, however, indicated Hispanic children comprise the largest minority group and are the second largest group of children in the country led only by non-Hispanic White children. It is important to recognize that immigration has played a small part in the overall increase of both Hispanic and Asian American children. According to the U.S. Bureau of the Census (2000b) less than 9% of all children were foreign born.

Changing Family Structure

Another important demographic trend affecting children and youth is the changing family environment. Increased labor force participation by women, lack of access to full-time employment for men, increased rates of divorce, separation, and increased rates of out-of-wedlock births are some of the trends that have contributed to the decline of traditional, two-parent families. For example, in 2000, 69% of children lived with two parents, representing a decline from 77% in 1980 (U.S. Census Bureau, 2000a). Female headed households overwhelmingly comprise the majority of one-parent families. Although all racial and ethnic groups have experienced a decline in two-parent families (Ventura & Bachrach, 2000), between group differences have been observed. The percentage of black children who live in two-parent homes (38%) is significantly lower than Hispanic children (65%) or non-Hispanic White children (77%). In general, separation and divorce account for about two-thirds of children living in mother-only families while out-of-wedlock childbearing accounts for about one-third of children living in mother-only families (Hernandez, 1993).

A direct and indirect impact of these trends, including increased labor force participation by mothers, and increase in female-headed households, has been on the environments in which children are raised. For example, children under the age of 6 are spending significant amounts of time in the care of someone other than their parents (Hofferth, 1996). The most common source of childcare is outside the home with a nonfamilial caregiver. Advantages of this arrangement include increased socialization with peers, a potential for exposure to different and stimulating environments, and support for parents with different child-rearing issues. Disadvantages include potential conflicts in child-rearing practices and expectations, and potential safety issues for children resulting from a lack of regulations or enforcement of childcare regulations. Although the research in determining the advantages and disadvantages of differing child care arrangements is not yet conclusive, this change in environment for developing children is an important consideration in designing interventions and formulating effective health and social policy.

Poverty

Poverty is a significant issue impacting children and families in the U.S. In 2000, 16.9% of children under 18 lived in families with incomes below the poverty level (U.S. Census Bureau, 2000b). Although this represents a slight but gradual decline since about 1995, children represent the largest proportion of any age group living in poverty. There are differences in poverty rates among diverse groups of children. Poverty among Black and Hispanic children is significantly higher than among White children (33%, 30%, and 9%, respectively) (U.S. Census Bureau, 2000b). Across all groups, it is important to note that there are a significant number of children from working families that comprise this group. Government policies have created a safety net for poor children. Traditionally, government programs including Aid to Families with Dependent Children (AFDC), Housing Assistance, and nutrition supplemental programs such as Food Stamps, and the Special Supplemental Food Program for Women, Infants, and Children (WIC) have augmented the household budgets of poor families and increased access to specific necessities, such as food and housing (Devaney, Ellwood, & Love, 1987).

Welfare reform initiatives undertaken in 1996 have produced mixed results in maintaining the viability of this safety net. These reforms have been successful in reducing the rolls of AFDC and other federal subsidies, as well as assisting recipients to obtain employment, and in a limited sense, reducing poverty. Despite the overall decline in childhood poverty, however, the number of children who were in working poor families increased from 4.9 million to 5.6 million (U.S. Census Bureau, 2000a). Further, there has been a decline in federal assistance to working poor families (Wertheimer, 2001), thus making children from working families even more vulnerable.

Summary

Several important trends about the environment or context of U.S. children can be discerned. First, children will continue to comprise a significant proportion of the U.S. population. Demographic trends indicate that there will be increasing racial and ethnic diversity among U.S. children brought on by a disproportionate increase in Hispanic and Asian American children relative to White children. The majority of children will live in single-parent households; most of those will be headed by females. Mothers of young children will continue to comprise a significant part of the workforce and as a result, children will be spending more of their time outside of the home and in the care of nonfamily members. A significant portion of children will be living in or near poverty. Many of these children are from working poor families and lack adequate assistance from employers, in terms of benefits, or from the government, in terms of food, housing, or health care subsidies. It is in this context that the health choices of children and family make must be viewed and that health and social policy must be considered. It is in this context that one health policy for children, the issue of health insurance coverage, will be considered.

HEALTH INSURANCE FOR CHILDREN: POLICY APPROACHES

One example of health policy necessitated by these changing demographics is the effort to assure adequate health care coverage for children. It has been well documented that across the life span, those who have health insurance are more likely to have a regular source of health care, higher rates of health care service use, and better health outcomes (Lieu, Newacheck, & McManus, 1993; Newacheck, Stoddard, Hughes, & Pearl, 1998; Spillman, 1992). Children's access to health care is largely dictated by the circumstances of their family. Children in families that have access to private health coverage obtained principally through offerings from the employer of the head of household are in the best position to receive health care services. In 1999 more than 69% of children received coverage through private health insurance, and enjoyed the concomitant access to health care services (U.S. Census Bureau, 2000c).

For those without private health coverage, Medicaid, the government's health insurance program for low-income individuals and families, has improved access to health care for millions more children (Newacheck et al.,

1995). Federal law requires Medicaid coverage for all children through age 5 in families with incomes below 133% of the federal poverty level (FPL), and children between the ages of 6–13 in families at 100% of FPL. Children aged 14–18 years are covered by Medicaid only if they would have been eligible under the former AFDC program rules (Weil, 1997). Eligibility for AFDC, and consequently Medicaid, was based on maximum family income standards set by each state and other select criteria, such as an incapacitated or unemployed parent. In 1999 23% of children had health care coverage from public-sponsored health insurance, chiefly through the Medicaid program (U.S. Census Bureau, 2000c). Medicaid covered 20% of all children and 77% of all children at or below the FPL. A variety of structural barriers, such as the lack of understanding of eligibility rules among the poor and inadequate outreach efforts, have prevented many eligible children from being enrolled in Medicaid.

Medicaid and private health insurance are not expansive enough to provide all children in the U.S. with health insurance. There exists a growing gap of children whose access to health care is hampered by a lack of health insurance. In 1999, nearly 14% of all children in the U.S., 10 million, were not covered by private health insurance and were either ineligible or did not receive publicly financed health insurance (U.S. Census Bureau, 2000c). This represents a slight decrease in numbers, though not percentage from previous years. The majority of uninsured children (70%) are in families whose income was below 200% of the FPL. Given the rates of poverty for employed and underemployed families, it is not surprising that nearly two thirds of uninsured children were in families in which the head-of-household was employed year round at either full-time or part-time levels with no periods of unemployment. There are also significant differences in health insurance among racial and ethnic groups. Hispanic and Black children are more likely to be uninsured as compared with White children (27%, 18%, & 9% respectively).

Health Insurance Initiatives for Children

In response to the persistent and growing problem of uninsured children, the Balanced Budget Act of 1997 created a new program and funding for states to provide health insurance to children, the State Children's Health Insurance Program (SCHIP). The purpose of SCHIP, enacted as Title XXI of the Social Security Act, is to provide funds to States to enable them to initiate and expand the provision of child health assistance to uninsured, low-income children (SCHIP, 1997). SCHIP was appropriated $24 billion of child health insurance over 5 years in federal and state matching grant funds (Keigher, 1997). Additional funding in 1999 expanded SCHIP's longevity from a 5-year to a 10-year program.

The program, targeting low-income children under 19 years of age, provided approximately $4 billion a year to the states beginning in fiscal year 1998. To obtain these federal funds, states had to contribute matching funds at rates that were 70% of their state share under Medicaid. An expenditure limit of 10% was set for administrative costs. Because SCHIP was not established as an entitlement, states could chose whether or not to participate (Markus & DeGraw, 1997).

The rules and regulations of SCHIP required states to follow very basic standards with room to negotiate terms to allow flexibility. States had substantial discretion on how aggressively funds would be utilized to decrease the number of uninsured children. Under SCHIP, states could choose to expand their existing Medicaid programs, establish a new program, or create a combination of both programs. Many states chose to create their own program to avoid expanding the Medicaid entitlement. States were given the jurisdiction to determine the percentage of federal poverty level (FPL) to qualify families (Markus & McGraw, 1997). By keeping the qualifying FPL low, fewer children are eligible to participate in the program; higher qualifying FPLs provide a greater number of children the opportunity to participate in the SCHIP. Among those states choosing to create their own program, the FPL eligibility ranges from 133% to 200%. Among states that chose to create a combination program, the FPL eligibility ranges from 133% to 350%. The states that opted to expand their Medicaid program only have a FPL eligibility range from 100% to 300%. The flexibility of states to establish qualifying FPL potentially limits the eligibility of children in need of health care insurance.

The federal government did establish several mandates. These included that: (1) children under 19 years of age be covered; (2) payments could not be used for abortions (except in the case of incest, rape, or if the life of the mother is in danger); (3) the program had to provide insurance at the same level as the current state employee benefits; and, (4) funds would be based on the proportion of the total number of low-income uninsured children multiplied by a geographic cost factor (Health Care Financing Administration [HCFA], 1997). This calculation was intended to provide an appropriate level of funding for each state based on their specific needs. Those states that had lower numbers of uninsured children or lower health care costs were subsequently given less funding.

To illustrate the successes and challenges with SCHIP, the experience of one state, Michigan, will be detailed.

The Michigan Program

The Michigan version of SCHIP, a combination of expanding Medicaid and creating a new program termed *MI Child*, was approved by the Michigan Department of Health and Human Services in April of 1998, almost 1 year after the SCHIP plan was approved. The state determined that the MI Child plan would be available to those who were 150%–200% of the FPL. Families below 150% of the FPL would be eligible for the Medicaid program. This expanded the scope of the Medicaid program by qualifying families from a 133% maximum FPL qualifying level to 150% of the FPL. The benefit package of the combination program mirrored the exact plan that Michigan state employees received, including the delivery of services by multiple managed care provider organizations.

When MI Child was proposed in 1998 it was estimated that 133,000 children who were 150–200% of the FPL would be enrolled over a 2-year period. At the end of the 2-year period, however, only 63,800 children were enrolled. One issue accounting for this low number is that many children that were enrolled during the first year were not being reenrolled for the second year (Michigan Council for Maternal and Child Health, 2000). Low enrollments have been attributed to difficulties in the renewal application, administrative difficulties in locating families in nonpermanent housing, and the frustrations parents experienced from participating in a new program that was initially not running smoothly.

The state of Michigan during this period received $91 million to allocate into the expanded Medicaid program and the new MI Child plan. At the end of the year 2000 Michigan had only utilized $42.7 million, while the number of uninsured children that qualified for SCHIP rose to 247,000 (Children's Defense Fund, 2000). Of the 247,000 uninsured children in Michigan, 69,200 were children not enrolled during 1998–1999, while 177,800 were newly uninsured children or children that were not accounted for in the original 1998 estimates. This alarming underutilization trend was witnessed across the country.

Many speculate that too much money was allocated at the start-up phase of the program when states had no use for large amounts of money. During the start-up phase many states were slow to enroll patients until other aspects of the programs were more developed. Another reason for the underutilization of funds was that the money was not distributed appropriately across the 10-year span of the program. The SCHIP was appropriated assuming that the costs of the program would not increase as the program developed (Kenney, Ullman, & Weil, 2000).

Three other factors that have contributed to the underutilization of the MI Child program. First, when MI Child was implemented, the State of Michigan underestimated the staff requirements relative to the demand of the program. This created long delays in the application process that hindered enrollment. Another potential reason for low enrollment was an extensive multipage application for new enrollees; renewal required an 8-page application. In addition, both the initial and renewal process required supplemental documents that could have delayed the enrollment process. Another problem related to the application process is the lack of continuity among government employees (Michigan Council for Maternal and Child Health, 2000). For example, one family may interact with multiple agencies and multiple contact persons to process one application. The development of comprehensive outreach strategies, adequate staffing, and simplification of enrollment processes might result in a greater number of children being enrolled.

Despite the best efforts of Medicaid and SCHIP, not every child will qualify for either program. It is estimated that 4 million uninsured children are in families whose income is too high for government programs and their employer does not provide insurance, or the cost of the provided insurance is too high (Kaiser Commission on Medicaid and the Uninsured, 2000). There are currently 69,000 children in Michigan who fall into this gap between government assistance programs and private insurance opportunities (Michigan Council for Maternal and Child Health, 2000).

A national survey of changes in health insurance coverage between 1996–1997 and 1998–1999 in fact confirm the persistence of a significant number of uninsured children. Although there have been gains in public coverage, as a result of SCHIP programs and Medicaid expansion, there has been a decline in private insurance (Cunningham & Park, 2000). Further, for those families with children below the poverty line, there was no change in public coverage. As SCHIP programs continue to expand, health care costs expand, and employer based benefits decrease, their effects on protecting children will need to be carefully monitored.

Summary

The changing demographics and socioeconomic environment of children and families today has necessitated a policy solution to the erosion of the health insurance safety net. New programs aimed at providing health care for the uninsured are one effort to improve the health and well-being of children. It is evident from early experiences with SCHIP that health care policies must be encompassing. Such initiatives must address issues such as transportation, outreach efforts for easy enrollment, child care, inadequate office hours, lengthy waiting times, and an absence of culturally competent care providers. Because racial and ethnic minorities are overrepresented among low-income and uninsured populations, outreach efforts and improved access to health care is viewed as a major step toward eliminating racial and ethnic disparities in children's health (USDHHS, 1997).

CONCLUSION

Ensuring health care coverage for children and equitable access to care are both important policy goals. As discussed in this chapter, however, the design and implementation of this policy goal is complex; both are dependent upon and will influence a number of health, social, and economic factors. There are many that contend that incremental changes in health care have shifted the focus from health reform to finance reform. Although one could effectively argue that health care coverage and equitable access to health care are important determinants of health, they are not sufficient to promote and support the health of our children.

As predicted by Smith and Wesley (1993), the outcome of the health care debate has focused narrowly on benefits, eligibility, financing, cost control, and administration as opposed to strengthening public health, prevention, and protection. Clearly, comprehensive strategies and health and social policies directed toward creating and supporting healthy environments, communities, and families are necessary to protect our most important resource—our children.

REFERENCES

Bronfenbrenner, U. (1979). *The ecology of human development*. Boston: Harvard University Press.

Children's Defense Fund. (2000). State of Michigan's Children: 2000. Retrieved June 12, 2000 from www.childrendefense.org/states/data_mi.htm

Cohall, A. T., Mayer, R., Cohall, K., & Walter, H. J. (1991). Teen violence: the reasons why. *Contemporary Pediatrics, 8,* 54–77.

Cunningham, P. J., & Park, M. H. (2000). Recent trends in children's health insurance coverage: No gains for low income children. *Issue Brief Cent Stud Health Syst Change,* April (29), 1–6.

De Leeuw, E. (1989). *The sane revolution health promotion: Backgrounds, scope, prospects.* Maastricht, The Netherlands: Van Gorcum, Assen.

Devaney, B. L., Ellwood, M. R., & Love, J. M. (1997). Programs that mitigate the effects of poverty on children. *The Future of Children, 7*(2), 88–112.

Earls, F. A. (1991). A developmental approach to understanding and controlling violence. *Theory and Methods in Behavioral Pediatrics, 5,* 61–88.

Health Care Financing Administration. (1997). *Children's Health Insurance Program.* Retrieved August 28, 2001 from www.hcfa.gov/init/kidssum.html

Hernandez, D. J. (1993). *America's children, resources from family, government, and the economy.* New York: Russell Sage Foundation.

Hofferth, S. L (1996). Child care in the U.S. today. *The Future of Children, 6*(2), 41–61.

Kaiser Commission on Medicaid and the Uninsured. (2000). Health insurance coverage in America: 2000 data update. http://www.kff.org/content/2002/4007/. Accessed 26 March 2002.

Keigher, S. M. (1997). The Medicaid sweater, children's health, and the tiny hole. *Health and Social Work, 22*(4), 306–311.

Kenney, G. M., Ullman, F. C., & Weil, A. (2000). *Three years into SCHIP: What states are and are not spending.* The Urban Institute, No A-44 (Assessing the New Federalism, Series A).

Kopelman, L. M., & Palumbo, M. G. (1997). The U.S. health delivery system: Inefficient and unfair to children. *American Journal of Law & Medicine, 23*(2&3), 319–337.

Lerner, R. M. (1992). Dialectics, developmental contextualism, and the further enhancement of theory about puberty and psychological development. *Journal of Early Adolescence, 12,* 366–388.

Li, J., & Bennett, N. (1998). *Young children in poverty: A statistical update.* March 1998 ed. Columbia University, New York: National Center for Children in Poverty.

Lieu, T. A., Newacheck, P. W., & McManus, M. A. (1993). Race, ethnicity, and access to ambulatory care among U.S. adolescents. *American Journal of Public Health, 83,* 960–965.

Link, B. G., & Phelan, J. C. (1996). Understanding sociodemographic differences in health—the role of fundamental social causes. *American Journal of Public Health, 86,* 471–472.

Markus, A. R., & DeGraw, C. (1997). Expanding health insurance coverage for uninsured children: The next step in health care reform? *The Journal of the American Board of Family Practice, 10*(5), 363–369.

Michigan Council for Maternal and Child Health. (2000). *Uninsured and newly insured children in Michigan.* Retrieved July 12, 2000 from www.mcmch.com/archives/uninsuredchildren5199.htm

National Institute of Nursing Research. (1993). *Health Promotion for Older Children and Adolescents.* (NIH Publication No. 93-2420). Bethesda, MD: National Institutes of Health.

Newacheck, P. W., Hughes, D. C., English, A., Fox, H. B., Perrin, J., & Halfon, N. (1995). The effect on children of curtailing Medicaid spending. *Journal of the American Medical Association, 274,* 1468–1471.

Newacheck, P. W., Stoddard, J. J., Hughes, D. C., & Pearl, M. (1998). Health insurance and access to primary care for children. *New England Journal of Medicine, 338*(8), 513–519.

Resinick, M. D., Bearman, P. S., Blum, R. W., Bauman, K. E., Harris, K. M., Jones, J., Tabor, J., Beuhring, T., Seiving, R. E., Shew, M., Ireland, M., Bearinger, L. H., & Udry, J. R. (1997). Protecting adolescents from harm—Findings from the National longitudinal study on adolescent health. *Journal of the American Medical Association, 278*, 823–832.

Sells, C. W., & Blum, R. W. (1996). Morbidity and mortality among U.S. adolescents: An overview of data and trends. *American Journal of Public Health, 86*, 513–519.

Singh, G. K., & Yu, S. M. (1996a). Trends and differentials in adolescent and young adult mortality in the United States, 1950 through 1993. *American Journal of Public Health, 86*, 505–512.

Singh, G. K., & Yu, S. M. (1996b). U.S. childhood mortality, 1950 through 1993: Trends and socioeconomic differentials. *American Journal of Public Health, 86*, 505–512.

Smith, G. R., & Wesley, R. L. (1993). Health promotion: Public policy goal. In R. Knollmueller (Ed.), *Prevention across the life span: Healthy people for the twenty-first century* (pp. 97–106). Washington, DC: American Nurses Publishing.

Spillman, B. C. (1992). The impact of being uninsured on utilization of basic care services. *Inquiry, 29*(4), 457–466.

U.S. Census Bureau. (2000a). *America's Families and Living Arrangements: Population Characteristics*. Retrieved August 28, 2001 from http://www.census.gov/population/www/socdemo/hhfam.html

U.S. Census Bureau. (2000b). *Foreign-Born Population in the United States: Population Characteristics Population by Nativity and Region of Residence*. Retrieved August 28, 2001 from www.census.gov/prod/2000pubs/p20-534.pdf

U.S. Census Bureau. (2000c). *Health Insurance Coverage—1999*. Retrieved August 28, 2001 from www.census.gov/hhes/www/hlthin99.html

U.S. Census Bureau. (2001a). *Population by Age, Sex, and Race and Hispanic Origin*. Retrieved August 28, 2001 from www.census.gov/population/socdemo/race/black/ppl-142/tab01.txt

U.S. Census Bureau. (2001b). *Poverty Status of the Population in 1999 by Age, Sex, Race and Hispanics*. Retrieved August 28, 2001 from www.census.gov/population/socdemo/race/black/ppl-142/tab16.txt

U.S. Department of Health and Human Services. (1997). *Eliminating racial and ethnic disparities in health*. Website at http://raceandhealth.hhs.gov/over.htm

U.S. Department of Health and Human Services Office of the Assistant Secretary for Planning and Evaluation. (2001). *Trends in the Well Being of America's Children and Youth*. Washington, DC: Government Printing Office.

Vaughan, R. D., McCarthy, J. F., Armstrong, B., Walter, H. J., Waterman, P. D., & Tiezzi, L. (1996). Carrying and using weapons: A survey of minority junior high school students in New York City. *American Journal of Public Health, 86*, 568–572.

Ventura, S. J., & Bacharac, C. A. (2000). Nonmarital childbearing in the United States, 1940–1999. *National Vital Statistics Reports, 48*(16). Hyattsville, MD: National Center for Health Statistics.

Weil, A. (1997). The new children's health insurance program: Should states expand
    Medicaid? The Urban Institute, No. A-13 (Assessing the New Federalism, Series A).
Wertheimer, R. (2001). *Working poor families with children: Leaving welfare doesn't
    necessarily mean leaving poverty.* Child Trends Research Brief. Retrieved August
    28, 2001 from www.childtrends.org/pdf/May_2001.pdf

Index

Pediatrician-provided counseling and information, 159
Pedometer, Amsterdam study, 130–131
Pedometers, 133
 for energy measurements, 126
Peer-related risk factors, 183
Peers, and social support, 48–50
Personality, relation to smoking and alcohol use, 25
Pharmacotherapeutic agents, substance
 abuse, 200
Pharmacotherapy, substance abuse, 199,
 200
Physical activity
 difficulties of analysis, 224–225
 effect of age on, 108–109
 future research outlook, 137
 importance of in childhood and adolescence, 105–142
 methods of training, 119–129
 nature of, 105–109
 relation to growth and health, 109
 relation to obesity, 224–225
 relation to weight loss, 214–215
 relationship with aerobic fitness,
  135–137
 and social support, 52–54
 support for relative to age and sex,
  53–54
Physical activity measured by interviews,
 133–134
Physical appearance domains, 42
Physical inactivity, risk factors of, 107
Physiologic functions, energy expenditure
 using, 127
Pittsburgh Adolescent Alcohol Research
 Center, 181
Planfulness in drug use studies, 14
Playground safety, 165
Poison Prevention Packaging Act, 164
Population attributable risk, 107
Portable accelerometers, for energy mea-
 surements, 126–127
Positive emotionality, 7

Possible selves, relation to social support,
 44
Post-treatment analysis, substance abuse,
 196–201
Poverty
 government funds available for, 265
 health risks caused by, 262–263
 impact of on children, 265
Pretreatment characteristics, substance
 abuse, 196–201
Prevalence of childhood injuries, 146–147
Prevention of substance abuse, 191–192
Preventive actions, child-oriented,
 160–163
Preventive health, media reports on, 91
Previous injuries, relation to childhood in-
 juries, 152
Private health insurance, role of, 267
Protective factors, relation to tempera-
 ment, 23
Psychiatric co-morbidity, 186–189
Psychiatric disorders, relation to SUDs,
 186–189
Psychopathology, 188
Psychotropic agents, substance abuse,
 200–201
Psychotropic medications, substance
 abuse, 199

Questionnaires and interviews for energy
 measurements, 125

Race
 effects of on physical activity, 225–226
 relation to overweight children, 215
Race variations in HIV risk-reduction
 studies, 243
Racial patterns
 changes of, 264
 of drug abuse, 181
Range of reaction, 8
Receiving social support, 44, 46–47
Regulations, limitations on, 166
Religious organizations, social support
 from, 50–51

Springer Publishing Company

Adolescent Pregnancy
Policy and Prevention Services
Naomi Farber, PhD, MSW

The author provides social work practitioners with research-based information necessary to develop prevention programs and policies that target young people according to their different levels of early sex, pregnancy, and parenthood experiences. The need to develop policies and services designed to reduce teenage pregnancy in ways appropriate for the social worker's specific client population is emphasized throughout.

Identifying and synthesizing the wide literature on prevention theory and practice, this book offers "best practice" applications for effective social work intervention.

Special issues of teens, such as the relation between alcohol, drug use, and early sex and pregnancy, and the needs of the children of teens are also explored.

Partial Contents:
• Dimensions of Adolescent Sexual Activity and Fertility
• Theories of Illegitimacy
• Contemporary Research: Sexual Risk Taking
• Conceptual Framework: A Continuum of Risk
• Approaches to Prevention of Adolescent Pregnancy
• Planning Prevention Services: An Assessment Framework
• Alcohol and Drug Use and Adolescent Pregnancy, *Nancy N. Brown*
• A Developmental Perspective on Adolescent Parenting *Janet R. Shapiro*
• Appendix A: State Laws on Minors' Access to Abortion
• Appendix B: State Policies for Sexuality and STD/HIV Education

Springer Series on Social Work
2002 238pp (est.) 0-8261-2372-4 hardcover

536 Broadway, New York, NY 10012 • Telephone: 212-431-4370
Fax: 212-941-7842 • Order Toll-Free: 877-687-7476 • Order On-line: www.springerpub.com

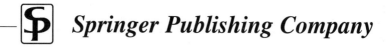

Springer Publishing Company

Health Promotion in Communities
Holistic and Wellness Approaches
Carolyn Chambers Clark, EdD, RN, ARNP, FAAN, HNC, DABFN, Editor

In her latest book, Dr. Clark applies a holistic wellness perspective to community health, focusing on community strengths and resilience—such as positive nutrition, healthy environment, fitness, and self-care skills—rather than risks and disease.

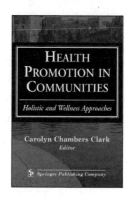

Practitioners and students will find this book a practical and comprehensive resource for creating community health programs and promoting wellness among individuals and groups.

Partial Contents:
- A Model for Health and Wellness Promotion in Communities, *C.C. Clark*
- Health Promotion with Changing and Vulnerable Populations, *G. Erickson*
- Community Self-Assessment, *C.C. Clark*
- Principles of Planning Effective Community Health Programs, *E. Erkel*
- Evaluating Community Health Programs, *S. MacDonald*
- Health Promotion in Rural Settings, *J.W. Aucoin and S.G. Rodgers*
- Fitness and Flexible Movement, *B. Resnick*
- Stress Management, *C.C. Clark*
- Smoking Cessation, *C. Long*
- Environmental Wellness, *C.C. Clark*
- Working with Groups, *C. Johnson and B. Keely*
- Working with Families, *J.U. Davidson*
- Violence Prevention in Schools, *P.P. DiNapoli*
- Health Promotion in a Homeless Center, *C.O. Helvie*

Nurse's Book Society Selection
2002   496pp   0-8261-1407-5   hardcover

536 Broadway, New York, NY 10012 • Telephone: 212-431-4370
Fax: 212-941-7842 • Order Toll-Free: 877-687-7476 • Order On-line: www.springerpub.com